Every Decker book is accompanied by a CD-ROM.

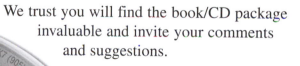

The disc appears in the front of each copy, in its own sealed jacket. Affixed to the front of the book will be a distinctive BcD sticker **"Book *cum* disc."**

The disc contains the complete text and illustrations of the book, in fully searchable PDF files. The book and disc are sold *only* as a package; neither is available independently, and no prices are available for the items individually.

BC Decker Inc is committed to providing high-quality electronic publications that complement traditional information and learning methods.

We trust you will find the book/CD package invaluable and invite your comments and suggestions.

Brian C. Decker
CEO and Publisher

Critical Decisions
in
Periodontology

FOURTH EDITION
with 250 illustrations

WALTER B. HALL, BA, DDS, MSD

Professor Emeritus
Department of Periodontics
University of the Pacific School of Dentistry
San Francisco, California

2003
BC Decker Inc
Hamilton • London

BC Decker Inc
P.O. Box 620, L.C.D. 1
Hamilton, Ontario L8N 3K7
Tel: 905-522-7017; 800-568-7281
Fax: 905-522-7839; 888-311-4987
E-mail: info@bcdecker.com
www.bcdecker.com

02 03 04 05/GSA/9 8 7 6 5 4 3 2 1

ISBN 1-55009-184-0
Printed in Spain

Sales and Distribution

United States
BC Decker Inc
P.O. Box 785
Lewiston, NY 14092-0785
Tel: 905-522-7017; 800-568-7281
Fax: 905-522-7839; 888-311-4987
E-mail: info@bcdecker.com
www.bcdecker.com

Canada
BC Decker Inc
20 Hughson Street South
P.O. Box 620, LCD 1
Hamilton, Ontario L8N 3K7
Tel: 905-522-7017; 800-568-7281
Fax: 905-522-7839; 888-311-4987
E-mail: info@bcdecker.com
www.bcdecker.com

Foreign Rights
John Scott & Company
International Publishers' Agency
P.O. Box 878
Kimberton, PA 19442
Tel: 610-827-1640
Fax: 610-827-1671
E-mail: jsco@voicenet.com

Japan
Igaku-Shoin Ltd.
Foreign Publications Department
3-24-17 Hongo
Bunkyo-ku, Tokyo, Japan 113-8719
Tel: 3 3817 5680
Fax: 3 3815 6776
E-mail: fd@igaku-shoin.co.jp

U.K., Europe, Scandinavia, Middle East
Elsevier Science
Customer Service Department
Foots Cray High Street
Sidcup, Kent
DA14 5HP, UK
Tel: 44 (0) 208 308 5760
Fax: 44 (0) 181 308 5702
E-mail: cservice@harcourt.com

Singapore, Malaysia,Thailand, Philippines, Indonesia, Vietnam, Pacific Rim, Korea
Elsevier Science Asia
583 Orchard Road
#09/01, Forum
Singapore 238884
Tel: 65-737-3593
Fax: 65-753-2145

Australia, New Zealand
Elsevier Science Australia
Customer Service Department
STM Division
Locked Bag 16
St. Peters, New South Wales, 2044
Australia
Tel: 61 02 9517-8999
Fax: 61 02 9517-2249
E-mail: stmp@harcourt.com.au
www.harcourt.com.au

Mexico and Central America
ETM SA de CV
Calle de Tula 59
Colonia Condesa
06140 Mexico DF, Mexico
Tel: 52-5-5553-6657
Fax: 52-5-5211-8468
E-mail:
editoresdetextosmex@prodigy.net.mx

Argentina
CLM (Cuspide Libros Medicos)
Av. Córdoba 2067 – (1120)
Buenos Aires, Argentina
Tel: (5411) 4961-0042/(5411) 4964-0848
Fax: (5411) 4963-7988
E-mail: clm@cuspide.com

Brazil
Tecmedd
Av. Maurílio Biagi, 2850
City Ribeirão Preto – SP – CEP: 14021-000
Tel: 0800 992236
Fax: (16) 3993-9000
E-mail: tecmedd@tecmedd.com.br

Contents

Preface

Earlier editions of this book, which were titled *Decision Making in Periodontology*, illustrated the thought processes used in determining optimal therapy for individual patients as conceived by various experts of the field. This fourth edition takes learning a step farther by providing readers with the means to use the knowledge they have already acquired in the practice of periodontics. Renamed *Critical Decisions in Periodontology*, this fourth edition describes common clinical problems and how practitioners go about deciding what should be done. The approach offers an algorithm (decision tree) for solving each clinical problem as it may be experienced in practice. Chapters describe common clinical problems and, guided by the thinking of experts, allow the reader to arrive at decisions that would take much longer to contrive if guided only by classical teaching texts. Several commonly available additional readings are provided for further details.

This updated and enhanced text should continue to serve the needs of several groups in the fields of dental care. Experienced clinicians may seek answers to specific problems and compare their methods with those outlined. Teachers of periodontology may use this text as a stimulus to rethink modes of presenting information and as a model to test whether students have grasped the concepts they have been taught and are able to use them in a practical manner. Undergraduate students will find this material useful in integrating concepts that they have been taught in a more conventional way, and postgraduate students may argue the merits of the decision-making process as outlined and rewrite the decision trees. Auxiliary personnel will find the material helpful in understanding why specific things happen in certain ways within the dental office. In the rapidly progressing and contentious field of periodontology, some of the decision making presented by our international group of authors may be controversial; however, if the decision trees presented here stimulate thought and discussion, the book will have fulfilled its purpose.

Many thanks to Brian Decker who conceived the idea of books that help dental care providers use their knowledge to make decisions in dental care, and to Charmaine Sherlock and Paula Presutti, who edited this text. Thanks also to all of those talented individuals who contributed chapters. Special thanks to Dr. Eric Curtis, who provided the illustrations, and to my family, Fran, Scott, and Greg, for their encouragement during the preparation of this book.

Walter B. Hall
October 2002

To my wife, Frencella, and my sons, Scott and Gregory,
for their love, support, and understanding during the
preparation of this text

Contributors

Donald F. Adams, DDS, MS
Professor and Director Emeritus
Department of Periodontology
School of Dentistry
Oregon Health Sciences University
Portland, Oregon

Edward P. Allen, DDS, PhD
Department of Periodontics
Baylor College of Dentistry
Dallas, Texas

Tamer Alpagot, DDS, PhD
Associate Professor of Periodontics
University of the Pacific School of Dentistry
San Francisco, California

Tiziano Baccetti, DDS
Department of Orthodontics
University of Florence
Florence, Italy

Roberto Barone, DDS
Private Practice
Florence, Italy

Antonio Bascones, MD, DDS, PhD
Professor of Periodontics, Oral Medicine, and Surgery
School of Dentistry
Universidad Complutense
Madrid, Spain

Carrie Berkovich, DDS, MS
Assistant Professor of Periodontics
University of the Pacific School of Dentistry
San Francisco, California

Burton E. Becker, DDS
Professor of Stomatology, Periodontics, Graduate Periodontics
University of Texas
Houston, Texas

William Becker, DDS, MSD
Private Practice
Periodontics
Tuscon, Arizona

Gretchen J. Bruce, DDS, MBA
Assistant Professor of Periodontics
University of the Pacific School of Dentistry
San Francisco, California

Francesco Cairo, DDS
Research Fellow of Periodontology
Dental School, University of Florence
Florence, Italy

Paulo M. Camargo, DDS, MS
Assistant Professor of Periodontics
UCLA School of Dentistry
Los Angeles, California

Jordi Cambra, MD, DDS, ME
Private Practice
Periodontics
Barcelona, Spain

Miguel Carasol, MD, DDS
Professor of Periodontology
European University School of Dentistry
Madrid, Spain

Carlo Clauser, MD
Private Practice
Florence, Italy

Pierpaolo Cortellini, MD
Department of Periodontology
Eastman Dental Institute
University College of London
London, United Kingdom

Mithridade Davarpanah, MD, DMD
Clinical Assistant Professor of Periodontology
University of Paris
Paris, France

Daniel Etienne, DCD, MS
Associate Professor of Periodontology
University of Paris
Paris, France

Lavin Flores-de-Jacoby, DDS
Professor
Department of Periodontology
Phillipps-Universität
Marburg, Germany

Craig Gainza, DDS, MSD
Private Practice
Periodontics
Vallejo, California

James Garibaldi, DDS, MA
Associate Professor of Oral Surgery
University of the Pacific School of Dentistry
San Francisco, California

Timothy F. Geraci, DDS, MSD
Private Practice
Periodontics
Oakland, California

William Grippo, DDS,
Private Practice
Periodontics
Napa, California

Walter B. Hall, DDS, MSD
Professor Emeritus of Periodontics
University of the Pacific School of Dentistry
San Francisco, California

Lisa A. Harpenau, DDS, MS, MBA
Assistant Professor of Periodontics
University of the Pacific School of Dentistry
San Francisco, California

Stephen K. Harrel, DDS
Private Practice
Periodontics
Dallas, Texas

Luther H. Hutchens Jr, DDS, MSD
Professor Emeritus of Periodontics
School of Dentistry
University of North Carolina
Chapel Hill, North Carolina

Brian J. Kenyon, BA, DMD
Assistant Professor of Oral Medicine
University of the Pacific School of Dentistry
San Francisco, California

Perry R. Klokkevold, DDS, MS
Associate Professor and Clinical Director of Periodontics
UCLA School of Dentistry
Los Angeles, California

John Y. Kwan, DDS
Private Practice
Periodontics
Oakland, California

Eugene E. LaBarre, BA, DMD, MS
Associate Professor and Chair of Removable Prosthodontics
University of the Pacific School of Dentistry
San Francisco, California

Alan S. Leider, DDS, MA
Professor Emeritus of Pathology
Department of Diagnostic Sciences
University of the Pacific School of Dentistry
San Francisco, California

Casimir Leknius, DDS, MBA
Associate Professor of Restorative Dentistry
University of the Pacific School of Dentistry
San Francisco, California

Vojislav Lekovic, DDS, PhD
Professor of Periodontics and Dean
University of Belgrade
Belgrade, Yugoslavia

Joseph Levy, BA, MS, PhD
Professor and Chair of Physiology and Pharmacology
University of the Pacific School of Dentistry
San Francisco, California

Larry G. Loos, DDS
Professor and Chair of Restorative Dentistry
University of the Pacific School of Dentistry
San Francisco, California

William P. Lundergan, DDS, MA
Professor and Chair
Department of Periodontics of the Pacific School of Dentistry
San Francisco, California

Benjamin J. Mandel, DDS
Chair and Founder
Santa Clara Periodontics Study Club
Tiburon, California

Alex R. McDonald, DDS, PhD
Associate Professor of Oral Surgery
University of the Pacific School of Dentistry
San Francisco, California

Reiner Mengel, DDS
Department of Periodontology
Phillipps-Universität Marburg
Marburg, Germany

Scott W. Milliken, DDS, MS
Assistant Professor of Periodontics
University of the Pacific School of Dentistry
San Francisco, California

Francisco Martos Molino, MD, DDS
School of Dentistry
Universidad Complutense
Madrid, Spain

Kathy I. Mueller, MS, DMD
Assistant Professor of Fixed Prosthodontics
University of the Pacific School of Dentistry
San Francisco, California

Leonardo Muzzi, DDS
Research Fellow in Periodontology
Dental School, University of Florence
Florence, Italy

Michael G. Newman, BA, DDS
Professor of Periodontics
UCLA School of Dentistry
Los Angeles, California

Giovan Paolo Pini-Prato, MD, DDS
Professor and Chair of Periodontology
Dental School, University of Florence
Florence, Italy

Mauricio Ronderos, DDS, MS, MPH
Assistant Professor of Periodontics
University of the Pacific School of Dentistry
San Francisco, California

Roberto Rotundo, DDS
Research Fellow in Periodontics
University of the Pacific School of Dentistry
San Francisco, California

Randal W. Rowland, DMD, MS
Professor of Clinical Periodontology
Director Postgraduate Periodontology
University of California
San Francisco, California

Richard S. Rudin, DDS
Assistant Professor of Oral Medicine
University of the Pacific School of Dentistry
San Francisco, California

Mariano Sanz, MD, DDS
Professor and Chair of Periodontology
University of Madrid School of Dentistry
Madrid, Spain

Thomas Schiff, MD, DDS
Professor and Chair of Dental Radiology
University of the Pacific School of Dentistry
San Francisco, California

Alberto Sicillia, MD, DDS
Associate Professor of Periodontics
School of Stomatology
University of Oviedo
Oviedo, Spain

E. Robert Stultz Jr, DMD, MS
Adjunct Professor of Periodontics
University of the Pacific School of Dentistry
San Francisco, California

Charles F. Sumner III, DDS, JD
Associate Professor of Periodontics
University of the Pacific School of Dentistry
San Francisco, California

Maurizio Tonetti, DDS, MS
Department of Periodontics
University of Bern School of Dentistry
Bern, Switzerland

Steven A. Tsurudome, DDS, MS
Assistant Professor of Periodontics
University of the Pacific School of Dentistry
San Francisco, California

Gonzalo Hernández Vallejo, MD, DDS, PhD
Professor of Periodontics, Oral Medicine, and Surgery
School of Dentistry
Universidad Complutense
Madrid, Spain

Ian Van Zyl, DDS, MS
Assistant Professor of Restorative Dentistry
University of the Pacific School of Dentistry
San Francisco, California

Vicki Vlaskalic, BDS, MDSc
Assistant Professor of Orthodontics
University of the Pacific School of Dentistry
San Francisco, California

Galen W. Wagnild, DDS
Associate Clinical Professor of Restorative Dentistry
University of California School of Dentistry
San Francisco, California

Borja Zabelegui, MD, DDS
Professor Titular
Estomatologia
Universidad Pais Vasco
Bilbao, Spain

Jon Zabelegui, MD, DDS
Visiting Professor in Postgraduate Periodontology
Universidad Complutense
Madrid, Spain

Mark Zablotsky, DDS
Adjunct Assistant Professor of Periodontics
University of the Pacific School of Dentistry
San Francisco, California

Giliana Zuccati, MD
Private Practice
Florence, Italy

Introduction

Each two-page chapter in this text consists of an algorithm or decision tree, which usually appears on the right-hand page, and a brief explanatory text with illustrations and additional readings, which begin on the left-hand page. The decision tree is the focus of each chapter and should be studied first in detail. The letters on the decision tree refer the reader to the text, which provides a brief explanation of the basis for each decision. Boxes have been used on the decision tree to indicate invasive procedures or the use of drugs. A combination of line drawings and halftones were selected to clarify the text. Cross-references have been inserted to avoid repeating information given in other chapters. Additional readings that are likely to be readily available to the practitioner have been selected.

Chapters have been grouped by general concepts in the order that follows the typical sequence of therapy in periodontal practice. An index is included to guide the reader further in locating specific information.

The decisions outlined here relate to typical situations. Unusual cases may require the clinician to consider alternatives; however, in every case, the clinician must consider all aspects of an individual patient's data. The algorithms presented here are not meant to represent a rigid guideline for thinking but rather a skeleton to be fleshed out by additional factors in each individual patient's case.

1 Medical History

Walter B. Hall

Before examining a new patient, the dentist should take a medical history. At each subsequent visit, a simple question such as "How have you been since I saw you last?" may elicit an important response, such as "I found out I'm pregnant," which the patient might consider unimportant to her dental treatment. At recall visits, before any dental examination, the dentist should question the patient more extensively regarding visits to a physician, any illnesses, and any changes in medication. In the treatment record the dentist should indicate the medical history was updated by noting, "No changes in medical history," or by recording specific changes that have occurred. The medicolegal importance of such notations cannot be overemphasized.

A A health questionnaire ("yes or no" format) is useful in making the patient responsible for the accuracy of the medical history. The patient may complete such a questionnaire while waiting to see the dentist. Usually, questions are grouped according to systems. The dentist uses this form as a guideline in questioning the patient further about positive answers and writes additional information in the chart.

B The new patient's age is important in developing a treatment plan and as a guide to certain age-related diseases. Note the date and findings of the patient's last physical examination. List the names and addresses of any physicians treating the patient, as well as medications the patient is currently taking and reasons for their use. Refer to important medications in an easily seen place, or use colored stickers to indicate these medications in a standard area on the chart.

C Note heart attacks, rheumatic heart disease, heart surgery, and replacement parts in the heart so that precautions such as antibiotic prophylaxis for patients with rheumatic heart disease or artificial valves can be taken. The patient may even require medication before periodontal probing. Many patients are aware of blood pressure abnormalities, but others are not. Many dentists obtain a baseline blood pressure reading at this time.

D Diabetes is a major problem in successful management of periodontal diseases. For a known diabetic, determine whether (1) the disease is controlled and (2) the patient has visited a physician within the past 3 to 6 months. If the patient is unaware of having diabetes, questions regarding a personal history of periodontal abscesses and blood relatives with diabetes may suggest a problem requiring medical evaluation.

E Infectious diseases such as hepatitis, acquired immuno-deficiency syndrome (AIDS), and tuberculosis (TB) should be included in the questionnaire. Establish whether a patient who has had hepatitis B is a carrier. Encourage the patient to be tested, for family safety if for no other reason. (The test is simple and inexpensive.) HIV+ often has an associated periodontal problem (see Chapters 32 and 33). Questioning regarding this disease must be managed discreetly. TB is uncommon among native-born Americans but quite prevalent among recent immigrants and increasingly common among patients in general.

F Hepatitis (see **E**) and cirrhosis are common problems that affect dental care. Cirrhosis may impair a patient's healing potential. Recurrent kidney infections may require antibiotic prophylaxis before periodontal treatment.

G Patients with seizure disorders may require additional medication before periodontal treatment. Those taking diphenylhydantoin sodium (Dilantin) often develop a "hyperplastic" gingival response (see Chapter 29).

H Asthma can complicate periodontal treatment, especially when anesthetics containing epinephrine are used. Sinusitis can complicate the differential diagnosis of periodontal pain in the maxillary posterior area.

I Avoid nonemergency periodontal treatment of any complexity throughout pregnancy but especially in the first and third trimesters. Pregnancy can modify gingivitis. Such "pregnancy gingivitis" often does not respond to treatment until several months after gestation.

J Gastric or duodenal ulcers may complicate periodontal healing because of dietary restrictions. Gingival changes may accompany colitis.

K Various types of cancer present complications in periodontal treatment. Leukemia may be accompanied by gingival enlargement. The prognosis for the more severe or advanced types of cancer can force modification of usual treatment plans. Radiation therapy may make surgical treatment inadvisable. The treating physician should be contacted if chemotherapy is being used or has been used recently.

L Many medicaments and drugs used in periodontal treatment are significant allergens that may have to be avoided with sensitized patients.

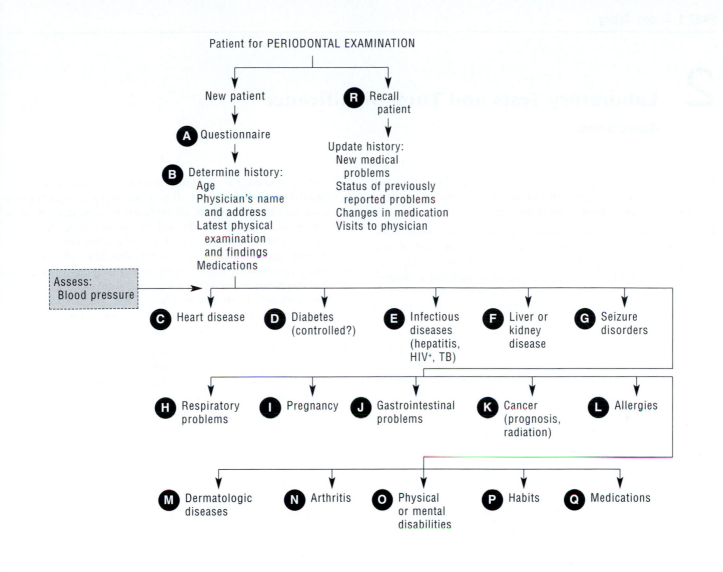

M Some dermatologic diseases, such as lichen planus, pemphigus, and pemphigoid, have periodontal components.

N Some types of arthritis can restrict dexterity required for plaque removal. Corticosteroid therapy often delays healing after periodontal treatment.

O Physical or medical disabilities may help explain the etiology of inflammatory periodontal disease if the patient is unable to perform adequate oral hygiene procedures. Disabilities may also influence the prognosis and treatment planning.

P Heavy smoking, excessive alcohol consumption or drug use influence the periodontal diagnosis, prognosis, and treatment planning. Vigorous tooth brushing, especially with a hard brush, may explain root exposure. Self-mutilating habits may alter gingival appearance.

Q Medications used for the treatment or management of any medical problem may affect periodontal treatment. Some medications, such as β-blockers, may require changes in anesthetics. Others, such as antibiotics, may produce temporary improvements in periodontitis. A dentist must have a recent edition of the *Physicians' Desk Reference* or a similar reference to determine possible effects of new medications on the treatment plan.

R Update the medical history of a recall or continuing patient at every visit. New medical problems, altered status of previously diagnosed medical problems, and changes in medications can affect periodontal treatment.

Additional Readings

Carranza FA Jr, Newman MG. Clinical periodontology. 8th ed. Philadelphia: WB Saunders; 1996. p. 344.

Genco RJ, Goldman HM, Cohen DW. Contemporary periodontics. St. Louis: Mosby; 1990. p. 203.

2 Laboratory Tests and Their Significance

Richard S. Rudin

A The patient initiates the examination process by completing a health questionnaire. This provides the basis for the dentist to initiate taking a health history.

B A complete and thorough health history is the most valuable source of necessary patient care information. Clinic laboratory testing is often a useful adjunct in the diagnosis and treatment process and must be considered a supplement to a complete history and physical examination. Occasionally, laboratory testing is necessary to confirm a diagnosis or uncover findings separate from the chief complaint.

The ordering of laboratory tests falls within the scope of practice of licensed general dentists and specialists. Many dentists fail to make use of this area of health analysis because of lack of training. Depending on the background and experience of the treating dentist, the patient will be referred either to a clinic laboratory or a physician for appropriate testing.

A large number of tests from body fluids and venous blood samples are of use to the practicing physician, and a limited number are of interest to the dentist. A positive answer or suggestive family history on a health questionnaire in conjunction with an oral examination may lead the practitioner to assess further for any of the following:

C Cardiovascular disease—The periodontist may request results of an electrocardiogram or echocardiogram, a Holter monitor, or any study evaluating cardiac function, especially to rule out a valvular problem, for which antibiotic prophylaxis may be needed. Analysis of creatine phosphokinase (CPK) or serum enzyme level is rarely ordered or used by dentists. CPK is the first enzyme level to rise in suspected myocardial infarction (MI). Release of CPK indicates tissue damage.

D Endocrine disease (diabetes)—Patients at high risk should be screened for their family history. Evaluate patients with a history of recurrent oral infection; periodontal disease in excess of observed local factors; or symptomatic polyuria, polydipsia, and polyphagia. An evaluation of the patient's level of control should include the following:

Fasting blood sugar
Clinitest tablets
Clinistix strips

E Infectious disease including acquired immunodeficiency syndrome (AIDS), hepatitis, and tuberculosis (TB)—It may be important to determine the infectivity of a patient with a positive history of hepatitis. Tests for core and antigen are relatively easy and inexpensive. Vaccination for hepatitis B has significantly decreased the risk for dental personnel, but it does *not* provide lifelong immunity. An *antibody titer* to the virus may be advisable. A test for bilirubin, which is responsible for the clinical manifestation of jaundice, is rarely used or ordered by dentists.

Numerous oral and periodontal findings are associated with human immunodeficiency virus (HIV) disease. If signs are discovered, the condition must be handled with confidentiality and sensitivity. Direct access to comprehensive medical care is required. Be prepared to refer the patient if an initial diagnosis is expected. If invasive procedures are planned, values including a CD4/CD8 platelet count, hemoglobin (Hgb), and hematocrit (HCT) should be obtained and must be relatively recent (within the past 3 months). Medical clearance is essential, and an antibiotic prophylaxis may be necessary. If an HIV test is ordered, written consent is necessary. If the treating periodontist orders the test (ELISA or Western blot), referral is necessary.

F Liver and kidney disease—Dentists rarely use or order serum enzyme levels to determine the presence of liver and kidney disease. From the dentist's perspective, the major importance of these values is for assessing a patient's status after hepatitis or other hepatic disease. Serum enzymes include the following:

Serum glutamic-pyruvic transaminase—associated with liver injury
Serum glutamic-oxaloacetic transaminase—increased by cell death in the liver, brain, or heart
Lactate dehydrogenase (LDH)—nonspecific
LDH_1—associated with MI
LDH_5—associated with liver damage and cell necrosis

Blood tests for *renal function* are rarely ordered. They include creatinine, which is increased in renal failure, and blood urea nitrogen, which is associated with changes in plasma volume.

G Cancer—A complete blood count is useful and inexpensive. It measures the HCT, which is based on Hgb and a platelet white blood count, important initially in some conditions. HCT increases in infection, inflammation, leukemia, and tissue destruction and decreases in aplastic anemia, drug toxicity, and viral infections. A differential white blood cell count determines the percentage of each kind of the following white blood cell types.

Polymorphonuclear neutrophil leukocytes
Increase: infection, inflammation
Decrease: aplastic anemia, cycle neutropenia, drug-induced myelosuppression
Lymphocytes
T cells—CD4/CD8 subpopulations
B cells
Monocytes
Important in subacute bacterial endocarditis TB, mononucleosis
Eosinophils
Increase in allergies, scarlet fever, hemolytic malignant disease—leukemia, Hodgkin's disease

H Habits—The dentist rarely uses urinalysis or venous samples to detect the presence of drugs. A biopsy specimen can be considered a laboratory test and may be ordered or performed for a variety of oral lesions.

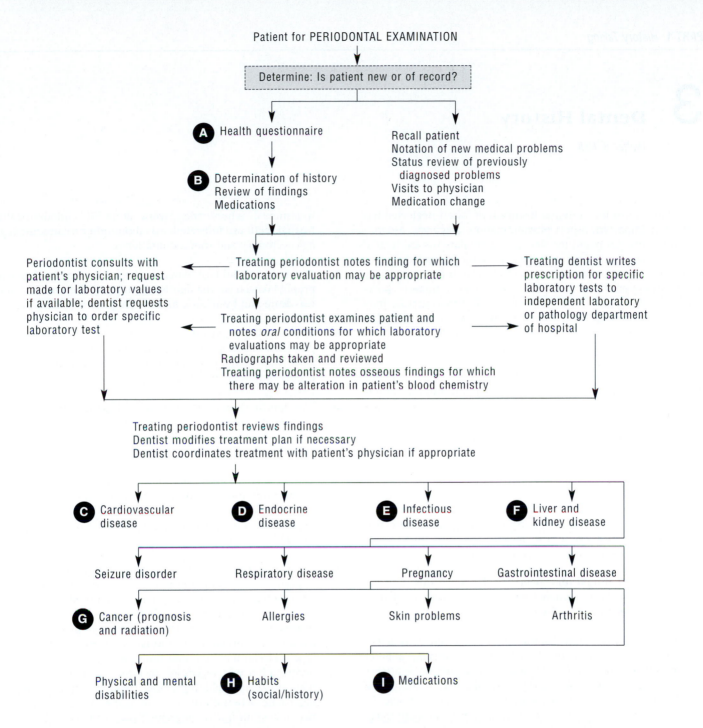

Patient for PERIODONTAL EXAMINATION

Determine: Is patient new or of record?

A Health questionnaire

B Determination of history
Review of findings
Medications

Recall patient
Notation of new medical problems
Status review of previously
  diagnosed problems
Visits to physician
Medication change

Periodontist consults with
patient's physician; request
made for laboratory values
if available; dentist requests
physician to order specific
laboratory test

Treating periodontist notes finding for which
laboratory evaluation may be appropriate

Treating periodontist examines patient and
notes *oral* conditions for which laboratory
evaluations may be appropriate
Radiographs taken and reviewed
Treating periodontist notes osseous findings for which
there may be alteration in patient's blood chemistry

Treating dentist writes
prescription for specific
laboratory tests to
independent laboratory
or pathology department
of hospital

Treating periodontist reviews findings
Dentist modifies treatment plan if necessary
Dentist coordinates treatment with patient's physician if appropriate

C Cardiovascular disease   **D** Endocrine disease   **E** Infectious disease   **F** Liver and kidney disease

Seizure disorder   Respiratory disease   Pregnancy   Gastrointestinal disease

G Cancer (prognosis and radiation)   Allergies   Skin problems   Arthritis

Physical and mental disabilities   **H** Habits (social/history)   **I** Medications

I Medications—Medications may alter a patient's hematologic profile. Drugs may significantly alter the bleeding profile.

Several tests are used to screen patients for potential bleeding disorders or measure current parameters if the patient is receiving anticoagulant medication. Bleeding problems can be caused by a decrease in the platelet count, abnormal function, or defects in the extrinsic, intrinsic, or common clotting pathways. Tests include the following:

Platelet count
Prothrombin time (PT)
Partial thromboplastin time (PTT)

PT is prolonged by anticoagulant therapy, aspirin, and deficiencies in factors I, II, V, VII, and X, as well as liver damage. PTT is prolonged in anticoagulant therapy with heparin and defects in the common and intrinsic pathways. Consultation with the treating physician is needed if the patient is receiving Coumadin, the international normalized ratio is unknown, and surgical procedures are planned.

Test for Disturbances of Bone

Periodontal (clinical) or radiographic findings may lead the dentist to order tests for serum calcium, phosphorus, or alkaline phosphatase. These tests may help in the diagnosis of the following:

Paget's disease of bone
Metastatic disease of bone
Hypoparathyroidism and hyperparathyroidism

Additional Readings

Carranza FA Jr, Newman MG. Clinical periodontology. 8th ed. Philadelphia: WB Saunders; 1996. p. 133.

Genco RJ, Goldman HM, Cohen DW. Contemporary periodontics. St. Louis: Mosby; 1990. p. 327.

Jolly D. Interpreting the clinical laboratory. J Can Dent Assoc 1995; 23:32.

Sonis ST, Fazio RC, Fang L. Principles and practice of oral medicine. 2nd ed. Philadelphia: WB Saunders; 1995. p. 17.

3 Dental History

Walter B. Hall

Taking and recording a dental history is an often-neglected but extremely important aspect of examination, diagnosis, prognosis, and treatment planning. Because many patients are treated by more than one dentist, this history should be updated regularly. The accuracy and reliability of facts from the dental history are always open to question. The patient's own answers, however, are important to record, because any inaccuracies may influence treatment. If the "facts" are not consistent with what is seen in the mouth or on radiographs or with the dentist's knowledge of periodontal problems and their treatment, more extensive questioning may be necessary.

A A questionnaire ("yes or no" format) is useful for gathering data. The patient can complete such a questionnaire while waiting to see the dentist. Provide space on the questionnaire for a new patient to indicate the date of the last dental visit and its purpose, the former dentist and reason for changing, and whether radiographs or other materials are available.

B Further questioning by the dentist is necessary to determine details such as the reason a certain procedure was done, the location in the mouth, and the time. Space should be available for such annotation in the chart.

C The patient should note which teeth are missing, and the dentist should ask when they were removed (or if they never appeared) and why.

D The patient may know that the third molars were extracted or are impacted. The dentist should ask about postsurgical problems if the molars were extracted, including when the surgery was done. If the molars are present, the dentist should ask whether the patient has ever been told they should be removed, and if so, the reason surgery was not performed. The dentist should ask about any symptoms (such as pain or swelling) that the patient has had in those areas.

E By asking a general question about other surgery, the dentist may learn about previous fractures of the jaw or oral tumors that have been removed. The dentist must use follow-up questions for details.

F The dentist should ask about restorations such as crowns, bridges, removable prostheses, and implants. If any are present, the dentist should ask the reason they were placed, when they were placed and by whom, and whether earlier restorations preceded them. A patient's knowledge of these events is likely to be unimpressive.

G The dentist should ask whether the patient has any endodontically treated teeth. If so, ask when they were treated and, in cases of atypical or inadequate root canal treatments, where they were done. If endodontically treated teeth are indicated, ask about other treatments (eg, apicoectomies and root amputations).

H The dentist should ask whether the patient has had regular prophylaxes. If so, the dentist should ask when the last one was done and by whom, and the frequency of cleanings.

I The dentist should ask whether the patient has had bite problems or jaw pain. If so, a detailed history of the problems, their diagnoses, treatments, and the dates of these events should be annotated.

J The dentist should ask whether the patient has had any orthodontic treatment. If so, the dentist should record its nature, times of treatment, extractions, the patient's satisfaction with the outcome, and any relapse.

K The dentist should ask about clenching and grinding (ie, bruxism, night grinding), record the patient's concept of the problem, and note whether the problem can be related to particular life or dental events. Prior use of a night guard should be noted.

L For a periodontal patient, the periodontal history is most important. An essential question is whether the patient has had a previous periodontal problem diagnosed. If not, questions regarding bleeding, swollen gingiva, pain, or gingival ulcerations may reveal that periodontal problems have existed. If a previous diagnosis was made, annotate the types of treatment and their times. If no previous treatment occurred but was suggested, ascertain the reason no treatment was performed. If previous treatment was performed, determine whether there were acute problems such as necrotizing ulcerative gingivitis (NUG) or necrotizing ulcerative periodontitis (NUP), human immunodeficiency virus (HIV) gingivitis or periodontitis, or a periodontal abscess. Also, establish when and how they were treated.

M A recall periodontal patient may have had dental problems or treatment by other dentists since the last visit. Update the dental history; specifically ask whether any problems have occurred, the response to earlier treatment, oral hygiene measures used, and dental treatment performed elsewhere.

Additional Readings

Carranza FA Jr, Newman MG. Clinical periodontology. 8th ed. Philadelphia: WB Saunders; 1996. p. 345.

Genco RJ, Goldman HM, Cohen DW. Contemporary periodontics. St. Louis: Mosby; 1990. p. 331.

Wlison TG, Kornman KS. Fundamentals of periodontics. Chicago: Quintessence Publishing; 1996. p. 206, 305.

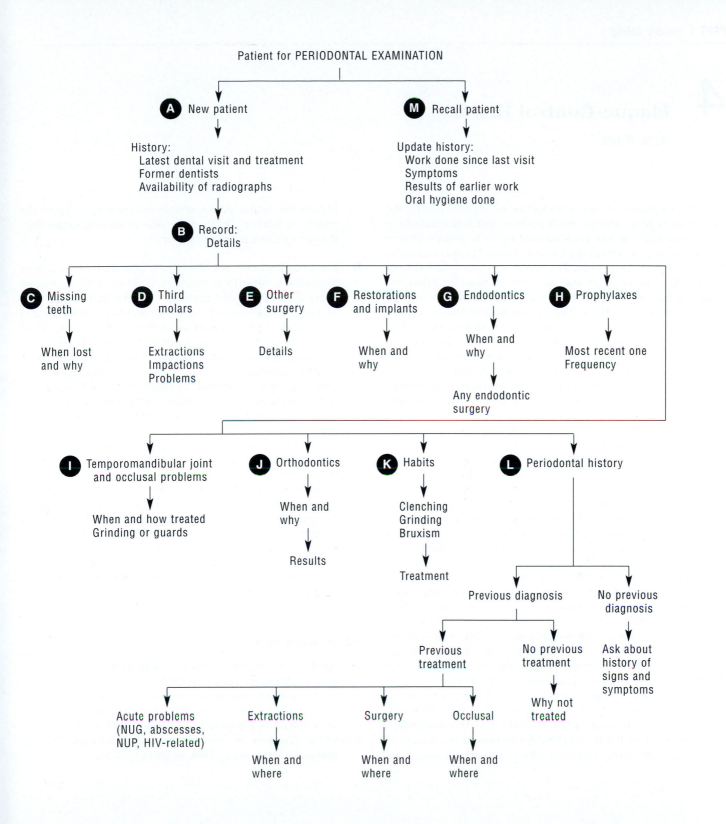

Patient for PERIODONTAL EXAMINATION

A New patient

M Recall patient

History:
Latest dental visit and treatment
Former dentists
Availability of radiographs

Update history:
Work done since last visit
Symptoms
Results of earlier work
Oral hygiene done

B Record:
Details

C Missing teeth

When lost and why

D Third molars

Extractions
Impactions
Problems

E Other surgery

Details

F Restorations and implants

When and why

G Endodontics

When and why

Any endodontic surgery

H Prophylaxes

Most recent one
Frequency

I Temporomandibular joint and occlusal problems

When and how treated
Grinding or guards

J Orthodontics

When and why

Results

K Habits

Clenching
Grinding
Bruxism

Treatment

L Periodontal history

Previous diagnosis

No previous diagnosis

Previous treatment

No previous treatment

Ask about history of signs and symptoms

Why not treated

Acute problems
(NUG, abscesses, NUP, HIV-related)

Extractions

When and where

Surgery

When and where

Occlusal

When and where

4 Plaque-Control History

Walter B. Hall

A history of plaque control is important to establish during the examination of a new or recall patient. What the patient is doing, has done, or has been advised to do to control plaque accumulation can explain the current status of plaque control at the time of the examination. The dentist can also collect data of a subjective nature. The way patients respond to questions regarding plaque-control efforts may be as important to helping them as the answers themselves. If the tone of the answers is negative, the dentist must expend a greater effort or find a new approach to sensitizing the patient to the need for personal effort. If the patient cannot be motivated or is unable to perform adequate plaque control, the dentist's responsibilities become greater and more frequent visits will be necessary. The patient should be made aware that the cost in money, time, and discomfort will be greater; this may help motivate the patient.

A   For a new patient, a history of plaque control regarding past and current practices is required. Past practices, such as using a hard or medium brush with a scrub stroke, may be the reason recession is present. Relating past brushing to current techniques may indicate when recession occurred and whether it is stable or ongoing. These are important factors in deciding whether gingival grafting is needed. It is important to ascertain how long the patient has been flossing, the way the floss is used, and what the patient is trying to accomplish. Improper use of floss with a "shoe-shining" motion may explain the origin of floss cuts. If adjuncts such as water spray or irrigation devices, interproximal brushes, wooden interproximal sticks, toothpicks, or a Perio Aide have been used, note the manner of their use and the patient's understanding of their rationale. Damage relating to the misuse of such devices also may be suggested. Note the reasons for discontinuing the use of a device.

Document the patient's current practices in regard to brushing, flossing, and use of adjunctive devices. Note the adequacy of the approaches as *satisfactory* or *needing changes* in regard to what is being used and how. If the patient is doing something different than instructed, note and explain this action. At the initial examination, compare the results of what is being done and explore discrepancies. Record a plaque index at that time.

B   For a recall patient, ask the person to demonstrate, at least by motions, the current practices. If the patient has stopped using all recommended devices or has changed the methods of their use, the reason for doing so should be explained and the degree of success with the revised approach should be evaluated. Occasionally, a patient may devise a better means of using a device than the method taught. If not harmful, it may be advisable to allow the patient to continue using the new approach. When the examination is performed, the stated practices can be compared with results and discrepancies explored. Record a plaque index at this time as well.

C   If a patient's plaque-control program needs to be changed, an electric brush may be helpful for physically impaired individuals. A sonic brush may be especially useful for those individuals. It cleans *even beyond* the contacts of bristle tips; therefore it is preferable to a hand or electric brush for patients who are missing interproximal areas. For patients whose flossing is inadequate, a change to an adjunctive device often works wonders. Where they fit between teeth or roots, interproximal brushes are best. If spaces are too narrow, various sticks can be an excellent alternative.

Additional Readings

Carranza FA Jr, Newman MG. Clinical periodontology. 8th ed. Philadelphia: WB Saunders; 1996. p. 347.

Schluger S, Yuodelis R, Page RC. Periodontal diseases: basic phenomena, clinical management, and occlusal and restorative interrelationships. 2nd ed. Philadelphia: Lea & Febiger; 1990. p. 349.

Wilson TG, Kornman KS. Fundamentals of periodontics. Chicago: Quintessence Publishing; 1996. p. 350, 353, 371–2.

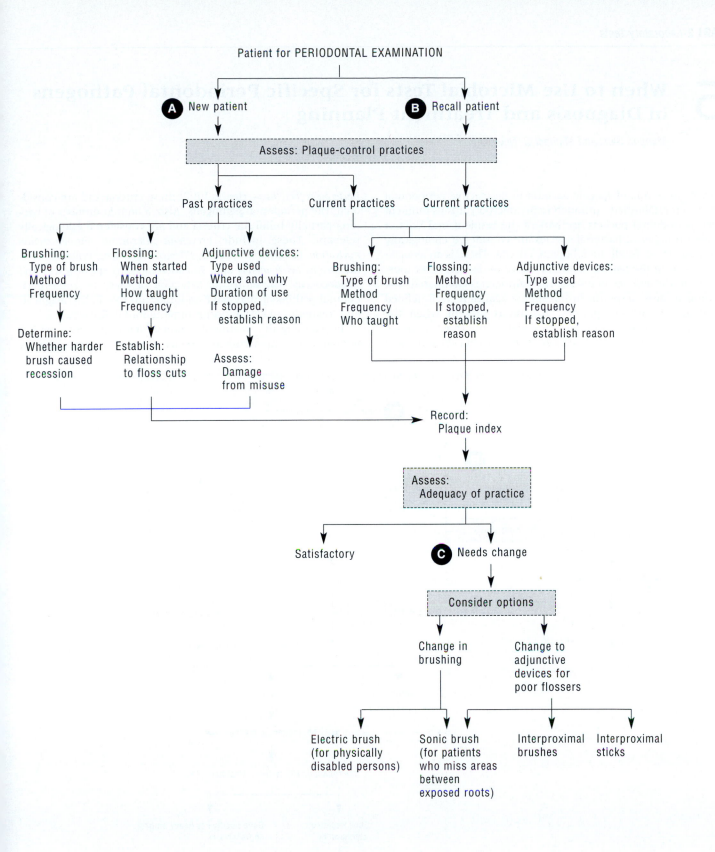

Patient for PERIODONTAL EXAMINATION

A New patient   **B** Recall patient

Assess: Plaque-control practices

Past practices   Current practices   Current practices

Brushing:
Type of brush
Method
Frequency

Flossing:
When started
Method
How taught
Frequency

Adjunctive devices:
Type used
Where and why
Duration of use
If stopped,
establish reason

Determine:
Whether harder
brush caused
recession

Establish:
Relationship
to floss cuts

Assess:
Damage
from misuse

Brushing:
Type of brush
Method
Frequency
Who taught

Flossing:
Method
Frequency
If stopped,
establish
reason

Adjunctive devices:
Type used
Method
Frequency
If stopped,
establish reason

Record:
Plaque index

Assess:
Adequacy of practice

Satisfactory   **C** Needs change

Consider options

Change in
brushing

Change to
adjunctive
devices for
poor flossers

Electric brush
(for physically
disabled persons)

Sonic brush
(for patients
who miss areas
between
exposed roots)

Interproximal
brushes

Interproximal
sticks

5 When to Use Microbial Tests for Specific Periodontal Pathogens in Diagnosis and Treatment Planning

Mariano Sanz and Michael G. Newman

The etiologic role of specific bacteria in destructive periodontal diseases is established. Although many microorganisms found in deep periodontal pockets are part of the resident oral flora, a limited number of bacterial species are considered etiologically relevant. These fulfill the following criteria: There is an association between the pathogen and presence of disease. After therapy or in the absence of disease the pathogen is eliminated. The pathogen causes a specific host response against it. Well-defined virulence factors are present. Disease is present when the pathogen is inoculated in animal models. Only three species—*Actinobacillus actinomycetemcomitans*, *Porphyromonas gingivalis*, and

Bacteroides forsythus—clearly fulfill these criteria and are considered true periodontal pathogens. Also, a limited number of bacteria partially fulfill the criteria and are considered etiologically relevant. These include *Prevotella intermedia*, *Fusobacterium nucleatum*, *Campylobacter rectus*, *Eikenella corrodens*, *Peptostreptococcus micros*, *Selenomonas* spp, *Eubacterium* spp, spirochetes, and strepococcus. Therefore the detection of these potential periodontal pathogens may have an important role in the diagnosis and treatment of certain forms of periodontal diseases.

In planning the treatment complex dental problems with a periodontal component, the results of microbial tests may be

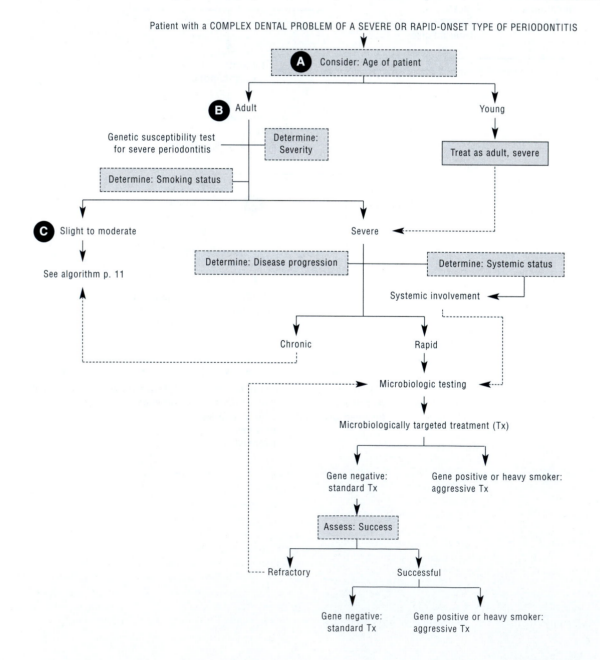

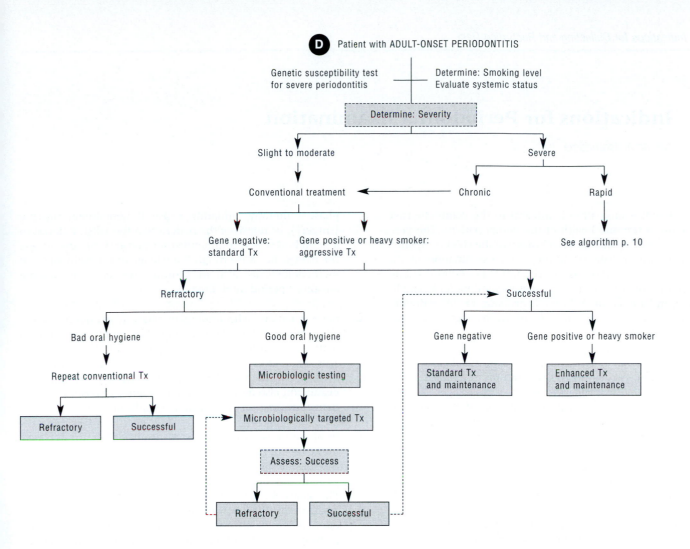

Patient with ADULT-ONSET PERIODONTITIS

Genetic susceptibility test
for severe periodontitis

Determine: Smoking level
Evaluate systemic status

Determine: Severity

Slight to moderate — Severe

Conventional treatment ← Chronic — Rapid

See algorithm p. 10

Gene negative: standard Tx — Gene positive or heavy smoker: aggressive Tx

Refractory — Successful

Bad oral hygiene — Good oral hygiene — Gene negative — Gene positive or heavy smoker

Repeat conventional Tx — Microbiologic testing — Standard Tx and maintenance — Enhanced Tx and maintenance

Refractory — Successful — Microbiologically targeted Tx

Assess: Success

Refractory — Successful

useful. In types of periodontitis that are severe or of rapid onset or that do not respond well to conventional periodontal therapy specific microorganisms may be causing the problem. Clinical measurements, radiographic evaluation, and monitoring for progression of disease will determine whether microbial tests can be useful. In many such cases, these tests determine the type and magnitude of the entire treatment plan. The following factors are applicable to all patients.

A   The age of the patient may determine the potential usefulness of microbial tests. In early-onset periodontitis, when periodontal disease is usually severe, identification of specific pathogens such as *A. actinomycetemcomitans* or *Porphyromonas gingivalis* is often valuable information that can be used to guide treatment. Elimination of these and other periodontopathic bacteria through adequate periodontal and/or antimicrobial therapy can be associated with improved clinical outcomes and a better periodontal prognosis.

B   In adult forms of periodontitis, the severity of the problem is assessed clinically and radiographically. For individual adults, the future course of the disease can be anticipated by knowing whether the patient is a heavy smoker (> 20 pack/year) or has a genetic predisposition to severe disease. Heavy smokers have a 4.2 times greater risk of severe disease, and those who have the interleukin-1 genetic predisposition have an 18.9 times higher risk of severe disease.

C   Adult patients with less severe conditions or genotype-negative individuals should be treated via conventional periodontal therapy. In most of these instances the disease

can be arrested and the patient successfully treated. However, a few individuals do not respond adequately to conventional methods despite good levels of oral hygiene. These patients may also benefit from microbial testing and, based on the results, institution of microbially targeted periodontal therapy.

D   Assessing the systemic health status of adult patients is also extremely important. Patients with associated systemic disease may have an altered host response. Opportunistic infections may appear as a result of impaired healing, an inability to tolerate certain treatments, potential drug interaction, or a compromised immune system. In these patients, it is especially important to perform a microbial test to ensure that the appropriate antimicrobial therapy is prescribed.

Additional Readings

Carranza FA Jr, Newman MG. Clinical periodontology. 8th ed. Philadelphia: WB Saunders; 1996. p. 714.

Haffajee A, Socransky SS. Microbial etiological agents of destructive periodontal diseases. Periodontology 2000 1994;5:78–111.

Kornman KS et al. The interleukin 1 genotype as a severity factor in adult periodontal disease. J Clin Periodontol 1995;22:258.

Lang NP, Karring T. Proceedings of the 1st European Workshop on Periodontology. London: Quintessence Publishing; 1994.

World Workshop in Clinical Periodontics. In: Newman MG, editor. Annals of periodontology. Vol 1. Chicago; ARP; 1997. p. 37.

Van Winkelhoff AJ, Rams TE, Slots J. Systemic antibiotic therapy in periodontics. Periodontology 2000 1996;10;45.

6 Indications for Periodontal Examination

Steven A. Tsurudome

The periodontal examination is integral to the comprehensive examination of the oral health of the dental patient. The periodontal examination includes the history of the chief complaint, the patient's medical-dental history, and examination of the extraoral and intraoral soft tissue. The initial periodontal examination (IPE) provides the baseline documentation, for example, of gingival inflammation and past destruction to the periodontium, from which the appropriate diagnosis, prognosis, and treatment plan are formulated.

A Each new dental patient should have an initial periodontal examination; periodontal disease can occur at any stage in life, although the incidence increases with age. The IPE involves assessment and documentation of the following clinical parameters: probing depth measurements, clinical attachment levels, bleeding on probing, furcation involvements, plaque index, gingival index, mucogingival anatomy, tooth mobility, occlusion, and full-mouth radiographic evaluation of the alveolar bone. The extent of presenting periodontal destruction is revealed by the IPE. Assessment of the clinical parameters just described does not predict future destruction. The IPE is essential, nevertheless, in bringing problem areas into focus.

B The problem areas may become recognizable by any of the following changes: (1) probing depths of more than 3 mm, (2) furcation involvement, (3) bleeding on probing, (4) loss of attachment (LOA), (5) gingival exudate or suppuration, and (6) radiographic evidence of loss of alveolar bone.

C After a diagnosis of periodontal disease has been made, periodontal therapy phase I should be initiated, appropriate to the severity of the disease. Then, phase I evaluation (ie, evaluation of the initial treatment) must be performed to ascertain the success of this initial periodontal therapy (to assess, eg, the control of inflammation, bacterial plaque, and occlusion). Typically, this is undertaken about 4 to 6 weeks after the completion of the treatment. Phase I evaluation includes remeasuring the probing depths and attachment levels and reassessing the bleeding on probing, tooth mobility, gingival and plaque indexes, and occlusion.

D If the phase I evaluation reveals a statistically significant LOA (a change of 2 to 3 mm), periodontal disease activity may be present. From an assessment of the clinical parameters documented during the phase I evaluation, the clinician can formulate an appropriate plan for repeating phase I therapy, initiating phase II periodontal therapy (surgery), or referring the patient to a specialist. Referral to a periodontist is recommended for phase II therapy, unless the dentist has a thorough knowledge of the rationale and methodology, as well as clinical experience in treating advanced periodontal diseases.

E For the patient who undergoes phase II periodontal therapy, a phase II reevaluation should be performed approximately 3 months after the completion of that treatment. This evaluation is similar to the phase I evaluation and assesses the success of the phase II therapy. The phase II evaluation also determines the frequency of recall (maintenance) evaluations which may be indicated.

F In phase I evaluation, any statistically significant decrease in the rate of LOA may be indicative of progress in the control of the periodontal disease. If this is the case, the patient may be placed in the recall (maintenance) phase. The goals for the recall visits are periodic longitudinal assessment of the periodontal status, maintenance of periodontal health through appropriate scaling and/or root planing, and reinforcement of oral hygiene instructions (OHI) as necessary. The frequency of the periodic recall evaluations may be determined by the severity of the past periodontal disease or dental history of periodontal surgery. Usually, an average frequency of 3 months is typical, with the examinations performed alternatively between the referring dentist and the periodontist. Appropriate radiographs may be taken once a year, as needed.

G After consecutive recall evaluations indicate that stable periodontal health has been achieved, with control of bacterial plaque, the recall evaluation frequency may be extended to a yearly examination with appropriate radiographs taken by the dentist.

Additional Readings

American Academy of Periodontology. Proceedings of the World Workshop in Clinical Periodontics. Chicago: The Academy; 1989.

Armitage G. Clinical evaluation of periodontal diseases. Periodontology 2000 1995;7:39.

Genco RJ, Goldman HM, Cohen DW. Contemporary periodontics. St. Louis: Mosby; 1990. p. 339.

Lang N, Karring T. Proceedings of the 1st European Workshop on Periodontology. London: Quintessence Publishing; 1994. p. 42.

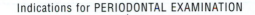

Indications for PERIODONTAL EXAMINATION

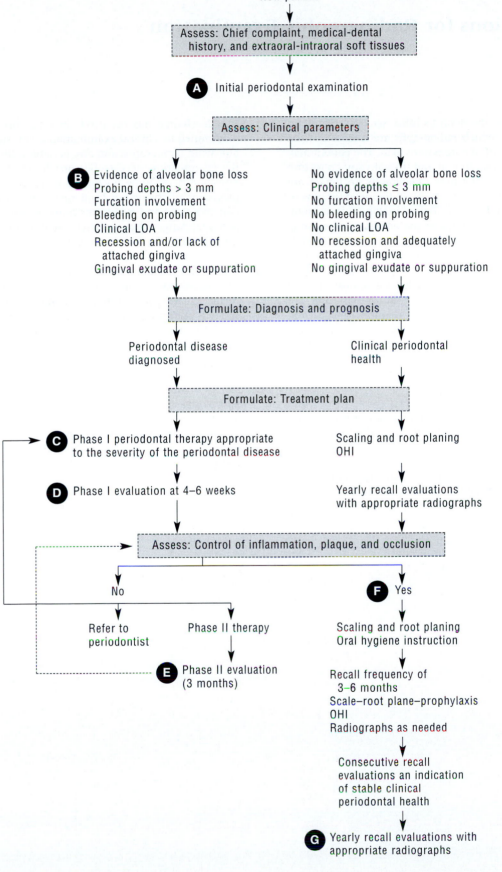

New patient

Assess: Chief complaint, medical-dental history, and extraoral-intraoral soft tissues

A Initial periodontal examination

Assess: Clinical parameters

B Evidence of alveolar bone loss
Probing depths > 3 mm
Furcation involvement
Bleeding on probing
Clinical LOA
Recession and/or lack of attached gingiva
Gingival exudate or suppuration

No evidence of alveolar bone loss
Probing depths ≤ 3 mm
No furcation involvement
No bleeding on probing
No clinical LOA
No recession and adequately attached gingiva
No gingival exudate or suppuration

Formulate: Diagnosis and prognosis

Periodontal disease diagnosed

Clinical periodontal health

Formulate: Treatment plan

C Phase I periodontal therapy appropriate to the severity of the periodontal disease

Scaling and root planing
OHI

D Phase I evaluation at 4–6 weeks

Yearly recall evaluations with appropriate radiographs

Assess: Control of inflammation, plaque, and occlusion

No

F Yes

Refer to periodontist

Phase II therapy

E Phase II evaluation (3 months)

Scaling and root planing
Oral hygiene instruction

Recall frequency of 3–6 months
Scale–root plane–prophylaxis
OHI
Radiographs as needed

Consecutive recall evaluations an indication of stable clinical periodontal health

G Yearly recall evaluations with appropriate radiographs

13

7 Indications for Radiographic Examination

Walter B. Hall

When a patient comes to the dentist's office seeking treatment, the dentist must decide which radiographs are needed for the diagnosis and development of a treatment plan. The patient may be new or returning for a recall visit and thus already on record. Temporal guidelines for taking new radiographs no longer are regarded as valid. The dentist's judgment on the need for new or additional films is accepted as valid. Before making this decision, the dentist must obtain and evaluate the adequacy of existing radiographs and weigh the potential value from new or additional films against the negative effects of cumulative radiation.

A   A full series of radiographs is needed for almost all new patients who have teeth. If earlier films exist and are obtained, assess the patient's age in relation to signs and symptoms. If the existing films are recent enough, assess their quality and adequacy in relation to current problems. Obtain new bite-wing and periapical films as necessary to evaluate specific problems. The routine taking of a new full series cannot be justified.

B   If the new patient has no recent radiographs or the existing films cannot be obtained expediently from the former dentist, take a new full series.

C   When a patient returns for a recall visit, the dentist must decide whether new or additional radiographs are required.

If little change has occurred since the preceding visit, as determined by clinical examination and histories, only new bite-wing radiographs and any periapical films indicated by the examination need to be considered. Annual taking of new bite-wing films no longer is indicated. The dentist's judgment of the value from new films suggested by the patient's signs and symptoms must be weighed against the potential danger of cumulative radiation from films that are not critical to diagnosis or treatment planning.

D   If no series has been obtained for many years, and a comprehensive radiographic evaluation seems necessary for further treatment planning or definite diagnosis, a new full series is indicated. The decision to take new films is the responsibility of the dentist.

Additional Readings

Carranza FA Jr, Newman MG. Clinical periodontology. 8th ed. Philadelphia: WB Saunders; 1996. p. 346.

Prichard JF. The diagnosis and treatment of periodontal disease. Philadelphia: WB Saunders; 1979. p. 67.

Wilson TG, Kornman KS. Fundamentals of periodontics. Chicago: Quintessence Publishing; 1996. p. 219–29.

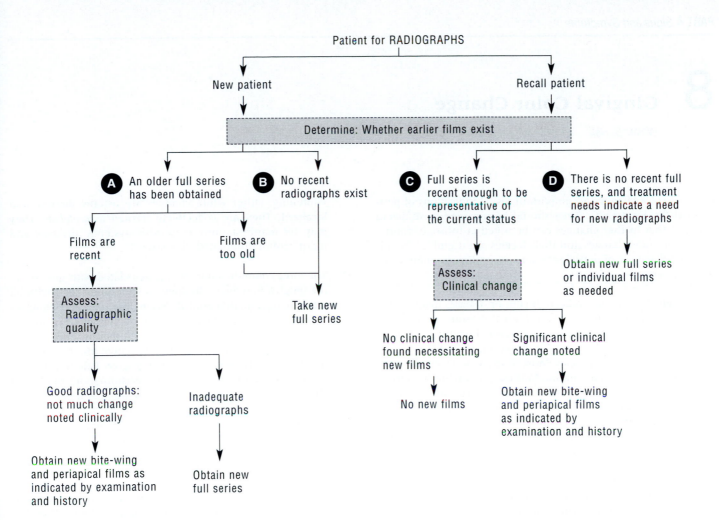

Patient for RADIOGRAPHS

New patient | Recall patient

Determine: Whether earlier films exist

A An older full series has been obtained

B No recent radiographs exist

C Full series is recent enough to be representative of the current status

D There is no recent full series, and treatment needs indicate a need for new radiographs

Films are recent | Films are too old

Assess: Radiographic quality

Take new full series

Assess: Clinical change

Obtain new full series or individual films as needed

Good radiographs: not much change noted clinically

Inadequate radiographs

No clinical change found necessitating new films

Significant clinical change noted

Obtain new bite-wing and periapical films as indicated by examination and history

Obtain new full series

No new films

Obtain new bite-wing and periapical films as indicated by examination and history

8 Gingival Color Change

Walter B. Hall

Gingival color changes are important visual indications of periodontal disease activity. They should be recorded in sufficient detail so that further changes can be noted at future examinations. The color changes and their locales are useful in the differential diagnosis of periodontal and other diseases manifested in the gingiva.

A Gingival color may indicate health or disease. Healthy gingivae vary in color depending on a person's racial background. American texts often describe healthy gingivae as being salmon pink; this color, however, is limited to many, but not all, white people. Most of the world's people have some melanin pigmentation to their gingivae in the normal or healthy state. Lighter coffee-colored, disseminated melanin pigment is typical of American Indians, Asians, and some white people. Darker tones, sometimes disseminated but more often discretely localized, are characteristic of black people.

B The effects of disease on the gingiva often are manifested by color changes. If the gingiva becomes whitened, the white may wipe away. If it wipes off, it is not a true white lesion but probably consists of sloughed cells and debris that have not been wiped away during cleaning. Such debris may accompany painful gingival lesions such as (1) herpetic gingivostomatitis, necrotizing ulcerative gingivitis (NUG), or necrotizing ulcerative periodontitis (NUP); or (2) human immunodeficiency virus (HIV) gingivitis or periodontitis, in which the patient avoids brushing or eating normally and the sloughed cell mass and detritus accumulate. Whitened gingiva that is not débridable by wiping often results from smoking. The problem is usually generalized; palatal changes are most common and most extensive, and changes on buccal mucosa or the tongue are often detectable. Trauma, such as occlusal function on an edentulous area, may produce localized areas of gingival whitening. Other white changes are usually discrete and localized. They are collectively termed *leukoplakias*. They may be manifestations of serious systemic diseases and merit careful differential diagnosis.

C The most common color change associated with diseases of the gingiva is redness. Redness is commonly seen with all inflammatory periodontal diseases. Marginal and papillary redness is a feature of various types of gingivitis, periodontitis, NUG and NUP, herpetic gingivostomatitis, and desquamative gingivitis. In desquamative gingivitis, the redness usually extends into the attached gingiva. Pale red changes are manifestations of less severe inflammation; bright red changes indicate a more severe or acute inflammation.

Linear marginal erythema is a narrow band of reddening affecting the marginal and papillary gingivae of patients with the classic immune deficiency gingivitis seen in people affected by HIV. A somewhat similar reddening may accompany pregnancy gingivitis.

D Changes to magenta are a manifestation of a chronic inflammatory situation in which stasis of blood flow has occurred as a result of fluid leakage and swelling. Such chronic changes are seen most often in patients with established gingivitis or periodontitis.

Additional Readings

Carranza FA Jr, Newman MG. Clinical periodontology. 8th ed. Philadelphia: WB Saunders; 1996. p. 350.

Genco RJ, Goldman HM, Cohen DW. Contemporary periodontics. St. Louis: Mosby; 1990. p. 339.

Grant DA, Stern IB, Listgarten MA. Periodontics. 6th ed. St. Louis: Mosby; 1988. p. 533.

Wilson TG, Kornman KS. Fundamentals of periodontics. Chicago: Quintessence Publishing; 1996. p. 159–64.

Patient for GINGIVAL COLOR ASSESSMENT

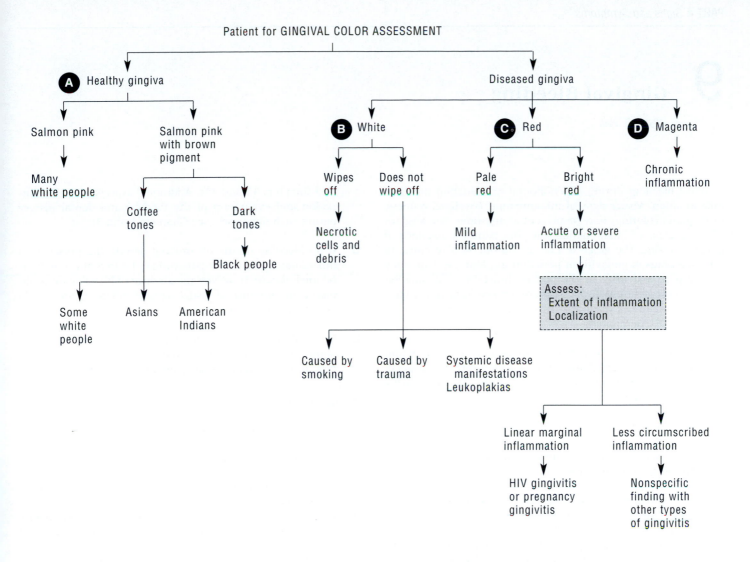

9 Gingival Bleeding

Walter B. Hall

Gingival bleeding during a periodontal examination indicates inflammation. Visual signs of inflammation (swelling, redness, or magenta coloring) may be present at any time. The absence of visual signs of inflammation does not permit a diagnosis of gingival health. The gingivae may be fibrotic as a response to repeated bouts of gingivitis or periodontitis, and the tissue may appear pink and firm. In the pocket, however, inflammation may be present, but its visual signs are masked from view superficially; therefore, a diagnosis of health cannot be made with only a visual examination.

A On probing, if no bleeding occurs and crevices are within normal limits, no inflammatory disease is present. If pockets are present but no bleeding occurs, the disease probably is in an inactive state.

B Bleeding may occur if inflammation is present in pocket areas. If bleeding does occur on probing, inflammatory periodontal disease is present and further examination permits an accurate diagnosis.

C When inflammatory signs are present, a short burst of compressed air may elicit "easy" bleeding, especially in interdental areas. "Easy" bleeding of this type is indicative of necrotizing ulcerative gingivitis (NUG) or necrotizing ulcerative periodontitis (NUP) (see Chapter 26) or of human immunodeficiency virus (HIV) gingivitis or periodontitis (see Chapters 32 and 33). Additional aspects of the examination and evaluation of the medical and dental history permit such diagnoses (see Chapters 1 and 3).

D If no bleeding occurs on probing despite the presence of inflammatory signs, the patient may be free of active periodontal disease; however, the absence of bleeding on probing in the presence of visual signs of inflammation would be a most unusual finding.

E When bleeding occurs on probing, active inflammatory periodontal disease is present. An additional evaluation of findings, history, and radiographs permits a definitive diagnosis.

Additional Readings

Abbas F et al. Bleeding plaque ratio and the development of gingival inflammation. J Clin Periodontol 1986;13:774.

Carranza FA Jr, Newman MG. Clinical periodontology. 8th ed. Philadelphia: WB Saunders; 1996. p. 353.

Grant DA, Stern JB, Listgarten MA. Periodontics. 6th ed. St. Louis: Mosby; 1988. p. 342.

Haffajee AD, Socransky SS, Goodson JM. Clinical parameters as predictors of destructive periodontal activity. J Clin Periodontol 1983;10:257.

Lindhe J. Textbook of clinical periodontology. 2nd ed. Copenhagen: Munksgaard; 1989. p. 362.

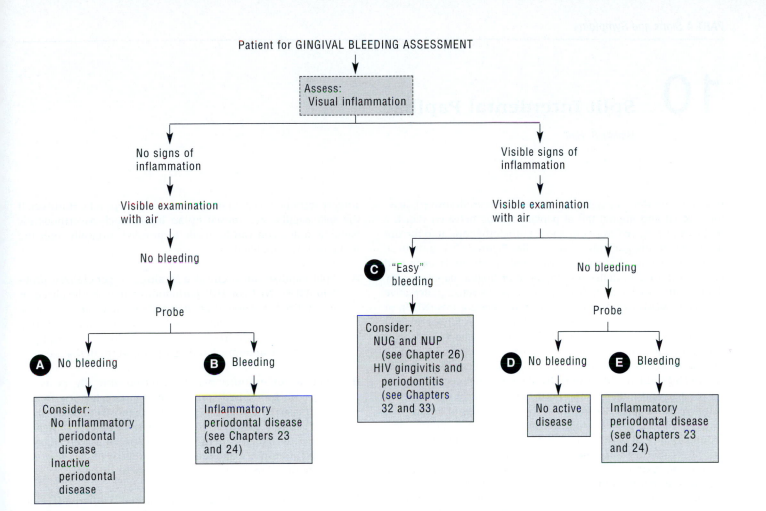

Patient for GINGIVAL BLEEDING ASSESSMENT

Assess:
Visual inflammation

No signs of
inflammation

Visible signs of
inflammation

Visible examination
with air

Visible examination
with air

No bleeding

C "Easy"
bleeding

No bleeding

Probe

Consider:
NUG and NUP
(see Chapter 26)
HIV gingivitis and
periodontitis
(see Chapters
32 and 33)

Probe

A No bleeding

B Bleeding

D No bleeding

E Bleeding

Consider:
No inflammatory
periodontal
disease
Inactive
periodontal
disease

Inflammatory
periodontal disease
(see Chapters 23
and 24)

No active
disease

Inflammatory
periodontal disease
(see Chapters 23
and 24)

10   Split Interdental Papillae

Walter B. Hall

In a split interdental papilla, the center has been destroyed, leaving a facial and lingual tab of papillary tissue between which a probe can be moved from one tooth to the other apical to the tips of the remaining portions of the papilla (Figures 10-1 and 10-2). Often, a split papilla can be visualized when air is expressed between the teeth, deflecting the facial or lingual papillary tabs. Split papillae are most often associated with necrotizing ulcerative gingivitis (NUG) or necrotizing ulcerative periodontitis (NUP), or they exist after NUP, creating a noncleansable area where adult periodontitis is likely to begin. NUG or NUP may be a localized or generalized problem. Similar split papillae may occur with human immunodeficiency virus (HIV) periodontitis and can be extremely severe and sudden. Orthodontic banding in which bands impinge on papillae and inflammation occurs as a result of difficulties in plaque control is the second most common cause of localized or generalized split papillae. Injuries caused during restorative procedures may also be a cause. Long-term heavy buildup of gross calculus is another common cause of split papillae, especially if the patient has never or rarely had dental cleaning. In the past decade the severe periodontitis associated with acquired immunodeficiency syndrome (AIDS) has been described; it has been termed *HIV periodontitis*. This must be differentiated from other lesions associated with split papillae, usually on the basis of history, membership in a high-risk group (eg, recreational drug users, homosexuals and bisexuals, hemophiliacs, dialysis patients, and sexually promiscuous people), antibody assay for the AIDS virus (HIV), T-cell lymphocyte assay (CD4 count), or high viral load counts. These problems and their etiologies are important to note during the development of a treatment plan. Surgical repair of split papillae can be a significant means of preventing the development or progress of tooth-endangering periodontitis. If the split papillae are caused by a disease with frequent recurrence (eg, NUG, NUP, or HIV periodontitis), the dentist must be certain that the patient is no longer highly susceptible to recurrence before a decision is made to proceed with surgery. Otherwise, the surgery must be repeated after a new disease episode. However, if the split papillae are caused by an injury, such as orthodontic banding, a decision can be made to proceed surgically after the movement is completed.

A   Split papillae can occur as a localized or generalized problem. NUG, NUP, or HIV periodontitis may be localized or generalized in their oral manifestations. Injuries may be (1) localized, especially if related to wounding during restorative procedures, or (2) generalized, especially if related to orthodontic banding or long-term dental neglect.

B   Evidence of an injury may be detected clinically, or its etiology can be elicited from an appropriate history. In this manner, most injury cases can be diagnosed and appropriate treatment planned. Surgical repair of defects caused by injuries, in which patient neglect or special susceptibility to disease does not make recurrence likely, is often preferable to repetitive instrumentation at frequent intervals.

C   When no history of injury can be elicited, a differential diagnosis must be made among gingivitis/periodontitis, NUG, NUP, recurrent NUG or NUP, periodontitis possibly following earlier lesions that caused nonrepaired split papillae, and HIV periodontitis. Redness and swelling may be signs of any of these lesions. Recurrent NUG or NUP may be masked visually by fibrotic repair after earlier episodes. HIV periodontitis usually exhibits marked redness and swelling with spontaneous bleeding and is characterized by sudden, severe episodes accompanied by generalized symptoms of illness, such as malaise, fever, and gastrointestinal upset.

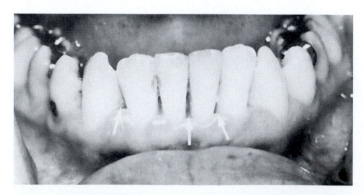

Figure 10-1 Split interdental papillae. Reproduced with permission from Hall WB, Roberts WE, LaBarre EE. Decision making in dental treatment planning. St. Louis: Mosby: 1994.

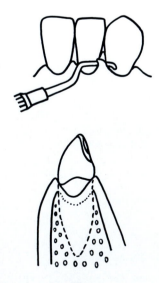

Figure 10-2 Split interdental papillae.

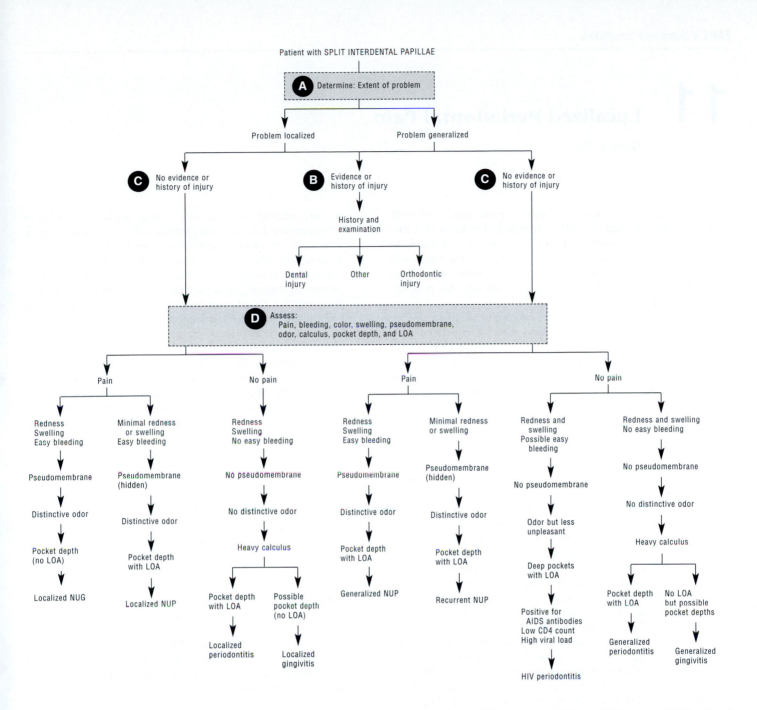

Patient with SPLIT INTERDENTAL PAPILLAE

A Determine: Extent of problem

Problem localized

Problem generalized

C No evidence or history of injury

B Evidence or history of injury

C No evidence or history of injury

History and examination

Dental injury

Other

Orthodontic injury

D Assess:
Pain, bleeding, color, swelling, pseudomembrane, odor, calculus, pocket depth, and LOA

Pain

No pain

Pain

No pain

Redness
Swelling
Easy bleeding

Minimal redness
or swelling
Easy bleeding

Redness
Swelling
No easy bleeding

Redness
Swelling
Easy bleeding

Minimal redness
or swelling

Redness and
swelling
Possible easy
bleeding

Redness and swelling
No easy bleeding

Pseudomembrane

Pseudomembrane
(hidden)

No pseudomembrane

Pseudomembrane

Pseudomembrane
(hidden)

No pseudomembrane

No pseudomembrane

Distinctive odor

Distinctive odor

No distinctive odor

Distinctive odor

Distinctive odor

Odor but less
unpleasant

No distinctive odor

Pocket depth
(no LOA)

Pocket depth
with LOA

Heavy calculus

Pocket depth
with LOA

Pocket depth
with LOA

Deep pockets
with LOA

Heavy calculus

Localized NUG

Localized NUP

Pocket depth
with LOA

Possible
pocket depth
(no LOA)

Generalized NUP

Recurrent NUP

Positive for
AIDS antibodies
Low CD4 count
High viral load

Pocket depth
with LOA

No LOA
but possible
pocket depths

Localized
periodontitis

Localized
gingivitis

HIV periodontitis

Generalized
periodontitis

Generalized
gingivitis

D "Easy" bleeding is especially associated with the initial episode of NUG, NUP, or their recurrences, but must be provoked by brushing or other minor trauma. Bleeding associated with HIV periodontitis may be spontaneous and unprovoked. Neither easy bleeding nor spontaneous, unprovoked bleeding is associated with gingivitis/periodontitis. The typical pseudomembrane (ie, white, tenaciously adherent mass of bacteria, dead cells, and fibrin) that fills the necrosed center of the split papilla is characteristic of NUG, NUP, or HIV periodontitis but not of gingivitis/periodontitis. A distinctive odor is associated with NUG or NUP, but a different, less unpleasant odor characterizes HIV periodontitis. Pocket depth with loss of attachment (LOA) can occur with any of these lesions, but it may not occur in the initial NUG episodes. Pain is a symptom especially related to NUG, NUP, and HIV periodontitis but not to gingivitis/periodontitis. Extremely heavy calculus that creates the appearance of split papillae may be indicative of gingivitis/periodontitis but may be found with any of these lesions; this necessitates the use of other criteria to make a differentiation. When AIDS or an AIDS-related syndrome (based especially on patient history) is suspected, an HIV antibody test, a low T-cell lymphocyte assay (CD4 count), and a raised viral load count can confirm or rule out this etiology with its sequelae.

Additional Readings

Carranza FA Jr, Newman MG. Clinical periodontology. 8th ed. Philadelphia: WB Saunders; 1996. p. 213.

Grupe HE, Wilder LS. Observations of necrotizing gingivitis in 870 military trainees. J Periodontol 1956;27:255.

Wilson TG, Kornman KS. Fundamentals of periodontics. Chicago: Quintessence Publishing; 1996. p. 159–64.

Winkler JR, Grassi M, Murray PA. Clinical description and etiology of HIV-associated periodontal diseases. In: Robertson RC, Greenspan JS, editors. Perspectives in oral manifestations of AIDS. Littleton (MA): PSG Publishing; 1988. p. 49.

11 Localized Periodontal Pain

Walter B. Hall

Localized pain is not a common sign directly associated with most periodontal diseases. Periodontal pain localized to a single tooth or area is usually associated with the development of a periodontal abscess, an endodontic problem, cracked tooth syndrome, or any combination of these. The differential diagnosis of these problems may be quite difficult and requires careful testing.

A Localized swelling and/or redness may be associated with localized periodontal pain. Probing the involved teeth for periodontal pockets is the first step in differential diagnosis. If no pocket depth with loss of attachment (LOA) is found, periodontitis can be eliminated as a possibility.

B If pocket depth is detected, inflammatory periodontal disease (most likely an abscess) is present. The next step would be electric pulp testing, examining for reaction to ice, ethylene oxide, or to hot gutta-percha applied to the tooth, and finally, radiographically evaluating for periapical radiolucencies. If no reaction to an electric pulp test occurs, an endodontic problem exists. Hot and cold tests are applied to clarify whether the pulp is vital. A radiograph showing a periapical radiolucency indicates a pulpal problem. The absence of such a radiolucency could indicate that no pulpal problem exists or that the pulpal problem is of insufficient duration to have destroyed enough bone periapically to be visible on the film at the time of the examination.

The dentist should evaluate all these findings together to decide whether a pulpal problem exists. If the tooth gives a positive pulp test electrically and reacts to hot and cold, and if the radiograph shows no periapical radiolucency, the problem should be treated as a periodontal abscess. If a pulp test is negative, reactions to hot or cold are negative, or if a periapical radiolucency is noted on the radiograph, endodontic treatment should be undertaken if the tooth is viewed as salvageable and useful in the overall treatment plan. If the endodontic treatment is successful, periodontal treatment follows. Whether or not pocket depth is present, endodontic treatment is usually performed before periodontal treatment. If a tooth with pain of periodontal or endodontic origin, or both, is nonessential to the overall treatment plan or nonsalvageable, it should be extracted.

C If no pocket depth is detected, the pain may be endodontic in origin, caused by a crack in the tooth (cracked tooth syndrome), or both. Electric pulp testing, application of ice or hot gutta-percha, and radiographic evaluation may be used, as already described, to determine whether the pulp is vital. If no endodontic problem can be diagnosed by these means, cracked tooth syndrome should be suspected. Investigate a history of trauma (eg, an automobile accident or a blow to the mouth). Visual examination for cracks, percussion to elicit sharp pain, and transillumination with fiberoptic light to indicate the depths of cracks can assist the diagnosis of cracked tooth syndrome. If the symptoms are not too severe, placing a fixed crown may resolve the problem for some time. More severe cracks may necessitate extraction of the tooth. When a pulpal problem is accompanied by deep cracks extending into the roots of teeth, the prognosis is guarded at best, and the patient should be informed that the tooth may be lost.

A vertical or spiral crack extending apically down the root usually is accompanied by deep, narrow pocket formation that is not characteristic in its width of typical periodontitis. Transillumination may disclose the crack extending into the pocket. Meticulous probing may elicit a sharp pain when probing is precisely at the crack position but not immediately on either side of it. If the pain is severe, the prognosis is hopeless.

D An additional cause of localized pain, which occurs often, is one caused by the lodging of a foreign body in the sulcus or pocket. Popcorn and sesame seeds are the most common causes of these localized, often very painful problems. They are resolved by removing the offending substance and allowing healing to occur. Long-time impactions of food can result in serious loss of periodontal support unless they are treated promptly.

Additional Readings

Cameron CE. The cracked tooth syndrome: additional findings. J Am Dent Assoc 1976;92:971.

Cohen S, Burns RC. Pathways of the pulp. 7th ed. St. Louis: Mosby; 1997. p. 750.

Hiatt WH. Incomplete crown-root fracture. J Periodontol 1973;44:369.

Pitts DL, Natkin E. Diagnosis and treatment of vertical root fractures. J Endodontics 1983;9:338.

Prichard JF. The diagnosis and treatment of periodontal disease. Philadelphia: WB Saunders; 1979. p. 117.

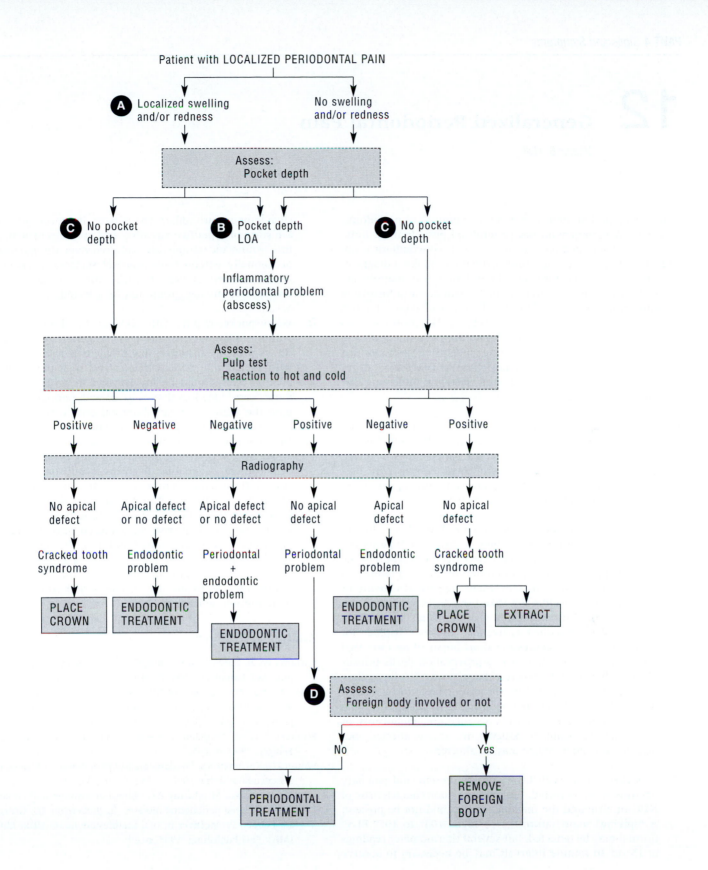

Patient with LOCALIZED PERIODONTAL PAIN

A Localized swelling and/or redness

No swelling and/or redness

Assess:
Pocket depth

C No pocket depth

B Pocket depth LOA

C No pocket depth

Inflammatory periodontal problem (abscess)

Assess:
Pulp test
Reaction to hot and cold

Positive

Negative

Negative

Positive

Negative

Positive

Radiography

No apical defect

Apical defect or no defect

Apical defect or no defect

No apical defect

Apical defect

No apical defect

Cracked tooth syndrome

Endodontic problem

Periodontal + endodontic problem

Periodontal problem

Endodontic problem

Cracked tooth syndrome

PLACE CROWN

ENDODONTIC TREATMENT

ENDODONTIC TREATMENT

ENDODONTIC TREATMENT

PLACE CROWN

EXTRACT

D Assess:
Foreign body involved or not

No

Yes

PERIODONTAL TREATMENT

REMOVE FOREIGN BODY

12 Generalized Periodontal Pain

Walter B. Hall

Generalized periodontal pain is not a symptom of periodontitis per se. A patient who has generalized periodontitis, however, may experience pain associated with concomitant problems affecting the periodontium, which can make a diagnosis difficult. Records and histories of old dental examinations are especially useful in establishing that a patient has a history of nonpainful periodontitis. The development of pain after this time indicates the onset of a new problem. The most common causes of generalized periodontal pain are necrotizing ulcerative gingivitis (NUG), necrotizing ulcerative periodontitis (NUP), human immunodeficiency virus (HIV) periodontitis, herpetic gingivostomatitis, and some systemic infections that may affect the gingiva.

A Generalized swelling and/or redness of the gingiva are found with most cases of NUG, NUP, or HIV periodontitis. With NUG, these changes affect the papillae most severely, but gingival margins often are affected as well. With herpetic gingivostomatitis, these changes are more generalized and not specifically associated with papillae.

B The absence of pocket depths with loss of attachment (LOA), as determined by probing, indicates that periodontitis is not involved. If papillary necrosis (destruction of the tips of papillae and pseudomembrane formation) is detected in multiple areas, evaluate the patient's breath for a distinctive, pungent odor. Take the patient's temperature. Question the patient regarding an unusual taste in the mouth (often described as *metallic*). Evaluate papillae for "easy" bleeding by expressing short bursts of air into each area to determine whether this provocation elicits unusually easy bleeding. The correct diagnosis is NUG if papillary necrosis is accompanied by the distinctive odor; a steady, but moderately raised temperature; a metallic taste; and easy bleeding. Such patients usually are adolescents or young adults. Younger patients are rarely affected, but occasionally older people may be affected.

C If pocket depths with LOA are not present and papillary necrosis is not detected, the pungent odor characteristic of NUG or NUP and the metallic taste should not be present. A "spiking" temperature that is high (104° to 105° F) to normal may be detected, but several thermometer readings at 15- to 30-minute intervals may be necessary to observe such temperature spikes. The patient, however, may reveal a history of repetitive sweating and episodes of malaise. If tiny, round ulcerations are scattered over the gingiva and occasionally extend onto mucosal surfaces, herpetic gingivostomatitis is indicated. Such patients usually are adolescent, but any age group may be affected.

D When pocket depths with LOA can be observed, with or without overt swelling and redness, generalized periodontitis is present, although this problem is rarely associated with periodontal pain. Other causes of generalized periodontal pain should be investigated. If probing produces more "easy" bleeding than is usual with periodontitis, evaluate the patient for an abnormal temperature and foul breath. NUP superimposed on periodontitis may be present. Papillary necrosis may not be obvious in such patients. In an adolescent or young adult, NUP may be an appropriate diagnosis; however, this diagnosis is unusual in an older patient. If the patient's history indicates sexual activity with multiple partners, significant drug use (especially intravenous), or the patient is in a group, such as homosexuals or bisexuals, at high risk for acquired immunodeficiency syndrome (AIDS), an evaluation for antibodies to HIV and T-cell lymphocyte assay (CD4 count) and viral load measurements are helpful in ruling out the severe, rapidly destructive, essentially irreversible periodontitis associated with immunodeficiency.

Additional Readings

Carranza FA Jr, Newman MG. Clinical periodontology. 8th ed. Philadelphia: WB Saunders; 1996. p. 249.

Grassi M et al. Management of HIV-associated periodontal diseases. In: Robertson PG, Greenspan JS, editors. Perspectives in oral manifestations of AIDS. Littleton (MA): PSG Publishing; 1988. p. 119.

Schluger S et al. Periodontal diseases. 2nd ed. Philadelphia: Lea & Febiger; 1990. p. 265.

Wilson TG, Kornman KS. Fundamentals of periodontics. Chicago: Quintessence Publishing; 1996. p. 252–5, 297, 442–4.

Winkler JR, Grasso M, Murray PA. Clinical description and etiology of HIV-associated periodontal diseases. In: Robertson PG, Greenspan JS, editors. Perspectives in oral manifestations of AIDS. Littleton (MA): PSG Publishing; 1988. p. 49.

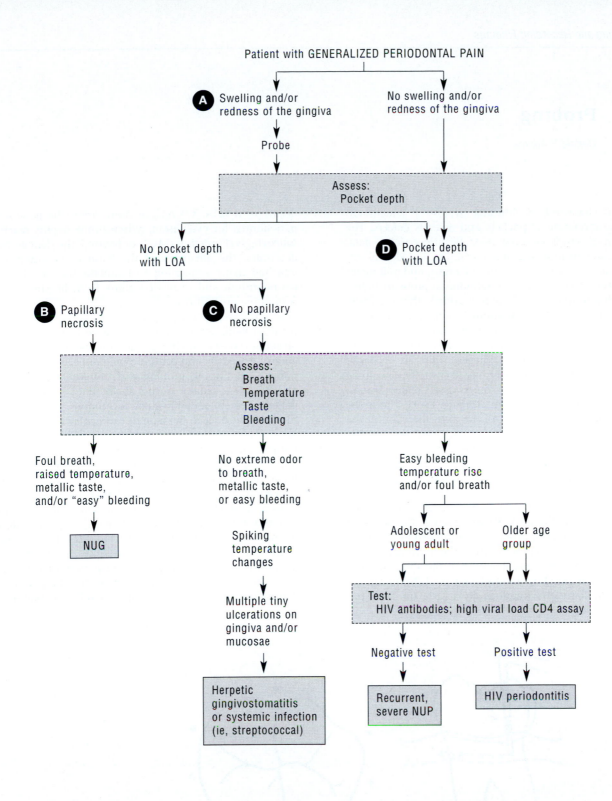

Patient with GENERALIZED PERIODONTAL PAIN

A Swelling and/or redness of the gingiva

No swelling and/or redness of the gingiva

Probe

Assess:
Pocket depth

No pocket depth with LOA

D Pocket depth with LOA

B Papillary necrosis

C No papillary necrosis

Assess:
Breath
Temperature
Taste
Bleeding

Foul breath, raised temperature, metallic taste, and/or "easy" bleeding

No extreme odor to breath, metallic taste, or easy bleeding

Easy bleeding temperature rise and/or foul breath

NUG

Spiking temperature changes

Adolescent or young adult

Older age group

Multiple tiny ulcerations on gingiva and/or mucosae

Test:
HIV antibodies; high viral load CD4 assay

Herpetic gingivostomatitis or systemic infection (ie, streptococcal)

Negative test

Positive test

Recurrent, severe NUP

HIV periodontitis

13 Probing

Donald F. Adams

Periodontitis is characterized clinically by loss of attachment (LOA) and the formation of pockets and osseous defects. The documentation of LOA is essential in establishing baseline data, monitoring treatment results, and determining periodontal stability. Probes vary in design by length, thickness, and millimeter markings. Characteristics of a good periodontal probe include a thin shaft with a rounded tip, durable markings that are easily read, and ease of sterilization. Commonly, six measurements are recorded per tooth, with each root of the molars treated as a single tooth. Therefore six facial and six lingual recordings are made for each mandibular molar, whereas there are six facial and three palatal recordings for each maxillary molar. The probe is inserted gently into the gingival sulcus and stepped around the tooth at about 1 mm increments (Figure 13-1). The probe should be kept as close as possible to the axial direction of the tooth while the tip remains in contact with the root surface. Measurements are made from the gingival margin for pocket depth and from the cementoenamel junction (CEJ), or a similar fixed point, to the gingival margin for recession.

A   The probing depth and recession measurements added together determine the LOA. Factors such as the health of the surrounding gingiva, probing force applied by the operator, and discomfort tolerance of the patient can make a difference of 1 to 2 mm in probe readings. Bleeding on probing of minimal pockets accompanied by LOA usually is managed similarly to situations in which no LOA has

occurred. If LOA is 5 mm or more, refer the patient to a periodontist for evaluation. When probe depths reach the mucogingival junction (MGJ) or beyond, the dentist should determine the adequacy of the band of keratinized and attached tissue remaining to maintain the health of the periodontium and to resist trauma from brushing and/or restorative procedures.

B   If the probing depth is up to 3 mm with no LOA, and no bleeding is observed after gentle probing, presume that the gingiva is healthy and continue regular periodontic maintenance. Bleeding on probing with minimal crevice depths and no LOA usually means inadequate hygiene by the patient. Review dental hygiene techniques, scale and polish the teeth, and place the patient on regular maintenance.

C   For patients with pockets that are deeper than 3 mm, evaluate the quality of their plaque control. Evidence of inadequate dental hygiene requires renewed efforts in patient education. Continued noncompliance or lack of patient skills may require referral for management and certainly is a contraindication to more definitive therapy. Bleeding in the presence of adequate hygiene indicates that the disease process is not being controlled despite the efforts of the patient. Because a principal goal of periodontal therapy is to create a manageable environment for the patient, the dentist can treat the affected area or refer the patient to a

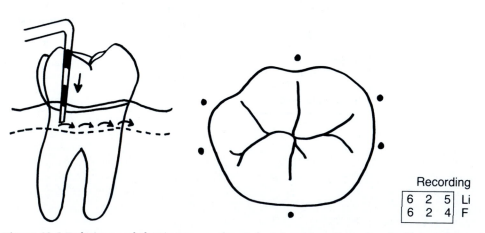

Figure 13-1 Technique and charting to record periodontal probings. Reproduced with permission from Hall WB, Roberts WE, Labarre EE. Decision making in dental treatment planning. St Louis: Mosby; 1994.

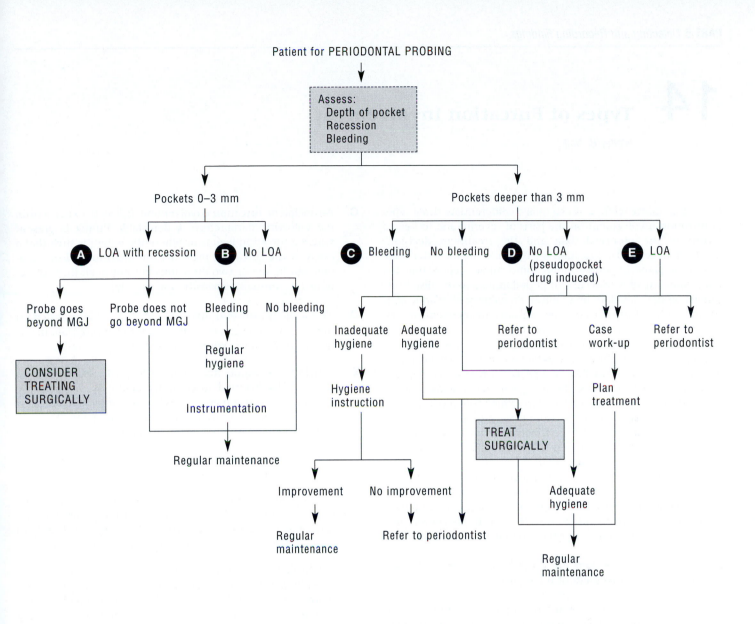

periodontist. If the choice is to maintain the area using nonsurgical means, it is crucial to monitor the patient regularly and document the treatment properly.

D Pseudopockets exist where probing depths are greater than 3 mm with no accompanying observable LOA are found; pseudopockets may be drug induced. A complete case work-up is required if the dentist chooses to manage the patient. Referral to a periodontist is also an option.

E When LOA is accompanied by probing depths greater than 3 mm, the options are referral or a comprehensive periodontal diagnostic work-up and the development of a treatment plan. In all instances, the patient must be informed of

the problem, the options available for management, and the consequences of each option. Collect and record adequate data, making periodontal probing an integral part of the findings.

Additional Readings

Listgarten MA. Periodontal probing: what does it mean? J Clin Periodontol 1980;7:165.

Listgarten MA, Mao R, Robertson PJ. Periodontal probing and the relationship of the probe tip to periodontal tissues. J Periodontol 1976;47:511.

Vander Velden U. Influence of periodontal health on probing depth and bleeding tendency. J Clin Periodontol 1980;7:120.

14 Types of Furcation Involvement

Walter B. Hall

In treating molar teeth, it is essential to differentiate three types of furcation involvement on the basis of severity and to keep a record of the observed data and the treatment decisions involved. In general, a furcation is a common site for active bone loss accompanying periodontitis. Some studies report that the most common sites of recurrent periodontitis are the distal furcations on the maxillary first molars. Problems with plaque control in involved furcations may be explained by these differences. A furcation is difficult for the dentist or dental hygienist to instrument because it is shaped like a gothic arch with internal flutings present on many roots. While the dentist may be able to get an instrument to the base of a pocket, it may prove impossible to move the instrument effectively without gouging adjacent root surfaces. Where maxillary molars exhibit root proximity, the roots of adjacent molars are so close to each other as to prevent the fit of an interproximal brush between the teeth, and thus neither the dentist nor patient is able to clean the distal furcation of the first molar. It is also impossible to insert an instrument into the furcation from the facial and palatal aspects so as to allow it to clear; therefore, the detection and recording of furcation involvements are extremely important steps in developing a treatment plan and for prognosis. The use of the newer fine ultrasonic tips for cleansing such areas may be a good option.

A   As periodontal pockets are probed and charted, note and record the involvement of furcations.

B   Explore all furcations with a no. 3 pigtail explorer or similar instrument (termed a *furca-finder*). Insert the instrument into the crevice or pocket, rotate it to the interradicular depth of the furcation involvement, and move it laterally and coronally to determine whether (1) a definite catch exists or (2) the instrument will slip out of the furcation in any or all directions.

C   An incipient furcation involvement (Class I) exists within the following parameters: A detectable fluting is present where a furcation begins or where the extent is such that a catch in the furcation prevents the instrument from slipping out in one or two directions but not in all three directions (ie, coronally, mesially, and distally).

D   An incipient furcation involvement (Class I) is recorded on the chart with a △ symbol placed in the appropriate furcation with the apex pointing coronally (Figure 14-1).

E   A definite furcation involvement (Class II) exists when a catch of the inserted furca-finder definitely prevents the instrument from slipping out when it is moved laterally or coronally while definitely stopping it from going "through and through" to another opening in the furca.

F   A definite involvement (Class II) is indicated by the symbol △ similarly positioned (see Figure 14-1).

G   A "through-and-through" furcation involvement (Class III) exists *only* where it is possible to insert the probe into one furca and at that same place the probe is apparently able to connect directly with one or more additional furcas.

H   A "through-and-through" involvement (Class III) is indicated by placing the symbol ▲ in two or more furcas on a tooth (see Figure 14-1). Class II furcation involvements may be treated for guided tissue regeneration when they involve 3 mm or more; the technique for guided tissue regeneration in "through-and-through" furcation involvements is now the standard of care in the United States.

Additional Readings

Carranza FA Jr, Newman MG. Clinical periodontology. 8th ed. Philadelphia: WB Saunders; 1996. p. 365.

Easley JF, Drennan GA. Morphological classification of the furca. Can Dent Assoc J 1969;35:12.

Genco RJ, Goldman HM, Cohen DW. Contemporary periodontics. St. Louis: Mosby; 1990. p. 344.

Grant DA, Stern JB, Listgarten MA. Periodontics. 6th ed. St. Louis: Mosby; 1988. p. 921.

Heins PJ, Carter SR. Furca involvement: a classification of bony deformities. Periodontics 1968;6:84.

Schluger S et al. Periodontal diseases. 2nd ed. Philadelphia: Lea & Febiger; 1990. p. 545.

Tarnow D, Fletcher P. Classification of the vertical component of furcation involvement. J Periodontol 1984;55:283.

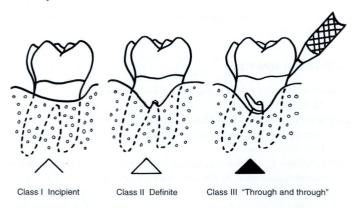

Class I Incipient   Class II Definite   Class III "Through and through"

Figure 14-1 Classes and appearance of furcation involvements, and their respective symbol.

Patient being examined for FURCATION INVOLVEMENT

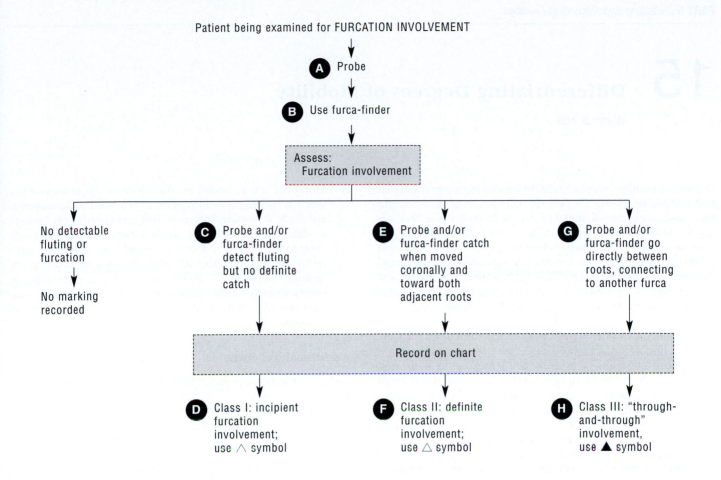

A Probe

B Use furca-finder

Assess:
Furcation involvement

No detectable
fluting or
furcation

No marking
recorded

C Probe and/or
furca-finder
detect fluting
but no definite
catch

E Probe and/or
furca-finder catch
when moved
coronally and
toward both
adjacent roots

G Probe and/or
furca-finder go
directly between
roots, connecting
to another furca

Record on chart

D Class I: incipient
furcation
involvement;
use △ symbol

F Class II: definite
furcation
involvement;
use △ symbol

H Class III: "through-
and-through"
involvement,
use ▲ symbol

15 Differentiating Degrees of Mobility

Walter B. Hall

Degrees of mobility may be useful in developing a treatment plan and making prognoses for periodontally involved teeth. Single-time measurements of mobility are of limited value (because slight mobilities may represent little more than clenching or pipe-stem chewing the night before the examination); however, when they are repeated at regular intervals and a change occurs, the alteration may be a significant finding that pinpoints a localized change or indicates an alteration in parafunctional habits (eg, bruxism) that may affect the overall prognosis greatly.

A   Mobility is evaluated by placing an instrument on the facial and lingual surfaces and a finger on the appearance side of a tooth and applying pressure while rocking the tooth (Figure 15-1). If the tooth being tested has no adjacent tooth, the instruments and pressure should be applied obliquely and mesiodistally. A "normal" tooth has a minute amount of "give" to it (ie, is not ankylosed). A tooth that moves more than this minute amount but in a total arc of less than 1 mm has Class 1 mobility. A tooth that moves in an arc of 1 mm or more but less than 2 mm has Class 2 mobility. A tooth that moves in an arc of 2 mm or more and can be depressed into its socket has Class 3 mobility.

When a tooth is adjacent to an empty space, mobility should be tested in oblique directions as well.

B   Mobilities are recorded on the chart in the crown of the tooth at the initial examination. If repeated measurements are made at various intervals, further records may be kept in different colors in the tooth form or in appropriately designated boxes. A marking should be made for each tooth, even if it is normal. With an assistant reading the findings, approach is more rapid and accurate; also, an empty space has more than one interpretation legally. Arabic numerals (0, 1, 2, 3) may be used to indicate degrees of mobility.

Additional Readings

Carranza FA Jr, Newman MG. Clinical periodontology. 8th ed. Philadelphia: WB Saunders; 1996. p. 349.

Hall WB. Clinical practice. In: Steele PF, editor. Dimensions of dental hygiene. 3rd ed. Philadelphia: Lea & Febiger; 1982. p. 153.

Miller SC. Textbook of periodontia. 2nd ed. Philadelphia: Blakiston; 1943. p. 103.

Ramfjord S, Ash MM. Occlusion. 3rd ed. Philadelphia: WB Saunders; 1983. p. 309.

Schulger S et al. Periodontal diseases. 2nd ed. Philadelphia: Lea & Febiger; 1990. p. 322.

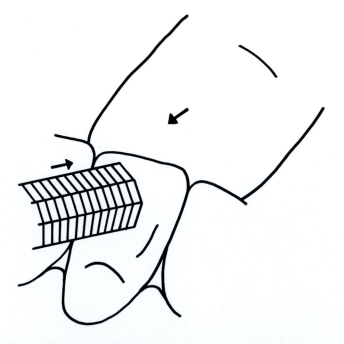

Figure 15-1 An instrument handle and a fingertip being used to determine the degree of mobility of a tooth.

Patient being examined for DEGREES OF MOBILITY

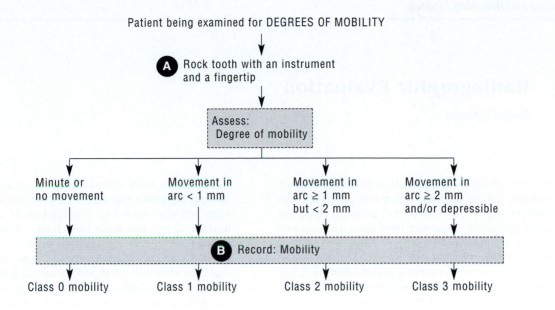

A Rock tooth with an instrument and a fingertip

Assess:
Degree of mobility

| Minute or no movement | Movement in arc < 1 mm | Movement in arc ≥ 1 mm but < 2 mm | Movement in arc ≥ 2 mm and/or depressible |

B Record: Mobility

| Class 0 mobility | Class 1 mobility | Class 2 mobility | Class 3 mobility |

16 Radiographic Evaluation

Donald F. Adams

Radiographs are an indispensable aid in identifying the presence of pathosis and the conditions that affect the prognosis and treatment of periodontosis. As with pocket probing, there are restrictions in interpretation. Exposure guidelines and processing procedures must be followed to achieve adequate contrast. Proper angulation of the film and of the head of the x-ray machine minimizes distortion. A properly placed radiograph has few overlapping contact areas, and the entire tooth is visible on periapical views. For periodontal purposes, it is useful to position bite-wing radiographs vertically so that both maxillary and mandibular bone crests are visible. Individual periapical radiographs are superior in detail to panographic radiographs and preferred for a more accurate analysis (Figure 16-1).

A   The bony crest is usually 1 to 2 mm apical to the cemento-enamel junction (CEJ) because of the attachment of collagen fibers immediately below the enamel. Clinical crown-to-root (C:R) ratios are determined according to the amount of root remaining in bone compared with the amount of tooth above the bone level. If the level of the bone is essentially equal across an interdental or interradicular area, it is called *horizontal bone loss* and measured as the percentage of bone lost (eg, 20% of the original bone height is lost). Angular bone loss occurs when one tooth

has lost more bone than its neighbor. A line is drawn connecting adjacent CEJs across an interdental space to determine whether tipped or extruded teeth have created the illusion of angular bone loss. Some clinicians consider a radiopaque interdental crest to be an indication of periodontal stability, whereas active disease results in a crest that appears moth-eaten with a loss of opacity. This observation is controversial and susceptible to variability in radiographic angulation. Radiographs cannot determine the activity of the disease, only its history. Changes in the continuity of the lamina dura and widening of the apical periodontal ligament indicate a possible endodontic involvement. Occlusal trauma can also result in a widened periodontal ligament (PDL) and thickened lamina dura, although the widening is also seen in the PDL along the lateral surfaces of the tooth. Trabeculation can also increase with hyperfunction. In hypofunction the PDL becomes atrophic and is narrower, along with a diminished lamina dura. Some conditions, such as hyperparathyroidism, may result in the loss of a distinct lamina dura. A variety of nonperiodontal conditions visible on radiographs may affect the prognosis and treatment, including the proximity of the maxillary sinuses to the alveolar crest, the proximity of the root, the oblique ridge, and the anatomy of the tuberosity.

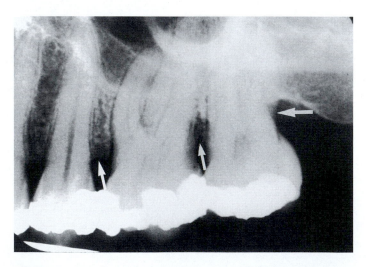

Figure 16-1 Radiograph suggesting two-walled defects (craters) between the first molar and adjacent teeth and distal furcation involvement on the second molar (arrows).

B   Radiographs indicate the integrity of restorations that could complicate periodontal maintenance. Discrepancies in the marginal ridge and open contacts can predispose to impaction of food. Improper margins and carious lesions frustrate the plaque-control efforts of the patient, whereas calculus and poor crown contours harbor plaque and perpetuate the periodontal problem. Use radiographs to assess the tooth position, the presence of caries in the crown or furcation areas and along root surfaces, and the condition of pulp chambers and canals. The size and shape of the anatomic crown are compared with root anatomy and the amount of bone support to determine the stability of the tooth.

C   The number, shape, and proximity of roots are closely related to the determination of prognosis and planning the treatment. A tooth with the normal complement of roots adequately spaced can more easily absorb occlusal loads. If the roots are fused or widespread, the maintenance of periodontal health is somewhat easier than if the roots are only slightly separated. On the contrary, widespread roots are

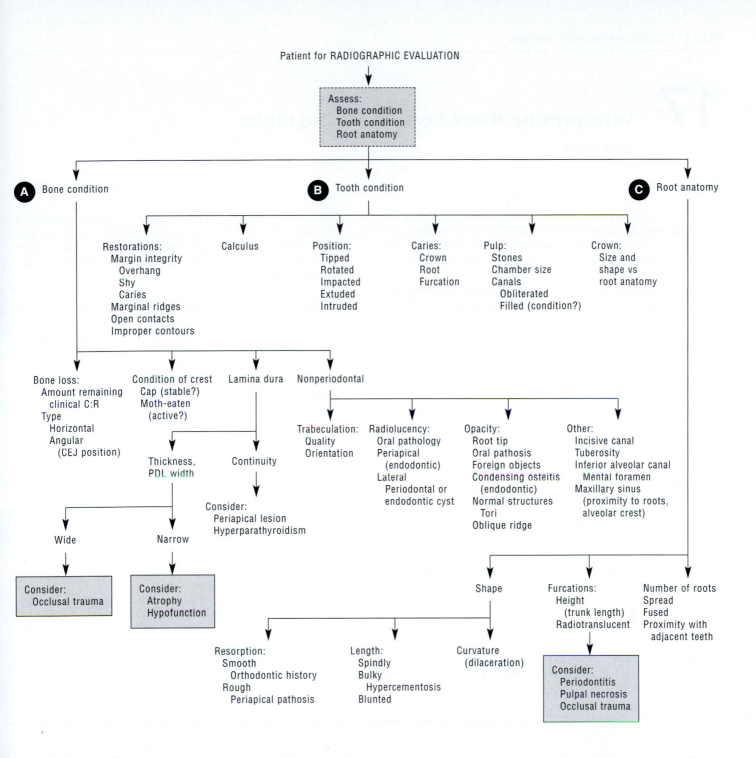

often close to roots of adjacent teeth, and this complicates disease management. A radiolucency in a furcation area may be the result of periodontitis, occlusal trauma, or pulpal necrosis draining through an accessory canal in the chamber floor. Long, bulky roots provide more adequate support in the presence of less bone than spindly, cone-shaped roots. Radiographs show whether a root has hypercementosis or is curved (dilacerated). A smooth blunting of root apices may be the result of orthodontic movement, whereas roughened apices may indicate the action of periapical pathosis.

Additional Readings

Carranza FA Jr, Newman MG. Clinical periodontology. 8th ed. Philadelphia: WB Saunders; 1996. p. 368.

Prichard JF. Advanced periodontal disease. 2nd ed. Philadelphia: WB Saunders; 1972. p. 142.

17 Interpreting Bone Loss on Radiographs

Walter B. Hall

A full series of radiographs from a patient should first be evaluated diagnostically, although no diagnoses of the bone status can be definitive on the basis of radiographs alone. Radiographs are only two-dimensional shadow pictures. Angulation, exposure time, and development time are factors that may influence suggestions of bone loss when it is not present, not show bone loss when it is present, or accurately portray the existing condition. Facial and lingual bone status is masked by the interposed teeth. Probing is the more definitive means of determining bony contours and is more likely to present an accurate picture than the radiograph. The more views that are present, the better the clinician can conceptualize the actual bony status. The angulation of individual films must be sufficient so that films can be read. Facial and lingual cusps should be close to being superimposed on the film if it is to be interpreted accurately. Roots should be sufficiently separated so that interproximal bone levels are not masked. If the existing films are inadequate, they should be retaken; however, if one correctly angulated picture is present, the value of retaking other views should be weighed against the dangers of excessive radiation.

A If the films are adequate, seek evidence of bone loss. If the crest of bone interproximally is more than 1 mm apical to the cementoenamel junction (CEJ), bone loss has occurred. Such a finding does not indicate the presence of periodontal disease. Bone loss may be actively occurring or may have occurred earlier and be in a static state at the time the picture is taken. Bone loss also may represent bone removed during osseous surgery.

B If the bone crest appears to be about 1 mm from the CEJ on the films, no radiographic evidence of bone loss can be described; however, bone loss may be present facially or lingually and not show or may be masked by existing cortical plates interproximally. Radiographs are only suggestive of existing bone status when the films were taken and are not diagnostic of disease.

C If bone loss is suggested on the films, it may be "horizontal" or "vertical" in character, as seen on a two-dimensional film. Horizontal bone loss is indicated when the bone loss interproximally on two adjacent teeth is equidistant from the CEJ on each tooth. Vertical bone loss is indicated when the bone crest is more apical to the CEJ adjacent to one tooth than to the other. A two-walled infrabony "crater" also is considered a vertical defect (see Chapter 100). When bone loss has occurred, periodontal disease has been and may be present at the time the film is taken. Use probing and the patient's dental history to determine whether bone loss is truly present and whether it represents existing or quiescent periodontal disease.

Additional Readings

Grant DA, Stern IB, Listgarten MA. Periodontics. St. Louis: Mosby; 1988. p. 552.

Prichard JF. Advanced periodontal disease. 2nd ed. Philadelphia: WB Saunders; 1972. p. 143.

Prichard JF. The role of the roentgenogram in the diagnosis and prognosis of periodontal disease. Oral Surg 1961;14:182.

Suomi JD, Plumbo J, Barbano JP. A comparative study of radiographs and pocket measurements in periodontal disease evaluation. J Periodontol 1968;89:311.

Worth HM. Radiology in diagnosis. Dent Clin North Am 1969;13:731.

Patient with RECENT FULL SERIES OF RADIOGRAPHS

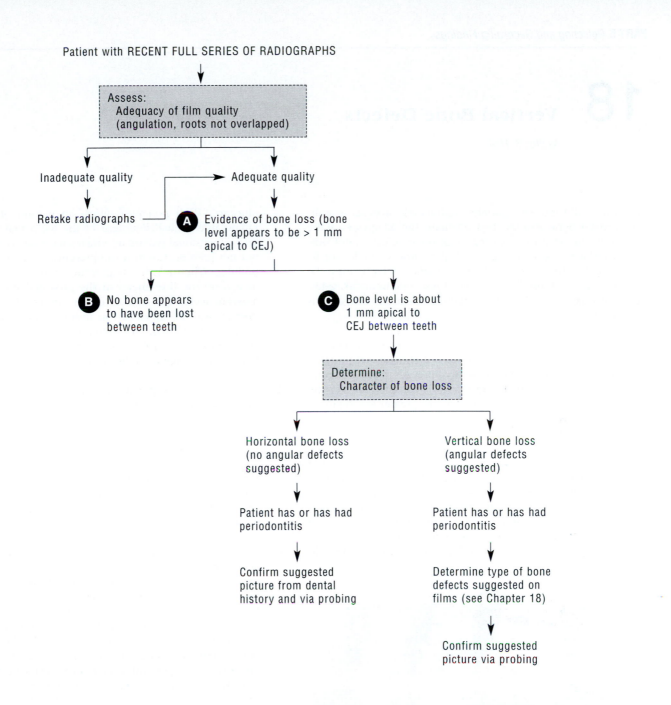

Assess:
Adequacy of film quality
(angulation, roots not overlapped)

Inadequate quality

Retake radiographs

Adequate quality

A Evidence of bone loss (bone level appears to be > 1 mm apical to CEJ)

B No bone appears to have been lost between teeth

C Bone level is about 1 mm apical to CEJ between teeth

Determine:
Character of bone loss

Horizontal bone loss (no angular defects suggested)

Patient has or has had periodontitis

Confirm suggested picture from dental history and via probing

Vertical bone loss (angular defects suggested)

Patient has or has had periodontitis

Determine type of bone defects suggested on films (see Chapter 18)

Confirm suggested picture via probing

18 Vertical Bone Defects

Walter B. Hall

When the full series of a patient's radiographs appears to indicate vertical bone defects, first evaluate the adequacy of the films to ensure that the appearance of these defects is not simply an artifact of poorly angulated films. Roots should not be overlapped; otherwise, existing angular defects may be obscured. If the films do not meet these requirements, additional adequate films should be obtained before any conclusions are drawn.

A Vertical (angular) bone defects are suggested when the bone crest is more apical to the cementoenamel junction adjacent to one tooth than to the other. An infrabony crater (a type of two-walled defect) also is considered a vertical defect, although bone loss may not be greater on one tooth than on the other.

B A typical infrabony crater is present when bone resorption has occurred between two adjacent teeth, with the greatest loss under the contact area. Facial and lingual cortical plates that extend more coronally remain. Viewed on a radiograph, two crestal heights are separated by a more radiolucent area. Periapical films are more likely to show such crests than are bite-wing radiographs, on which superimposed facial and lingual cortical plates may obscure the radiolucency. With periapical films, angulation of individual radiographs or malalignment of the teeth may result in a two-dimensional picture in which such a defect is suggested but not present. Confirm the presence of such a defect via probing. When a crater is present, probing shows shallow depths on the line angles of the proximal surfaces of the adjacent teeth with greater depth interproximally. If such findings are not apparent on probing, accept the probing findings rather than the radiographic conclusions (eg, no crater present). If probing confirms the radiographic suggestions, a two-walled infrabony crater is most likely present.

C When bone loss is greater on one tooth than on the other (adjacent) one, a hemiseptal or one-walled defect may be present. The radiograph will suggest that half the septum is missing, as seen in Figure 18-1. No suggestion of a remaining facial or lingual wall coronal to the greatest bone loss will be seen. Probe to confirm the suggested condition. Bone loss is not more apical under the contact area than at the line angles if a hemiseptal defect is present. Accept the probing findings as correct if they differ from the picture suggested by the radiographs.

D When additional facial or lingual walls or both are suggested on the film, a two- or three-walled infrabony defect may be present. If a third wall is present, two crestal heights may be suggested, superimposed over the area of vertical bone loss. The final differentiation of the two types of defects must be made via probing. When pocket depth is less on the facial or lingual line angle of the affected tooth, but the bone loss under the contact area and at the other line angle is deeper and similar, a two-walled defect is present. When the pocket depth at both line angles is less than under the contact area, a three-walled defect is present. Regard the findings on probing as correct if they differ from the suggested radiographic picture.

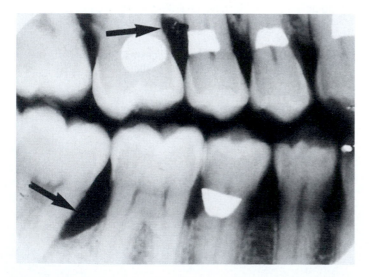

Figure 18-1 Hemiseptal (one-walled) defects are indicated by the arrows on this radiograph.

Additional Readings

Friedman N. Reattachment and roentgenograms. J Periodontol 1958;29:98.

Prichard JF. Advanced periodontal disease. 2nd ed. Philadelphia: WB Saunders; 1972. p. 175.

Prichard JF. The diagnosis and treatment of periodontal disease in general practice. Philadelphia: WB Saunders; 1979. p. 78.

Schluger S et al. Periodontal diseases. 2nd ed. Philadelphia: Lea & Febiger; 1990. p. 299.

Patient whose RADIOGRAPHS SUGGEST PRESENCE OF ANGULAR DEFECTS

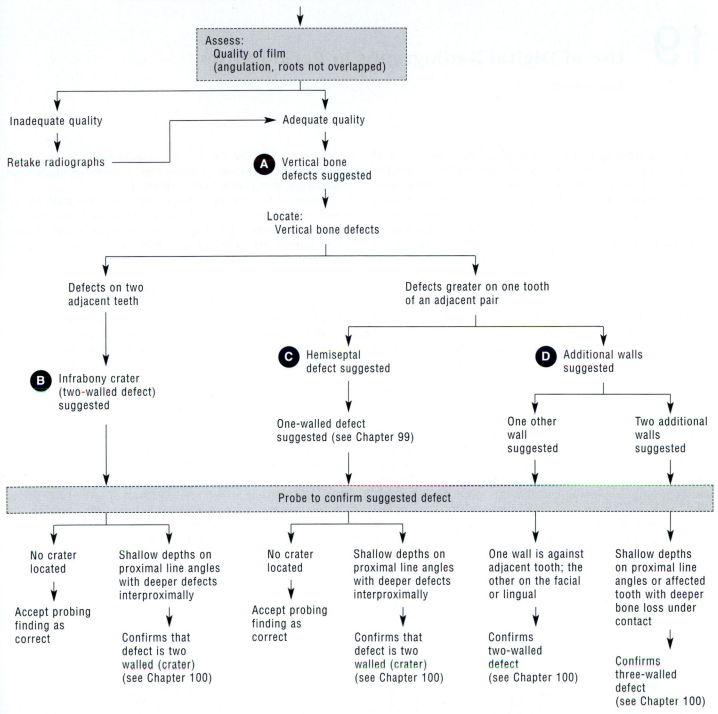

Assess:
Quality of film
(angulation, roots not overlapped)

Inadequate quality

Retake radiographs

Adequate quality

A Vertical bone
defects suggested

Locate:
Vertical bone defects

Defects on two
adjacent teeth

Defects greater on one tooth
of an adjacent pair

B Infrabony crater
(two-walled defect)
suggested

C Hemiseptal
defect suggested

D Additional walls
suggested

One-walled defect
suggested (see Chapter 99)

One other
wall
suggested

Two additional
walls
suggested

Probe to confirm suggested defect

No crater
located

Accept probing
finding as
correct

Shallow depths on
proximal line angles
with deeper defects
interproximally

Confirms that
defect is two
walled (crater)
(see Chapter 100)

No crater
located

Accept probing
finding as
correct

Shallow depths on
proximal line angles
with deeper defects
interproximally

Confirms that
defect is two
walled (crater)
(see Chapter 100)

One wall is against
adjacent tooth; the
other on the facial
or lingual

Confirms
two-walled
defect
(see Chapter 100)

Shallow depths
on proximal line
angles or affected
tooth with deeper
bone loss under
contact

Confirms
three-walled
defect
(see Chapter 100)

19 Use of Digital Radiographs in Periodontics

Thomas Schiff

The newest development in radiology is the replacement of films with a sensor system. Two systems are available today, the so-called CCD system (charged coupled devices) and the phosphorous storage plate system. The CCD system is attached directly to a computer and thus gives instant images on a screen, while the phosphorous storage plate system requires the plate to be scanned into the computer and therefore takes extra time for the formation of the image. This extra time is minimal, however, and in most cases it only takes between one and two minutes for the picture to develop. Use of the actual sensor is cumbersome because of its thickness and its attachment to wires, whereas the phosphorous storage plates are thinner and easier to place into the oral cavity.

The manufacturers of the CCDs provide positioning devices that make their use easy and comfortable to patients.

This system utilizes a sensor connected to a computer with a wire and allows instant imaging after exposure to minimal radiation. Due to the sensitivity of the CCD, the exposure time has been continuously reduced, allowing patient exposure to be minimal indeed. New technologies now making super high-speed films have reduced the CCD system's advantage of low exposure to radiation. These new films are the Kodak F speed films (INSIGHT). With no remaining differences between the films and sensors as to the amount of radiation they need, the digital system is no longer a great advantage over the CCD. The one real advantage is that the CCD image is viewable instantly on the computer screen and its enhancement is possible utilizing the software provided by the various manufacturers, allowing the application of sophisticated technology to view the images and adjust them to maximize correct diagnosis.

Printing of the images is critical, and only a few manufacturers of digital systems couple their system to good quality imaging. Kodak medical printing systems using their high-quality paper provide acceptable images. Printing the images on plain paper, however, will result in unacceptable images.

A In an office that has both digital and traditional radiographic capability, a decision must be made whether the product will be for in-office use only or for use in another office, upon referral, as well. If the images are solely for use in office, only digital systems offer the advantage of immediate viewing (no developing time needed) and enhancement of images as needed.

B If the product is to be sent elsewhere, the quality of the available digital image printer is a consideration. Unless that printer will produce excellent images, the radiographic system should be used, because only the very highest quality images are useful in periodontics.

C If the available printer produces ideal images, the choice of which capability to use would be up to the operator. For example, some operators prefer to have all their images stored in one system in their offices.

Patient for RADIOGRAPHIC OR DIGITALIZED IMAGES FOR PERIODONTAL USE

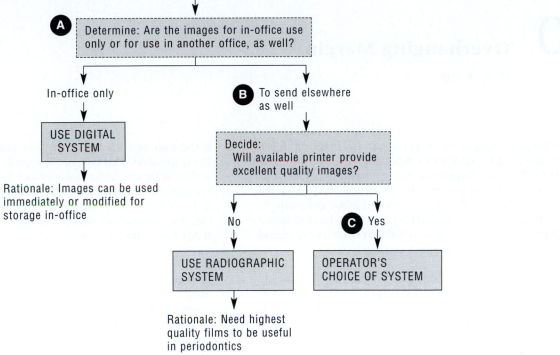

A Determine: Are the images for in-office use only or for use in another office, as well?

In-office only

B To send elsewhere as well

USE DIGITAL SYSTEM

Decide: Will available printer provide excellent quality images?

Rationale: Images can be used immediately or modified for storage in-office

No

C Yes

USE RADIOGRAPHIC SYSTEM

OPERATOR'S CHOICE OF SYSTEM

Rationale: Need highest quality films to be useful in periodontics

20 Overhanging Margin

Walter B. Hall

An overhanging margin on a periodontally involved tooth makes plaque removal difficult to impossible (Figure 20-1). The material of which the restoration was constructed is crucial in deciding the best way to resolve this type of problem. Generally, replacement of the defective restoration is the best approach. If, however, the overhang is minimal and accessible, less expensive alternatives such as smoothing out of the overhang or marginal repairs may be acceptable options.

A If the defective restoration is an amalgam that is basically adequate and no new caries is involved, smoothing out the overhang is the approach of choice. If the restoration is grossly defective, involves new caries, or is inaccessible for repair, it should be replaced.

B If the restoration is a composite and the defect is minimal, the overhang may be smoothed out and polished. If there is a gross defect or new caries, the restoration should be replaced because of the difficulty in doing acceptable repairs to existing composites.

C If the restoration is a gold inlay or onlay, it is cast in relatively soft gold. This type of gold "pulls" or flows when burnished with a rotating stone or polishing bur. If the defect is minimal, the discrepancy can be burnished out; however, if the defect is major and accessible for preparation and filling, the restoration should be replaced or a repair performed with foil or alloy.

D If the overhanging margin is on a gold crown, the gold used is harder and more difficult to pull. Only minimal discrepancies on gold crown margins are amenable to this approach. If the defect is greater and the area is accessible for preparation and filling, a repair may be performed. Replacement of gold crowns with defective margins is the approach of choice, but it is extremely expensive.

E If the overhanging margin is on a gold-alloy crown, this material is even harder and usually cannot be pulled. If the defect is accessible, an alloy repair may be adequate; if not, the crown should be replaced.

Additional Readings

Bjorn AL, Bjorn H, Grcovic B. Marginal fit of restorations and its relation to periodontal bone level. Odont Rev 1974;20:311.

Gilmore N, Sheiham A. Overhanging dental restorations and periodontal disease. J Periodontol 1971;42:8.

Renggli HH, Regolati A. Gingival inflammation and plaque accumulation by well-adapted supragingival and subgingival proximal restorations. Helv Odontol Acta 1972;16:99.

Roderiques-Ferrer HJ, Stroham JD, Newman HN. Effect on gingival health of removing overhanging margins of interproximal subgingival amalgam restorations. J Clin Periodontol 1980;7:457.

Schluger S, Yuodelis RA, Page RC. Periodontal disease. Philadelphia: Lea & Febiger; 1977. p. 589.

Wilson TG, Kornman KS. Fundamentals of periodontics. Chicago: Quintessence Publishing; 1996. p. 473–80.

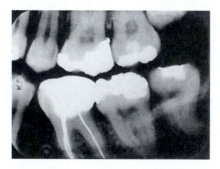

Figure 20-1 An overhang on the distal surface of the maxillary first molar.

Patient with OVERHANGING MARGIN ON TOOTH

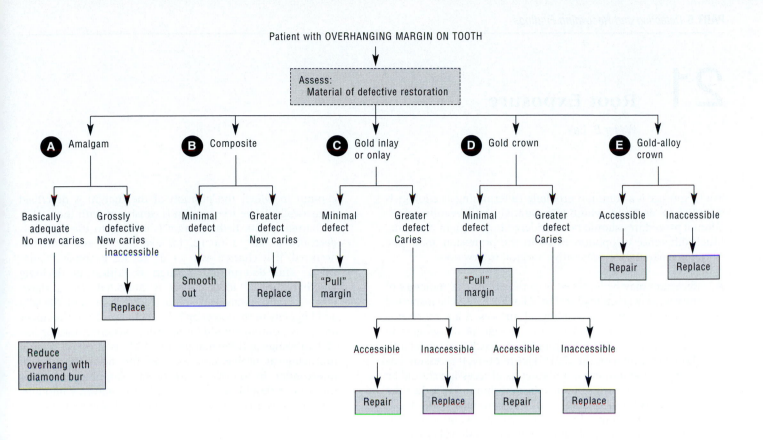

Assess:
Material of defective restoration

A Amalgam

Basically adequate
No new caries

Reduce overhang with diamond bur

Grossly defective
New caries inaccessible

Replace

B Composite

Minimal defect

Smooth out

Greater defect
New caries

Replace

C Gold inlay or onlay

Minimal defect

"Pull" margin

Greater defect
Caries

Accessible

Repair

Inaccessible

Replace

D Gold crown

Minimal defect

"Pull" margin

Greater defect
Caries

Accessible

Repair

Inaccessible

Replace

E Gold-alloy crown

Accessible

Repair

Inaccessible

Replace

21 Root Exposure

Walter B. Hall

Root exposure is a common problem. Determining its etiology is essential in deciding whether reparative or preventive periodontal procedures should be considered in treatment planning. Much difference of opinion exists in the profession about the need for reparative or preventive surgical intervention.

A Recession may be localized or generalized. The etiologies of the two may be quite different. All teeth should be inspected for recession on facial and lingual surfaces. A line representing the true position of the free margin of the gingiva in relation to the cementoenamel junction (CEJ) on each tooth should be drawn on the chart (Figure 21-1). If recession has occurred, the number of millimeters of recession should be recorded for future reference in determining whether the recession is active or stabilized. This determination often is critical in deciding whether surgical intervention is indicated. Some newer charting methods designed for computerization do not use tooth diagrams; instead, there is a

column in which the position of the margin is described numerically. If the free margin is consistent with the CEJ, it is charted as a 0. If the margin is coronal to the CEJ, it is described as an 11 or 12, for example. If recession has occurred, it is charted as a 21 or 22, for example (Figure 21-2). This determination often is critical in deciding whether surgical intervention is indicated. On surfaces where a mucogingival junction (MGJ) is present (facially and lingually in the lower arch but only facially in the upper arch), its position should be recorded. Where 2 mm or less of total gingiva (free margin to MGJ) is present, a pure mucogingival problem exists, and the need for surgical intervention in the overall treatment planning process for the patient should be considered. In the newer, computer-compatible charts, a line is used on which total millimeters of gingiva can be entered (see Figure 21-1).

B The skill of the dentist in eliciting the facts of a patient's dental history and the temporal placement of the events in that history often are clues to the sequential development of recession. Frequently, the dentist must glean a patient's recollection of these events and their temporal sequence through repetitive and incisive questioning. The dentist's knowledge of the typical sequencing of events in the process of recession may be used to guide the patient's recollections (see Figure 21-2).

C Injuries may occur in areas predisposed to recession by the presence of inadequate attached gingiva (Figure 21-3) or where adequate attached gingiva is present. Such injuries may be the result of a direct wound (eg, from crusty bread) or repeated bouts of gingivitis. Where inadequate attached gingiva is present, root exposure frequently results. Where

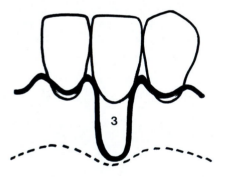

Figure 21-1 A chart recording an area of recession on a lateral incisor.

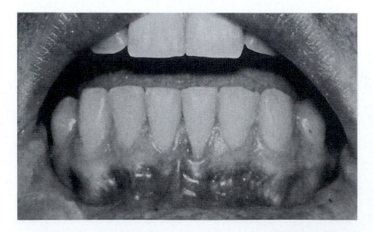

Figure 21-2 A central incisor with inadequate attached gingiva and recession.

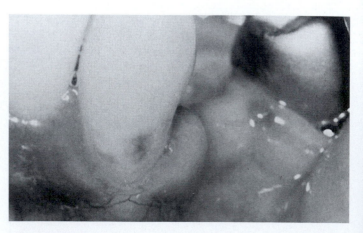

Figure 21-3 Recession in an area of inadequate attached gingiva has resulted in root exposure.

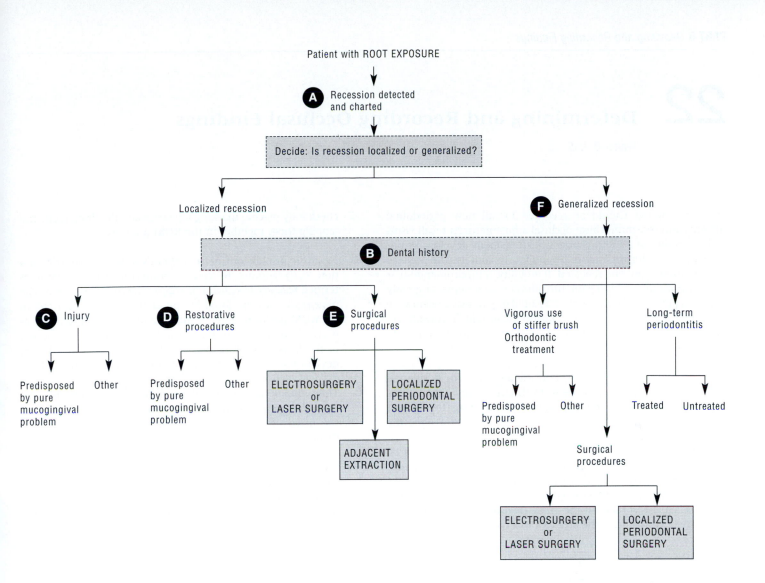

Patient with ROOT EXPOSURE

A Recession detected and charted

Decide: Is recession localized or generalized?

Localized recession

F Generalized recession

B Dental history

C Injury
- Predisposed by pure mucogingival problem
- Other

D Restorative procedures
- Predisposed by pure mucogingival problem
- Other

E Surgical procedures
- ELECTROSURGERY or LASER SURGERY
- LOCALIZED PERIODONTAL SURGERY
- ADJACENT EXTRACTION

Vigorous use of stiffer brush Orthodontic treatment
- Predisposed by pure mucogingival problem
- Other

Long-term periodontitis
- Treated
- Untreated

Surgical procedures
- ELECTROSURGERY or LASER SURGERY
- LOCALIZED PERIODONTAL SURGERY

an adequate band of attached gingiva is present (unless the wound is quite severe), healing usually occurs without much, if any, recession.

D Restorative procedures such as subgingival use of a diamond bur, taking of an impression subgingivally, or cementation and polishing of a restoration often result in recession when inadequate attached gingiva is present, but far less frequently do so when a broad band is present.

E Surgical procedures such as subgingival root planing, soft-tissue curettage, periodontal flap approaches, or gingivectomy may produce localized recessions. Electrosurgery and laser surgery often are a direct cause and may even create pure mucogingival problems where none existed before the procedure. The extraction of an adjacent tooth, especially if tissue displacement extends to adjacent teeth, often is followed by localized recession on adjacent teeth. Often it is dramatic when the adjacent tooth has little attached gingiva. The dentist's skills in drawing such information from the patient's dental history are most important in this situation.

F Generalized root exposure may result not only from events similar to those already described but also from additional factors. Vigorous use of a toothbrush, especially a stiffer one, frequently results in generalized recession, which may be much more extensive on teeth with little attached gingiva (especially canines, first premolars, and mandibular central incisors). Orthodontic treatment and consequent changes in brushing technique may do the same. Most periodontal flap and gingivectomy procedures produce some degree of root exposure with healing. So do electrosurgery or laser surgery. Generalized root exposure usually is seen after all pocket-elimination procedures. Repeated root planing and the modified Widman flap also usually result in root exposure. Long-term periodontitis, whether treated or untreated, often results in generalized root exposure as pocket formation progresses apically. The dentist's skill in eliciting these facts and placing them in a chronologic sequence is important.

Additional Readings

Gartrell JR, Mathews DP. Gingival recession: the condition, process and treatment. Dent Clin North Am 1976;20:199.

Gorman WJ. Prevalence and etiology of gingival recession. J Periodontol 1976;38:316.

Hall WB. Pure mucogingival problems. Berlin: Quintessence Publishing; 1984. p. 29.

Moscow BS, Bressman E. Localized gingival recession: etiology and treatment. Dent Radiograph Photograph 1965;38:3.

Wilson TG, Kornman KS. Fundamentals of periodontics. Chicago: Quintessence Publishing; 1996. p. 210–11.

22 Determining and Recording Occlusal Findings

Walter B. Hall

Occlusal findings should be recorded for all new periodontal patients and rerecorded after occlusal adjustment. At recall visits, if the mobility of a tooth changes or the patient develops symptoms of discomfort in a tooth in premature contact, the occlusal examination should be repeated. If mobility, temporomandibular joint symptoms, occlusal pain, furcation involvements, or grossly widened periodontal ligaments are noted or extensive restorative treatment is planned, occlusal adjustment should be considered. There are several approaches to occlusal evaluation, but only one is presented in this chapter.

A   The rearmost, uppermost, and midmost (RUM) position is obtained by placing the dentist's thumb on the incisal edges of the lower teeth and tapping the teeth together first against the thumb several times and then mandibular against the maxillary teeth while exerting gentle posterior and upward pressure against the chin. Alternatively, the dentist can sit behind the patient and grasp the mandible with both hands, gently retracting it and moving it occlusally with the thumbs until two or more teeth can be tapped together. This initial contact is recorded on the chart (Figure 22-1). Usually, the patient can indicate the area of initial contact. The dentist can

check it by placing marking tape between the dried teeth and tapping them together in the RUM position.

B   Next, the dimensions of the patient's slide from centric relation (CR) contact to centric occlusion (CO), sometimes termed *maximum occlusion* or *acquired centric,* is recorded. The patient's mouth is closed by the dentist to initial contact in the RUM position, and the movement to CO in three planes is recorded. The vertical, horizontal, and lateral translation of the jaws in millimeters and the direction of any lateral deviation of the mandible are recorded (see Figure 22-1).

C   Then the patient is asked to close in CO and slide the mandible to the right while the teeth are in contact, until the facial cusp tip to facial cusp tip position is reached. Cross-arch "balancing" (nonworking) side contacts are detected by placing tape on the "balancing" side and having the patient slide the dried teeth from CO to the cusp-to-cusp position on the working side. Then the tape is placed on the right side and the process repeated, indicating working side contacts and "cross-tooth" contacts. These contacts are recorded (see Figure 22-1).

INITIAL OCCLUSAL FINDINGS

| CENTRIC RELATION: Initial tooth contact | 1 2 3 4 5 6 7 8   9 10 11 12 13 14 15 16 |
| | 32 31 30 29 28 27 26 25   24 23 22 21 20 19 18 17 |

CENTRIC RELATION—CENTRIC OCCLUSION DISCREPANCY:
Forward slide .... mm
Vertical slide .... mm
Lateral slide .... R( ) .... L( ) .... mm

| CENTRIC OCCLUSION: Canine classification | Right Side   I   II   III | Left Side   I   II   III |

Vertical overlap (overbite) .... mm
Horizontal overlap (overjet) .... mm

EXCURSIVE MOVEMENTS

RIGHT LATERAL	1 2 3 4 5 6 7 8 9 10 11 12 13 14 15 16
	32 31 30 29 28 27 26 25 24 23 22 21 20 19 18 17
LEFT LATERAL	1 2 3 4 5 6 7 8 9 10 11 12 13 14 15 16
	32 31 30 29 28 27 26 25 24 23 22 21 20 19 18 17
PROTRUSIVE	1 2 3 4 5 6 7 8 9 10 11 12 13 14 15 16
	32 31 30 29 28 27 26 25 24 23 22 21 20 19 18 17

MAXIMUM OPENING .... mm
TMJ _____
MUSCLES _____

Figure 22-1 A typical occlusal analysis charting form. Courtesy University of Pacific. Reproduced with permission from Hall WB, Roberts WE, Labarre EE. Decision making in dental treatment planning. St. Louis: Mosby; 1994.

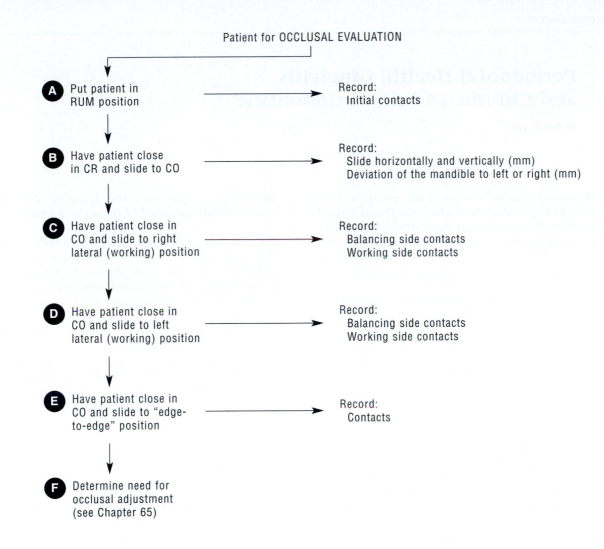

Patient for OCCLUSAL EVALUATION

A Put patient in RUM position → Record: Initial contacts

B Have patient close in CR and slide to CO → Record: Slide horizontally and vertically (mm) Deviation of the mandible to left or right (mm)

C Have patient close in CO and slide to right lateral (working) position → Record: Balancing side contacts Working side contacts

D Have patient close in CO and slide to left lateral (working) position → Record: Balancing side contacts Working side contacts

E Have patient close in CO and slide to "edge-to-edge" position → Record: Contacts

F Determine need for occlusal adjustment (see Chapter 65)

D Left lateral contacts are determined and recorded by repeating the previous procedure but having the patient slide from CO to the left lateral position. These findings are recorded (see Figure 22-1).

E Finally, the patient is asked to close in CO with tape between the dried anterior teeth and to slide anteriorly until the incisal edges of the mandibular anterior and maxillary anterior teeth are in contact in the "edge-to-edge" position. If the maxillary anteriors are quite mobile, gentle stabilizing pressure may be applied to their facial surfaces with the fingers of the left hand so that they move facially, leaving no contact marks from the marking tape to indicate heavy contacts. These contacts are recorded (see Figure 22-1).

F The occlusal findings are used by the dentist, along with all other examination findings, to determine whether any occlusal adjustment would be beneficial (see Chapter 65).

Additional Readings

Grant DA, Stern IB, Listgarten MA. Periodontics. 6th ed. St. Louis: Mosby; 1988. p. 1003.

O'Leary JJ. Tooth mobility. Dent Clin North Am 1969;13:567.

Ramfjord S, Ash MM. Occlusion. 3rd ed. Philadelphia: WB Saunders; 1983. p. 298.

Schluger S et al. Periodontal diseases. 2nd ed. Philadelphia: Lea & Febiger; 1990. p. 318.

Wilson TG, Kornman KS. Fundamentals of periodontics. Chicago: Quintessence Publishing; 1996. p. 491–4.

23 Periodontal Health, Gingivitis, and Chronic (Adult) Periodontitis

Walter B. Hall

A differential diagnosis among periodontal health, gingivitis, and periodontitis is begun by evaluating medical and dental histories. Older dental records and radiographs are especially helpful in establishing current disease activity as gingivitis or periodontitis.* Because these diseases are active in spurts, past findings are most helpful.

A A visual examination usually follows history taking. The gingiva may be inflamed, in which case there is marginal and papillary swelling and redness, or magenta coloring, or the gingiva may seem healthy, appearing pink, firm, and probably stippled. Such an appearance, however, may mask severe periodontitis. Gingiva that has become fibrotic as a result of frequent episodes of inflammation and healing may appear visibly healthy adjacent to deep pockets.

B Probing should be performed regardless of the visual signs. When the gingiva appears visibly inflamed, probing usually reveals pockets with depths of 3 mm or more and bleeding. Pocket depth alone is insufficient to make a diagnosis between gingivitis and periodontitis. Swelling alone may create pockets of considerable depth that bleed on probing.

C A diagnosis of gingivitis can be made when redness and swelling are present without loss of attachment (LOA). If the probe reaches the root, LOA has occurred. When the gingiva is red and swollen, pocket depths are present, and LOA has occurred, a diagnosis of chronic adult periodontitis is most likely to be correct. However, when earlier LOA and new localized swelling and redness have occurred, creating pocket depths, gingivitis could be a correct diagnosis. Such situations often apply when patients are recalled after successful treatment. Recurrent inflammation may be present unless the patient makes ideal oral-hygiene efforts.

D When radiographs do not suggest active bone loss and pockets are of minimal depth with evidence of swelling, gingivitis may be an acceptable diagnosis. Fortunately, in instances in which a decision is difficult to make, the differentiation may be more academic than practical, because treatment would be the same anyway.

E For a diagnosis of chronic adult periodontitis to be made, three concurrent findings must exist: pocket depth, LOA, and active bone loss. Radiographs can be helpful, but they are susceptible to aberrations in film placement, machine-head angulation, exposure time, kilovoltage used in taking the radiograph, and variability in developing technique. Radiographs alone, therefore, are never diagnostic; other findings must be considered. Fuzzy crestal bone may indicate active bone loss, but fuzziness can be created easily on radiographs from healthy patients, as already described. Series of radiographs taken at different times are more likely to yield a correct diagnosis; they should, however, be taken and prepared identically to be diagnostic. If inflammation, pocket depth, and LOA are present and radiographs suggest active bone loss, periodontitis is most likely the correct diagnosis.

F In instances with no visible signs of inflammation, periodontal health can be differentiated from chronic adult periodontitis on the basis of the absence of pocket depths greater than 3 mm. If the probe does not extend to the roots and radiographs indicate no bone loss, periodontal health is an appropriate diagnosis. LOA may result from earlier periodontitis, and radiographic evidence of bone loss may exist, but the combination of no pocket depth and no signs of inflammation suggests periodontal health. Without the visible signs of inflammation, gingivitis would not be a correct diagnosis.

Additional Readings

American Academy of Periodontology. Proceedings of World Workshop in Clinical Periodontics. Princeton: The Academy; 1989. p. 1–33.

Carranza FA Jr, Newman MG. Clinical periodontology. 8th ed. Philadelphia: WB Saunders; 1996. p. 58.

Parr RW. Examination and diagnosis of periodontal disease. Washington (DC): Dept. of Health, Education and Welfare (US); 1977. DHEW Pub. No. (HRA) 74–36.

Prichard JF. Advanced periodontal disease. 2nd ed. Philadelphia: WB Saunders; 1972. p. 116.

Worth HM. Radiology in diagnosis. Dent Clin North Am 1969;13:731.

---

*Periodontitis occurs in at least six subgroups: adult, prepubertal (mixed dentition), juvenile, rapidly progressive, necrotizing ulcerative, and human immunodeficiency virus (HIV) periodontitis.

Patient needing DIFFERENTIAL DIAGNOSIS AMONG PERIODONTAL HEALTH, GINGIVITIS, AND CHRONIC (ADULT) PERIODONTITIS

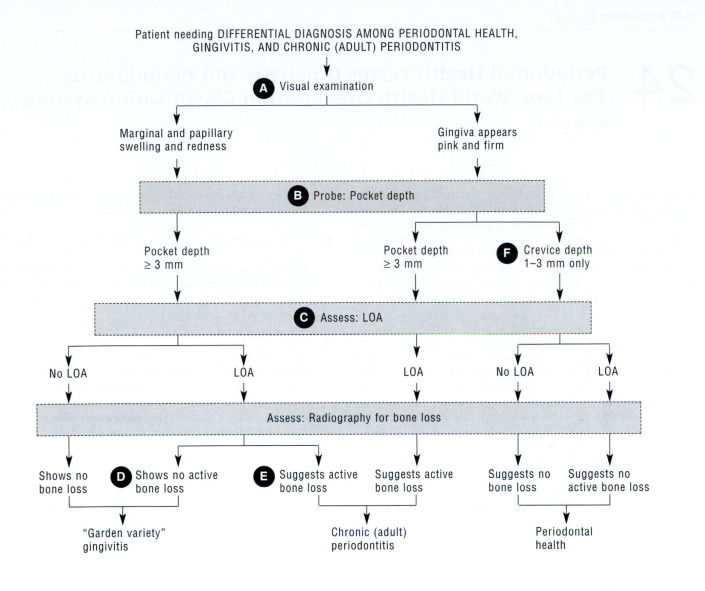

24 Periodontal Health versus Gingivitis and Periodontitis: The New World Health Organization Classification System

Walter B. Hall

In the new World Health Organization (WHO) classification of periodontal diseases, loss of attachment (LOA) has replaced pocket depth as the most pertinent finding, along with the presence or absence of clinical signs of inflammation, in making a differential diagnosis among periodontal health, gingivitis, and periodontitis. Systemic disease and specific infections can modify the subgroupings of each diagnostic situation. The differentiation process described herein deals only with a systemically healthy individual.

A   Clinical signs of inflammation include color change (from pink to reddish or magenta color), swelling (edema), and bleeding or suppuration on probing. When none of these findings is present, a tooth, a segment of teeth, or an entire dentition can be termed "healthy." When any of these findings is present, either gingivitis or periodontitis is present.

B   Attachment loss may be assessed visually, radiographically, or tactilely (by probing or exploring). Measuring and recording pocket depths remain critical means of chronicalling periodontal disease status, but measurements (estimates) of LOA are the means by which gingivitis and periodontitis are differentiated in the WHO system. When inflammation is present but LOA has not occurred, the diagnosis is gingivitis. When both LOA and inflammation are present, the diagnosis is periodontitis.

C   Periodontal health exists when clinical signs of inflammation are absent. When LOA is absent as well, the diagnosis would indisputably be "health." However, when LOA has occurred but inflammation is absent, to many the correct diagnosis would be periodontal health with a history of previous periodontal disease.

D   In the WHO classification system, periodontitis in systemically healthy patients may be chronic or aggressive in nature. At an initial examination, the rate of progression of the disease cannot be determined and must be deduced. Patient history, age, and various dental findings on radiographs may be helpful in making the differentiation. Repeated examinations are the means of proving the deduction.

Additional Readings

Wilson TG, Kornman KS. Fundamentals of periodontics. Chicago: Quintessence Publishing; 1996. p. 195–200, 204, 205, 212, 225–8.

World Workshop in Periodontics. Ann Periodontol 1996;1:216.

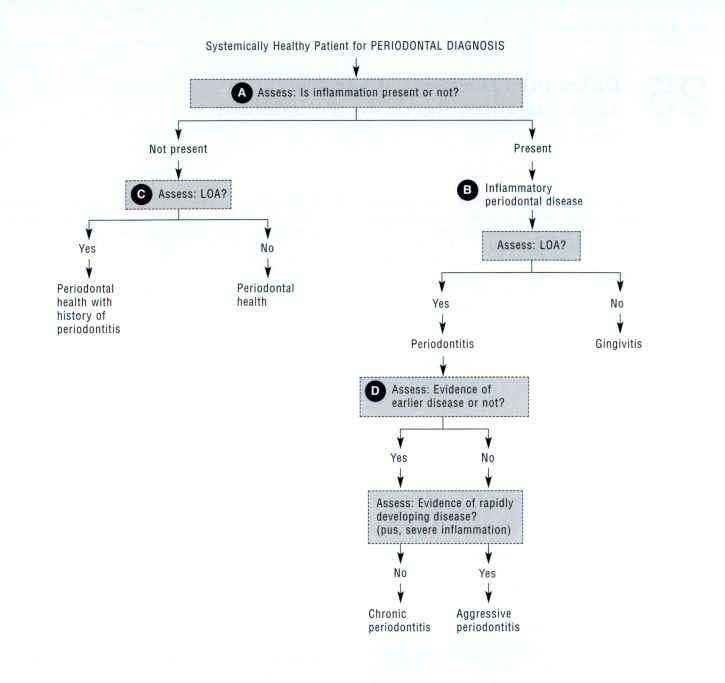

25 Differential Diagnosis of Localized and Generalized Aggressive Periodontitis

Steven A. Tsurudome

Aggressive periodontitis continues to be an evolving classification of periodontitis as a result of advances in the areas of microbiology and immunology. Due to the recent changes in the classification system for the periodontal diseases and conditions, the terms *juvenile periodontitis* and *rapidly progressive periodontitis* have been discarded because they are considered to be age dependent or require knowledge of rates of progression.

The clinical criteria that represented the disease category of *generalized juvenile periodontitis* and *localized juvenile periodontitis* are now classified as *generalized aggressive periodontitis* and *localized aggressive periodontitis,* respectively. The clinical criteria that represented the disease category of *rapidly progressive periodontitis* are now classified as *generalized aggressive periodontitis* or *chronic periodontitis*.

Even though the terms have changed, the distinguishing factors between these new categories still involve the age of onset, the rate and severity of the destruction of periodontal tissue, differences in host response, and the types of subgingival bacterial flora that are characteristic to this group.

A Radiographically, patients with localized aggressive periodontitis usually show bilaterally symmetric, rapid severe vertical bone loss and loss of attachment (LOA) of 4 mm or greater in the permanent first molar and incisor regions (Figure 25-1). Generalized aggressive periodontitis is characterized by rapid severe bone loss and LOA of 4 mm or greater around most of the teeth.

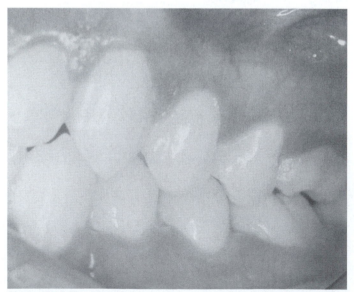

Figure 25-1 Deep, vertical bone defects mesial to first molars are typical of localized aggressive periodontitis (formerly juvenile periodontitis).

B In aggressive periodontitis cases, the onset of this disease usually occurs around puberty and is more prevalent in females than males (3:1). Aggressive periodontitis may have a familial distribution in that it may be inherited as an X-linked dominant or an autosomal recessive trait.

C In localized aggressive periodontitis, the bacterial flora may be dominated by *Actinobacillus actinomycetemcomitans* in combination with *Bacteroides intermedius, Capnocytophaga ochraceus,* and *Eikenella corrodens*. In generalized aggressive periodontitis, the bacterial flora may also include *B. gingivalis*.

D In aggressive periodontitis the patient's host response may be expressed in terms of a depressed neutrophil chemotaxis response to bacterial infections or as a random migration of neutrophils.

E Classically, aggressive periodontitis is characterized as a disease process whereby the rapid rate and severity of the periodontal destruction is not consistent with the clinical findings of minimal plaque accumulation and scarcity of clinically visible severe gingival inflammation.

F The diagnosis of generalized or localized aggressive periodontitis requires immediate modification to the periodontal treatment plan. Because of the significance of the bacterial flora in aggressive periodontitis, systemic antibiotic therapy in conjunction with scaling and root planing is recommended. Surgery may be considered for greater access for root débridement. The tetracyclines have been effective in treating both forms of aggressive periodontitis, as has a combination of amoxicillin and metronidazole; however, antibiotic susceptibility testing of the subgingival bacterial flora is recommended if there is any uncertainty regarding which antibiotics to prescribe. Because of the aggressive, complex, and advanced nature of both localized and generalized aggressive periodontitis, referral to a periodontal specialist is recommended.

Additional Readings

American Academy of Periodontology. Proceedings of the World Workshop in Clinical Periodontics. Princeton: The Academy; 1989.

Armitage GC. Development of a classification system for periodontal diseases and conditions. Ann Periodontol 1999;4:1.

Carranza FA, Newman MG. Clinical periodontology. 8th ed. Philadelphia: Saunders; 1996. p. 338–41.

Kornman KS, Robertson PB. Clinical and microbiological evaluation of therapy for juvenile periodontitis. J Periodontol 1985;56:443.

Krill DB, Fry HR. Treatment of localized juvenile periodontitis (periodontosis): a review. J Periodontol 1987;58:1.

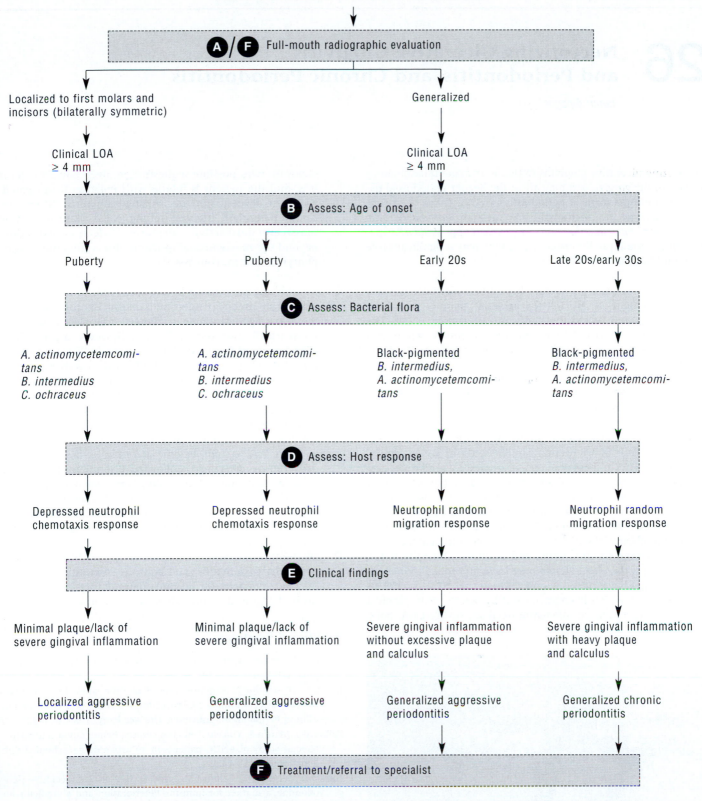

Patient with EVIDENCE OF SEVERE RAPID BONE LOSS

A / F Full-mouth radiographic evaluation

Localized to first molars and incisors (bilaterally symmetric)

Generalized

Clinical LOA ≥ 4 mm

Clinical LOA ≥ 4 mm

B Assess: Age of onset

Puberty | Puberty | Early 20s | Late 20s/early 30s

C Assess: Bacterial flora

| *A. actinomycetemcomitans* *B. intermedius* *C. ochraceus* | *A. actinomycetemcomitans* *B. intermedius* *C. ochraceus* | Black-pigmented *B. intermedius,* *A. actinomycetemcomitans* | Black-pigmented *B. intermedius,* *A. actinomycetemcomitans* |

D Assess: Host response

| Depressed neutrophil chemotaxis response | Depressed neutrophil chemotaxis response | Neutrophil random migration response | Neutrophil random migration response |

E Clinical findings

| Minimal plaque/lack of severe gingival inflammation | Minimal plaque/lack of severe gingival inflammation | Severe gingival inflammation without excessive plaque and calculus | Severe gingival inflammation with heavy plaque and calculus |

| Localized aggressive periodontitis | Generalized aggressive periodontitis | Generalized aggressive periodontitis | Generalized chronic periodontitis |

F Treatment/referral to specialist

Mandell RL, Socransky SS. Microbiological and clinical effects of surgery plus doxycycline on juvenile periodontitis. J Periodontol 1983;59:373.

Page RC et al. Clinical and laboratory studies of a family with a high prevalence of juvenile periodontitis. J Periodontol 1985;56:602.

Page RC et al. Rapidly progressive periodontitis: a distinct clinical condition. J Periodontol 1983;54:197.

Suzuki JB. Diagnosis and classification of the periodontal diseases. Dent Clin North Am 1988;32:195.

26 Necrotizing Ulcerative Gingivitis and Periodontitis, and Chronic Periodontitis

Tamer Alpagot

Necrotizing ulcerative gingivitis (NUG) is an acute inflammatory disease of the gingiva and may affect the deeper periodontal tissues, becoming a form of periodontitis (NUP). It has been suggested that specific microorganisms such as *Bulleidia extructa, Dialister* spp, *Fusobacterium* spp, *Streptococcus* spp, *Veillonella* spp, as well as certain predisposing factors may play a significant role in the pathogenesis of NUG/NUP.

A   Several predisposing factors have been identified for the development of NUG/NUP; bacterial plaque, poor oral hygiene, and preexisting gingivitis are among them. The prevalence of NUG/NUP is higher in patients with poor oral hygiene than in individuals who have good oral hygiene. Stress conditions, socioeconomic status, smoking, and altered host resistance are contributing factors in the pathogenesis of NUG/NUP. Assess the signs and symptoms associated with these diseases.

B   NUG is characterized by rapid-onset, gingival pain, crater-like necrosis of interdental papillae without loss of attachment (LOA) and covered by a gray pseudomembrane, gingival hemorrhage, metallic taste, and bad breath (fetor oris) (Figure 26-1). The gingival lesions may be localized or generalized. The lesions are more common in the anterior than the posterior region of the mouth. Early in the course of the disease, the ulceration in the tip of the papillae may be obscured by the edema and swelling. Once the lesion develops, the affected area may have an eroded, punched-out appearance. It has been proposed that NUG progresses into NUP, which is characterized by severe pain, gingival bleeding, extensive soft-tissue necrosis, severe LOA, bone

exposure with possible sequestration, deep jaw ache, fetor oris, and the patient is febrile with malaise. If untreated, NUP can develop into necrotizing stomatitis (NS), which can be potentially life threatening. NS is characterized by massively destructive, ulcerative infection extending beyond the mucogingival junction into contiguous palato-pharyngeal or mucous tissues.

C   As with any periodontal lesions, the removal of plaque and debris from the site of infection is critical. Because the patient may have significant pain, a complete root planing and scaling is usually not initially feasible. However, a generalized débridement of the affected areas can be facilitated by irrigation with 3% peroxide diluted 50% with warm water. The next phase of the office treatment is to evaluate the need for chemotherapeutic agents as adjunctive therapy. If fever, severe necrosis, and exposure of bone or severe pain are present, antibiotic coverage is usually required. Metronidazole, 250 mg four times daily for 5 days, is the drug of choice. In addition, 0.12% chlorhexidine oral rinse for home use twice daily can be prescribed. Following resolution of the acute inflammation, meticulous scaling and root planing can be instituted in several visits. Finally, after therapy is completed, the long-term management of these patients must be considered including the pocket-elimination procedures.

D   Differential diagnosis must be made among NUG/NUP, herpetic gingivostomatitis, and aphtous stomatitis. NUG/NUP may be a predictor for immune deterioration and the diagnosis of acquired immunodeficiency syndrome (AIDS).

Additional Readings

Carranza FA Jr, Newman MG. Clinical periodontology. 8th ed. Philadelphia: WB Saunders; 1996. p. 59.

Caton J. Periodontal diagnosis and diagnostic aids. In: American Acdemy of Periodontalogy. Proceedings of the World Workshop in Clinical Periodontics. Princeton: The Academy; 1989. p. 1–22.

Falker WJ, Martin S, Vincent J, et al. A clinical, demographic and microbiologic study of ANUG patients in an urban dental school. J Clin Periodontol 1987;14:307.

Glick M, Muzyka BC, Salkin LM, Lurie D. Necrotizing ulcerative periodontitis: a marker for immune deterioration and a predictor for the diagnosis of AIDS. J Periodontol 1994;65:393.

Melnick SL, Roseman JM, Engel D, Cogen RB. Epidemiology of acute necrotizing gingivitis. Epidemiol Rev 1988;10:191–211.

Russell MK, Alpagot T, Boches SK, et al. Bacterial species and phylotypes in necrotizing ulcerative periodontitis [abstract #1050]. J Dent Res 2001;80:167.

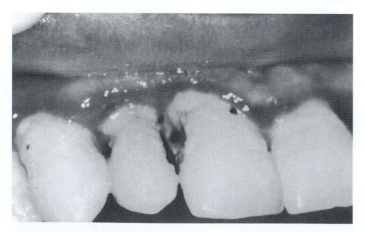

Figure 26-1 Severe, necrotizing ulcerative periodontitis (NUP).

Patient with PAIN, GINGIVAL REDNESS, AND SWELLING

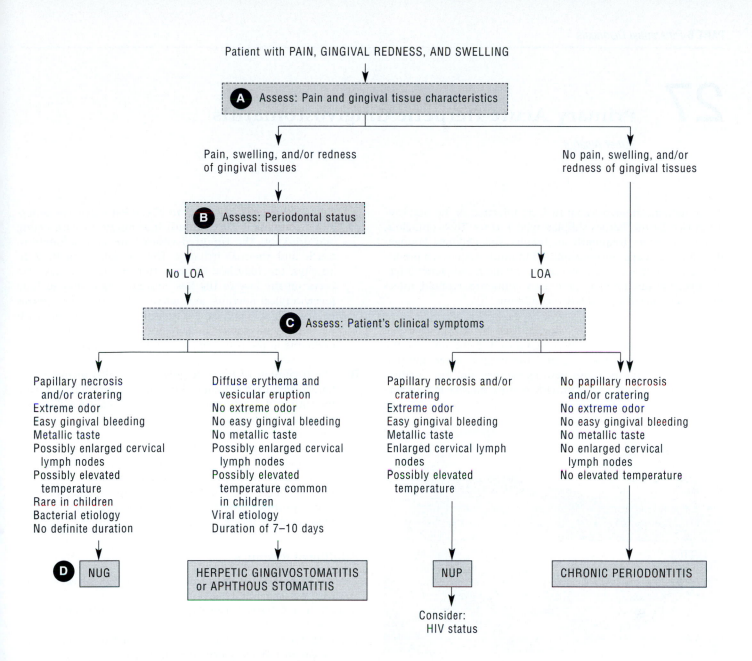

27 Primary Acute Herpetic Gingivostomatitis

Tamer Alpagot

Acute herpetic gingivostomatitis is an infection of the oral cavity caused by the herpes simplex type 1 virus. This contagious condition occurs frequently in infants and children younger than 6 years of age. A compromised immune system is a predisposing factor. It is commonly seen following recent acute infections such as pneumonia, meningitis, influenza, typhoid, infectious mononucleosis, and stress conditions.

A   In its early stage, it is characterized by the presence of spherical gray vesicles on the gingiva, the oral mucosa, the soft palate, the pharynx, and the tongue. After approximately 24 hours, these vesicles rupture and form painful ulcers, which appear as grayish-white craterlike lesions sur-

rounded by a red halo (Figure 27-1). Patients have generalized soreness in their mouth that interferes with eating and drinking. The ruptured vesicles are very sensitive to touch and thermal irritants. They usually remain 7 to 10 days, but may last 14 days. Herpetic lesions may also occur on the face or the lips. Systemic signs may include fever, cervical adenitis, and malaise. Differential diagnosis of acute herpetic gingivostomatitis must be made with necrotizing ulcerative gingivitis/periodontitis (NUG/NUP), erythema multiforme, and aphthous stomatitis.

B   The treatment of herpetic gingivostomatitis includes palliative measures to make the patient comfortable during the course of the disease. Supragingival scaling will reduce gingival inflammation. Extensive periodontal therapy should be postponed until the acute symptoms subside. Topical anesthetic mouthwashes enable the patient to eat comfortably. Some limited success with the use of acyclovir ointment has been reported. Supportive measures include intake of liquid nutritional supplements and systemic antibiotic therapy for the treatment of toxic systemic complications.

Additional Readings

Carranza FA Jr, Newman MG. Clinical periodontology. 8th ed. Philadelphia: WB Saunders; 1996. p. 255, 481.

Grant D, Stern I, Everett F. Periodontics. 6th ed. St. Louis: Mosby; 1988. p. 413.

Regezi JA, Sciubba JJ. Oral pathology: clinical-pathologic correlations. Philadelphia: WB Saunders; 1989. p. 255, 481.

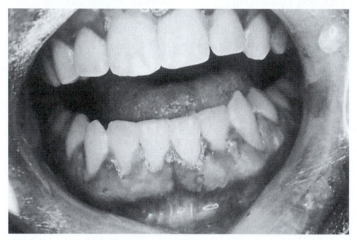

Figure 27-1 Gingival lesions of acute primary herpetic gingivostomatitis.

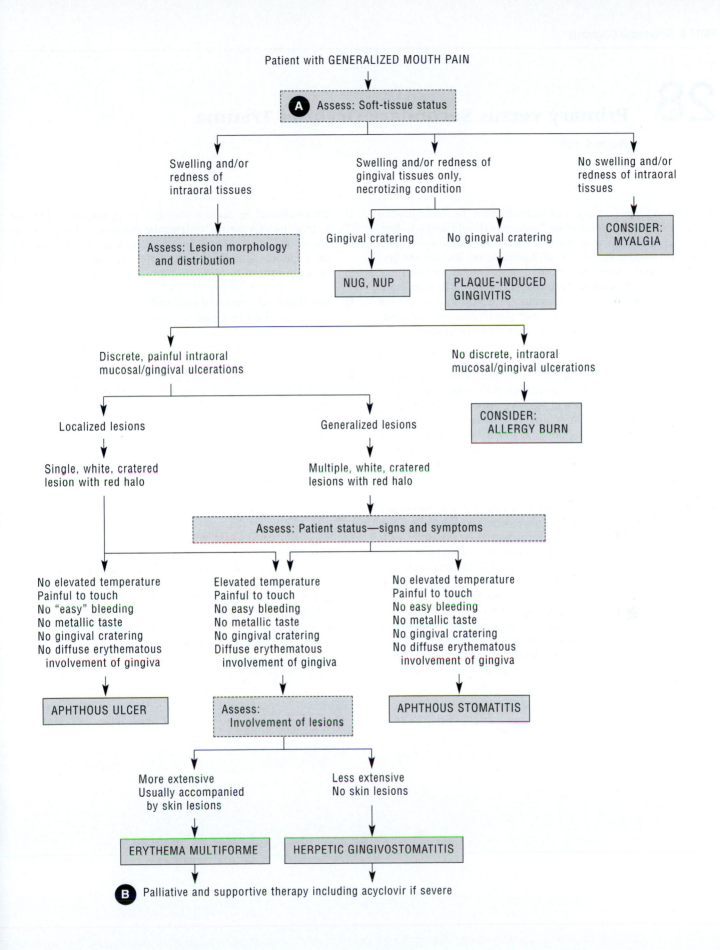

Patient with GENERALIZED MOUTH PAIN

A Assess: Soft-tissue status

Swelling and/or redness of intraoral tissues

Swelling and/or redness of gingival tissues only, necrotizing condition

No swelling and/or redness of intraoral tissues

CONSIDER: MYALGIA

Assess: Lesion morphology and distribution

Gingival cratering

No gingival cratering

NUG, NUP

PLAQUE-INDUCED GINGIVITIS

Discrete, painful intraoral mucosal/gingival ulcerations

No discrete, intraoral mucosal/gingival ulcerations

CONSIDER: ALLERGY BURN

Localized lesions

Generalized lesions

Single, white, cratered lesion with red halo

Multiple, white, cratered lesions with red halo

Assess: Patient status—signs and symptoms

No elevated temperature
Painful to touch
No "easy" bleeding
No metallic taste
No gingival cratering
No diffuse erythematous
  involvement of gingiva

Elevated temperature
Painful to touch
No easy bleeding
No metallic taste
No gingival cratering
Diffuse erythematous
  involvement of gingiva

No elevated temperature
Painful to touch
No easy bleeding
No metallic taste
No gingival cratering
No diffuse erythematous
  involvement of gingiva

APHTHOUS ULCER

Assess: Involvement of lesions

APHTHOUS STOMATITIS

More extensive
Usually accompanied
by skin lesions

Less extensive
No skin lesions

ERYTHEMA MULTIFORME

HERPETIC GINGIVOSTOMATITIS

B Palliative and supportive therapy including acyclovir if severe

28 Primary versus Secondary Occlusal Trauma

Walter B. Hall

Two general types of occlusal trauma must be distinguished before making a treatment plan. Primary occlusal trauma is diagnosed when a tooth or teeth with "normal" support are overloaded, producing symptoms of looseness or discomfort. Secondary occlusal trauma is diagnosed when a tooth or teeth that have lost support develop symptoms of looseness or discomfort when overloaded or loaded normally (ie, a load that would not produce symptoms if normal support were present). The treatment differs with the type of occlusal trauma diagnosed.

A   Several signs and symptoms are indicative of occlusal trauma. Primary among them is tooth looseness. Others include vague to severe pain, especially when faceting of occlusal surfaces is present and the muscles of mastication are sensitive to digital manipulation. Generalized tooth sensitivity often relates to clenching and grinding habits (bruxism). Faceting is indicative of hyperfunction; however, after a facet has developed, it remains even if one of the antagonistic teeth is lost.

B   The key means of differentiating primary and secondary occlusal trauma is determining whether bone loss has occurred (secondary) or not (primary). If an exposed root is evident visually, bone has been lost. Where a probe is able to touch the root of an affected tooth, bone has been lost. Radiographically, evidence of bone loss is speculative unless the loss of bone is quite advanced; this is because of variations in factors such as angulation, film development time, and the kilovoltage applied that may give misleading impressions of bone loss or its absence. If bone loss has occurred around involved teeth, the correct diagnosis is secondary occlusal trauma.

C   Other clinical findings at the time of examination may be helpful in making the differential diagnosis. If the patient has or has had moderate-to-severe periodontitis or is aware of a clenching-and-grinding habit (bruxism), secondary occlusal trauma is the more likely diagnosis.

D   If a "high" restoration (particularly a new one) is present, a periapical abscess is diagnosed. If the patient admits to a habit such as nail biting or pipe-stem clenching and bone loss is not evident, primary occlusal trauma is the more likely diagnosis.

E   Both types of occlusal trauma may be localized or generalized. Primary occlusal trauma is more likely to be localized, whereas secondary occlusal trauma is more likely to be generalized. Localized problems can be treated with minimal effort (eg, selective grinding, splinting). Generalized, moderate-to-severe, secondary occlusal trauma might benefit from occlusal correction, but a bite guard or extensive splinting may be necessary.

Additional Readings

Carranza FA Jr, Newman MG. Clinical periodontology. 8th ed. Philadelphia: WB Saunders; 1996. p. 314.

Genco RJ, Goldman HM, Cohen DW. Contemporary periodontics. St. Louis: Mosby; 1990. p. 195.

Schluger S et al. Periodontal diseases. 2nd ed. Philadelphia: Lea & Febiger; 1990. p. 125.

Wilson TG, Kornman KS. Fundamentals of periodontics. Chicago: Quintessence Publishing; 1996. p. 448.

Patient with PRIMARY AND/OR SECONDARY OCCLUSAL TRAUMA

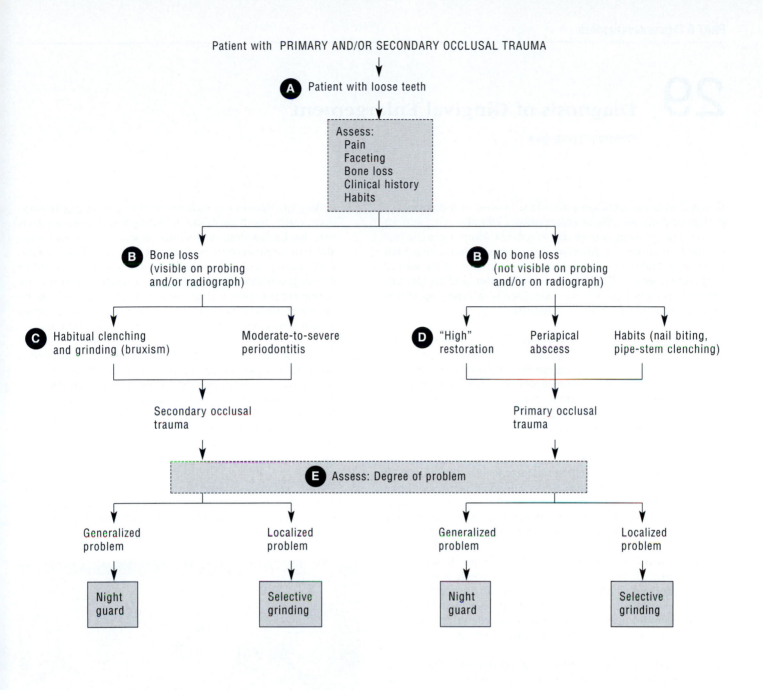

A Patient with loose teeth

Assess:
Pain
Faceting
Bone loss
Clinical history
Habits

B Bone loss
(visible on probing
and/or radiograph)

B No bone loss
(not visible on probing
and/or on radiograph)

C Habitual clenching
and grinding (bruxism)

Moderate-to-severe
periodontitis

D "High"
restoration

Periapical
abscess

Habits (nail biting,
pipe-stem clenching)

Secondary occlusal
trauma

Primary occlusal
trauma

E Assess: Degree of problem

Generalized
problem

Localized
problem

Generalized
problem

Localized
problem

Night
guard

Selective
grinding

Night
guard

Selective
grinding

29 Diagnosis of Gingival Enlargement

William P. Lundergan

Gingival enlargements are a common feature of inflammatory periodontal disease. These enlargements can also represent an endodontic problem, a response to a medication or genetic factor, or a neoplasia. A differential diagnosis requires thorough medical and dental histories, a careful evaluation of the nature of the enlargement (inflammatory vs fibrotic), and an identification of the etiologic factors. Occasionally, a biopsy specimen may be required to confirm a diagnosis.

A   Inflammatory gingival enlargements are characterized by swelling or edema, redness, and a tendency to bleed upon periodontal probing. Longstanding inflammatory enlargements can have a fibrotic component as well. A patient history helps establish the inflammatory enlargement as acute or chronic. Chronic enlargements are generally painless and slow to progress, whereas acute enlargements are characterized by a painful, rapid onset.

B   Localized gingival swelling characterized by acute pain of rapid onset suggests an abscess. Involved teeth should be probed for periodontal pocket formation and loss of attachment (LOA). Radiographic evaluation and pulp testing should accompany the periodontal examination. If no pocket formation with LOA is detected, and the tooth is vital, treat the problem as a gingival abscess. If pocket formation with LOA is detected, and the tooth is vital, treat the problem as a periodontal abscess. If the tooth is nonvital or partially nonvital, an endodontic problem exists. Endodontic therapy is indicated if warranted by the periodontal prognosis and overall treatment plan.

C   A localized or generalized gingival enlargement that is relatively painless and gradual in developing may be classified as a chronic inflammatory gingival enlargement. Chronic inflammatory gingival enlargements are generally associated with identifiable systemic or local factors. The primary local factor associated with these enlargements is plaque. Sec-

ondary local factors can include calculus, poor dental restorations, caries, tooth crowding or misalignment, open contacts with food impaction, orthodontic braces, mouth breathing, and removable appliances. Systemic factors include vitamin C deficiency, leukemia, and hormonal changes that occur during pregnancy or puberty or are associated with the use of oral contraceptives. If no local or systemic factors can be identified, the enlargement may be neoplastic and a biopsy should be considered to establish or confirm a diagnosis.

D   A gingival enlargement that is inflammatory and fibrotic can represent an enlargement that was initially fibrotic with secondary inflammation or an enlargement that was initially inflammatory but has become secondarily fibrotic. Medical and dental histories should suggest or rule out hereditary and drug-induced fibrotic enlargements. If the family and drug histories are negative, the clinician can assume that the enlargement is inflammatory.

E   Fibrotic gingival enlargements are characterized by pink, firm, and lobulated gingivae; however, secondary inflammation can result in a red coloration and an increased ten-

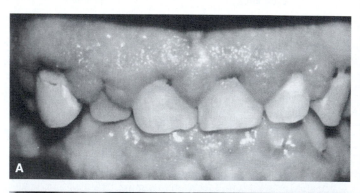

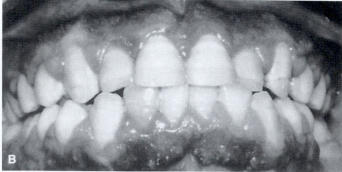

Figure 29-2 *A,* Gingival enlargement related to taking cyclosporine. *B,* Gingival enlargement related to taking Dilantin sodium. Clinically these two gingival enlargements cannot be differentiated. The patient's history permits the diagnosis.

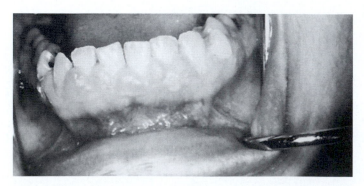

Figure 29-1 Phenytoin sodium hyperplasia.

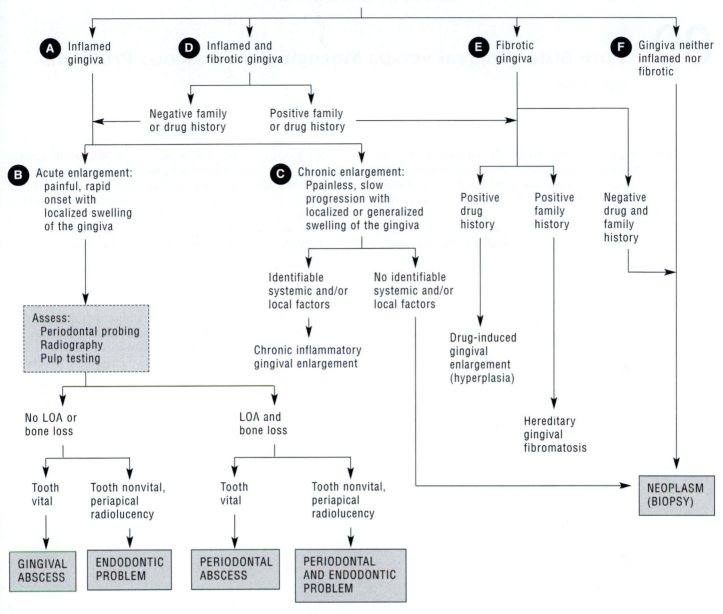

Patient with GINGIVAL ENLARGEMENT

A Inflamed gingiva

D Inflamed and fibrotic gingiva

E Fibrotic gingiva

F Gingiva neither inflamed nor fibrotic

Negative family or drug history

Positive family or drug history

B Acute enlargement: painful, rapid onset with localized swelling of the gingiva

C Chronic enlargement: Ppainless, slow progression with localized or generalized swelling of the gingiva

Positive drug history

Positive family history

Negative drug and family history

Identifiable systemic and/or local factors

No identifiable systemic and/or local factors

Assess:
Periodontal probing
Radiography
Pulp testing

Chronic inflammatory gingival enlargement

Drug-induced gingival enlargement (hyperplasia)

Hereditary gingival fibromatosis

No LOA or bone loss

LOA and bone loss

Tooth vital

Tooth nonvital, periapical radiolucency

Tooth vital

Tooth nonvital, periapical radiolucency

NEOPLASM (BIOPSY)

GINGIVAL ABSCESS

ENDODONTIC PROBLEM

PERIODONTAL ABSCESS

PERIODONTAL AND ENDODONTIC PROBLEM

---

dency to bleed. A definitive diagnosis can generally be established with thorough medical and dental histories. Drug-induced gingival enlargements (Figures 29-1 and 29-2) have been associated with phenytoin. The incidence varies from less than 1% and as high as 50% for these medications. There is evidence that concurrent administration of nifedipine and cyclosporine has a synergistic effect on the incidence of gingival enlargement. A diagnosis of drug-induced gingival enlargement can be made if the development of the fibrotic enlargement coincided with the administration of one of these medications and the family history is negative for hereditary gingival fibromatosis.

A rare fibrotic gingival enlargement of unknown etiology is hereditary gingival fibromatosis. The diagnosis is suggested by a positive family history of gingival enlargement, which generally begins with the eruption of the primary or permanent dentition. A fibrotic gingival enlargement that does not

seem to be drug induced or familial may be neoplastic or a secondarily fibrotic inflammatory enlargement. If a definitive diagnosis cannot be established from the patient history and clinical examination, a biopsy specimen may be required.

F An enlarged gingiva that is neither inflammatory nor fibrotic and does not have identifiable systemic or local etiologic factors may represent a neoplasm. A biopsy specimen with microscopic evaluation is needed to establish or confirm a diagnosis.

Additional Readings

Lundergan WP. Drug-induced gingival enlargements—dilantin hyperplasia and beyond. J Calif Dent Assoc 1989;17:48.

Newnan MG, Carranza FA Jr, Takei HH. Carranza's clinical periodontology. 9th ed. Philadelphia: WB Saunders; 2001.

30   Pure Mucogingival versus Mucogingival-Osseous Problems

Walter B. Hall

Mucogingival problems, which involve the relationship of alveolar mucosa and gingiva, may be divided into pure mucogingival problems and mucogingival-osseous problems. Pure mucogingival problems are caused by a tooth erupting into prominence at or near the mucogingival junction (MGJ) so that little or no attached gingiva is present over the prominence of the fully erupted tooth. These may be existing problems, where recession has already occurred, or potential problems, where they are predisposed to recession only. Mucogingival-osseous problems are caused by pockets so deepened with periodontitis that little or no attached gingiva remains. These problems have different etiologies, and their treatment may be different; it is therefore most important to differentiate between them properly at diagnosis.

A   Determine and record the position of the free margin of the gingiva for all teeth. If the free margin is on the crown of the tooth, no visible recession has yet occurred. If the free margin is on the root of the tooth, recession has occurred already. In probing for the location of the free margin on the crown, the probe may reach only to the cemento-enamel junction (CEJ) or may extend to the root surface, in which case loss of attachmen has occurred already.

B   Determine and record the location of the MGJ on all facial surfaces and on the lingual surface of mandibular teeth. The distance from the free margin of the gingiva to the MGJ is a measure of the total amount of gingiva on the surface of a tooth. If 2 mm or less of total gingiva is on a surface, a pure mucogingival or potential problem is present, whether the free margin of the gingiva is on the crown or root of the tooth because there is always a crevice of at least 1 mm. If more than 2 mm of total gingiva is present, a differential diagnosis cannot be made with only these data.

C   If more than 2 mm of total gingiva is present, measure the pocket depth to differentiate further between pure mucogingival and mucogingival-osseous problems. If the crevice depth is less than 3 mm, arbitrarily (but with reasonable accuracy) diagnose the problem as an existing or potential pure mucogingival problem and treat it as such. If the pocket depth is 3 mm or greater, diagnose the problem as inflammatory and treat it as a mucogingival-osseous problem. If more than 2 mm of total gingiva and more than 1 mm of attached gingiva are present, and the free margin is still on the crown, it is not a mucogingival problem of either type.

Additional Readings

Hall WB. Pure mucogingival problems. Chicago: Quintessence Publishing; 1984. p. 61.

Patient with PURE MUCOGINGIVAL OR MUCOGINGIVAL-OSSEOUS PROBLEM

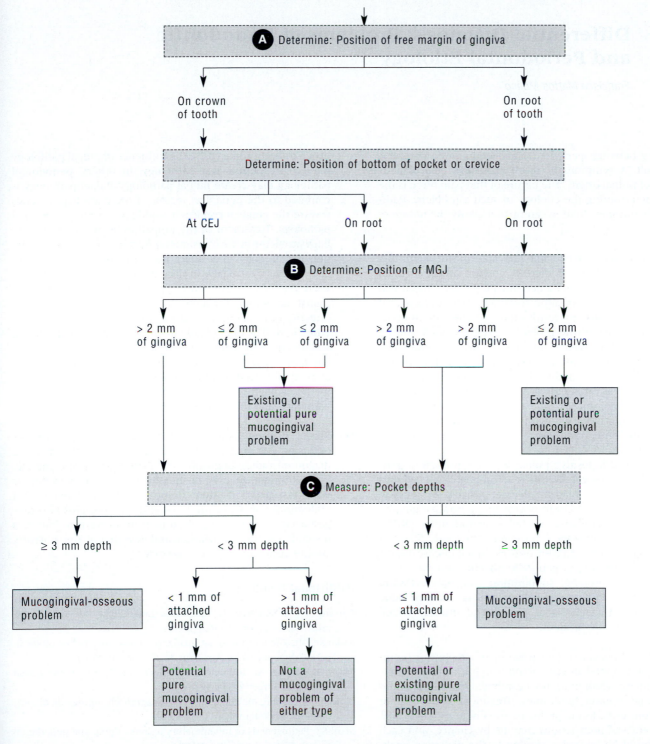

31 Differential Diagnosis: Problems of Endodontic and Periodontal Etiology

Francisco Martos Molino

Differentiating between periodontal and endodontic problems can be difficult. A symptomatic tooth may have pain of periodontal and/or pulpal origin. The nature of that pain often is the first clue in determining the etiology of such a problem. Radiographic and clinical evaluation can further clarify the nature of the problem.

A   A sharp pain that is irreducible indicates, in the beginning, a diagnosis of pulpitis. If there is no pain and the pulpal vitality tests are negative, a necrotic pulp exists, and it will be susceptible to endodontic treatment. The presence of large carious lesions and restorations may help in differentiating the nature of the problem. Cellulitis noted during exploration of the alveolar mucosa and the vestibulae may mean that there is an abscess whose origin is pulpal pathology. A fistula in the gingival crevice or vestibular zone usually indicates pulpal pathology. In the radiologic evaluation, a radiolucent zone at the apex or in the area of the furca in the molars suggests a pulpal problem susceptible to endodontic treatment.

B   Sharp pain and a positive pulpal test may indicate a periodontal abscess, especially if it is accompanied by cellulitis or a fistula in the adjacent alveolar mucosa or gingiva. Sharp pain may also exist in necrotizing ulcerative gingivitis (NUG) or necrotizing ulcerative periodontitis (NUP). NUG or NUP usually affects more than one tooth. Slight or no pain suggests periodontitis or periodontal disease associated with pocket depth generally affecting several teeth. Bleeding upon probing, suppuration, gingival recession, diastema, and radiographic evidence of generalized bone loss establish a diagnosis of periodontal disease, which needs periodontal treatment.

C   A periodontal pocket accompanied by other signs or symptoms of periodontal disease accompanying a pulpal alteration (pulp not vital) indicates a combined lesion (the endo-perio or perio-endo syndrome). Treatment is needed for each lesion; endodontic problems usually are treated first. The presence of both lesions may be by chance, and each lesion should be treated according to the diagnosis estab-

lished for it. In some cases, the influence of pulpal pathology may create periodontal pathology. In others, periodontal pathology may create pulpal pathology. Pulpal pathology is confined to the periapical region. If the pathology extends toward the gingival crevice, it could give rise to periodontal pathology. Treatment of the pulpal problem may eliminate both problems in such instances. Another way in which the pulpal pathology may affect the periodontium is through lateral canals, especially in the furcas of the molars. Controversy remains as to whether periodontal disease can cause pulpal pathology through the lateral canals. When the integrity of the dentinal tubes is violated, bacteria can penetrate here. The opening of lateral canals during periodontal scaling and root planing is another way that pulpal pathology may occur. Pulpal pathology can originate through the apex in advanced periodontal disease and may be reflected in the radiographs. In combined lesions, treat the pulpal pathology and then the periodontal problem.

D   Sharp, fleeting pain increasing with lateral pressure or occlusion is a sign of a fracture in the tooth that may be diagnosed radiographically when the fracture is complete. Transillumination may be helpful if the root is visible or with visualization after tissue has been flapped. Old endodontics or big restorations with posts or pins also suggest a radicular fracture. Treatment of the vertical fractures depends on the localization and severity of the fracture. Tooth extraction may be necessary.

Additional Readings

Carranza FA Jr, Newman MG. Clinical periodontology. 8th ed. Philadelphia: WB Saunders; 1996. p. 870.

Kirkman DB. The location of an incidence of accessory pulpal canals in periodontal pockets. J Am Dent Assoc 1975;91:353.

Mazur B, Massler M. Influences of periodontal disease on the dental pulp. Oral Surg 1964;17:592.

Simring M, Golberg M. The pulpal pocket approach: retrograde of periodontics. Periodontology 1964;35:22.

Stahl SS. Pathogenesis of inflammatory lesions in pulp and periodontal tissues. Periodontics 1966;4:190.

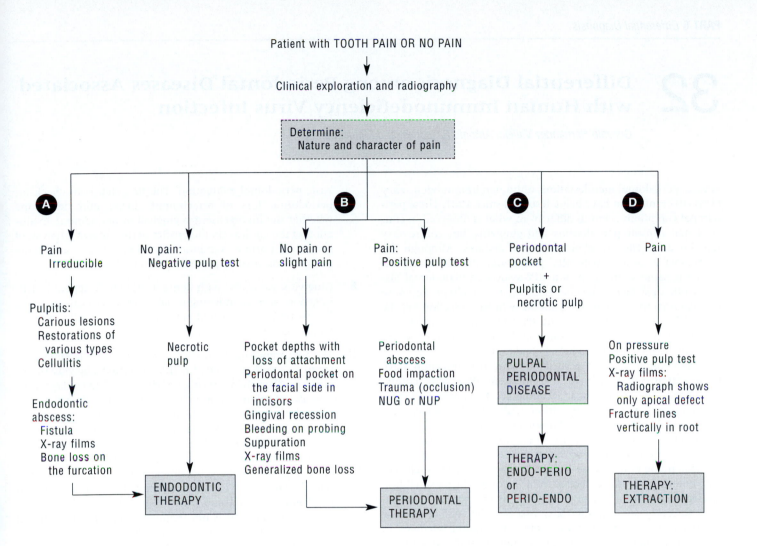

Patient with TOOTH PAIN OR NO PAIN

↓

Clinical exploration and radiography

↓

Determine:
Nature and character of pain

A

Pain
Irreducible

↓

Pulpitis:
  Carious lesions
  Restorations of
    various types
  Cellulitis

↓

Endodontic
abscess:
  Fistula
  X-ray films
  Bone loss on
    the furcation

No pain:
Negative pulp test

↓

Necrotic
pulp

↓

ENDODONTIC
THERAPY

B

No pain or
slight pain

↓

Pocket depths with
  loss of attachment
Periodontal pocket on
  the facial side in
  incisors
Gingival recession
Bleeding on probing
Suppuration
X-ray films
Generalized bone loss

Pain:
Positive pulp test

↓

Periodontal
  abscess
Food impaction
Trauma (occlusion)
NUG or NUP

↓

PERIODONTAL
THERAPY

C

Periodontal
pocket
+
Pulpitis or
necrotic pulp

↓

PULPAL
PERIODONTAL
DISEASE

↓

THERAPY:
ENDO-PERIO
or
PERIO-ENDO

D

Pain

↓

On pressure
Positive pulp test
X-ray films:
  Radiograph shows
  only apical defect
Fracture lines
  vertically in root

↓

THERAPY:
EXTRACTION

32 Differential Diagnosis among Periodontal Diseases Associated with Human Immunodeficiency Virus Infection

Gonzalo Hernández Vallejo, Antonio Bascones, and Miguel Carasol

Several periodontal manifestations of human immunodeficiency virus (HIV) infection have been described since 1987. These periodontal conditions seem to differ from what is observed in conventional chronic periodontitis and gingivitis, but controversy remains as to the prevalence of these diseases. Although the microbiota associated with HIV periodontal disease are essentially the same as those in non-HIV-associated periodontal diseases, other pathogenic mechanisms, such as an altered response in inflammatory mediators in patients with HIV infection may be responsible for their development. Elevated viral load levels correlate with oral disease prevalence, and CD4 cell counts also are associated with some periodontal conditions.

Periodontal changes associated with HIV infection have been extensively reviewed, and different diagnostic criteria have been used or proposed, accompanied by constant changes in the nomenclature and definitions. Although it is widely recognized that these periodontal lesions may have clinical characteristics that differentiate them from conventional diseases, the lack of specific criteria to accurately define them has delayed the understanding of their true nature. The occurrence of such specific criteria and the predictive value of some of these clinical characteristics would be of great value as indicators of the disease. Recently, some studies have assessed the validity of some diagnostic criteria for HIV-associated periodontal changes in order to distinguish between this condition and conventional periodontitis, although these new criteria need to be validated in wider samples.

According to the classification and diagnostic criteria used for oral lesions in HIV infection, several periodontal entities may be considered as lesions strongly associated with HIV. These include the HIV gingivitis (linear gingival erythema), HIV necrotizing ulcerative gingivitis (NUG), and HIV necrotizing ulcerative periodontitis (NUP). Plaque-associated gingivitis and chronic periodontitis may also be observed in HIV infections, but they are indistinguishable from those conditions in noninfected patients.

A The HIV-infected patient complaining of a periodontal problem must be evaluated according to the principles of basic periodontal evaluation. The first step is to check for periodontal loss of attachment (LOA) and determine whether the involvement is gingival or periodontal. Evaluation of the clinical characteristics of the gingiva, analysis of several important symptoms, general status, and bone examination usually provide enough information.

B Gingivitis associated with dental plaque may appear in HIV infection and is indistinguishable from typical gingivitis appearing in noninfected patients. Response to local treatment is good.

C The appearance of gingiva with atypical clinical features constitutes a condition defined as HIV-associated gingivitis, or linear gingival erythema (LGE), which is associated today with a *Candida* infection. Clinical characteristics include a fiery red band along the border of the gingiva 2 to 3 mm apical to the gingival margin, accompanied in some instances by a petechial or diffuse erythema affecting the attached gingiva. No ulceration, pocketing, or LOA is observed (Figure 32-1). These lesions may be generalized, or they can be limited to one or two teeth. No correlation exists between the amount of plaque observed and the severity of the inflammation. Bleeding on probing is not frequent. LGE does not respond effectively to standard periodontal therapy. Antifungal therapy may be prescribed if *Candida* is identified. Progression to HIV-associated periodontitis has been observed, although longitudinal studies do not support this progression.

D Involvement of the gingiva with necrosis or destruction of one or more interdental papillae and no LOA can be an early feature in HIV infection and should alert the clinician to a diagnosis of NUG, which is quite similar to that observed in noninfected patients. Clinically, the gingiva appears red and swollen, with a white-yellow band of necrosis limited to the marginal gingiva. Destruction of the papillae and gingival necrosis lead to crater formation in the interdental areas, spontaneous bleeding, severe pain, and typical fetor oris.

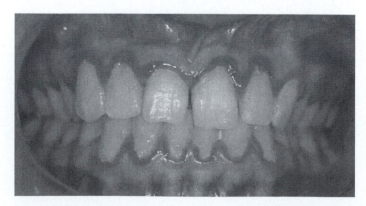

Figure 32-1 LGE in a young, female HIV-seropositive intravenous drug abuser.

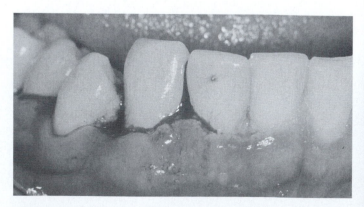

Figure 32-2 NUP affecting the lower anterior teeth in a 29-year-old, female HIV-seropositive intravenous drug abuser receiving triple antiviral therapy.

HIV-positive patient with a PERIODONTAL PROBLEM

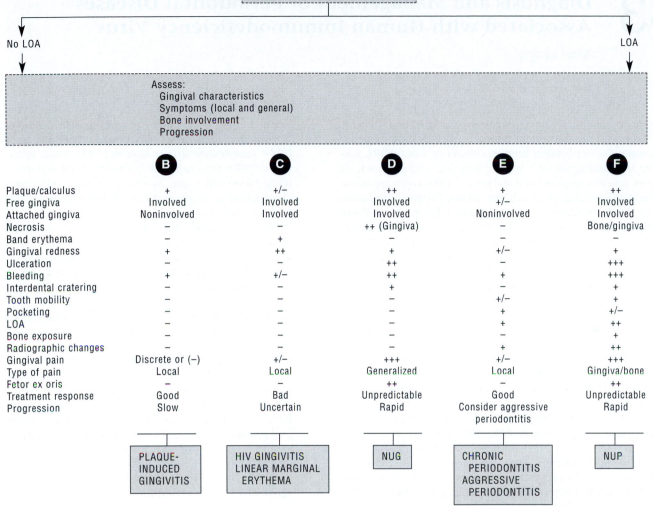

A Assess: Periodontal attachment

No LOA — LOA

Assess:
Gingival characteristics
Symptoms (local and general)
Bone involvement
Progression

	B	**C**	**D**	**E**	**F**
Plaque/calculus	+	+/−	++	+	++
Free gingiva	Involved	Involved	Involved	+/−	Involved
Attached gingiva	Noninvolved	Involved	Involved	Noninvolved	Involved
Necrosis	−	−	++ (Gingiva)	−	Bone/gingiva
Band erythema	−	+	−	−	−
Gingival redness	+	++	+	+/−	+
Ulceration	−	−	++	−	+++
Bleeding	+	+/−	++	+	+++
Interdental cratering	−	−	+	−	+
Tooth mobility	−	−	−	+/−	+
Pocketing	−	−	−	+	+/−
LOA	−	−	−	+	++
Bone exposure	−	−	−	−	+
Radiographic changes	−	−	−	+	++
Gingival pain	Discrete or (−)	+/−	+++	+/−	+++
Type of pain	Local	Local	Generalized	Local	Gingiva/bone
Fetor ex oris	−	−	++	−	++
Treatment response	Good	Bad	Unpredictable	Good	Unpredictable
Progression	Slow	Uncertain	Rapid	Consider aggressive periodontitis	Rapid

B PLAQUE-INDUCED GINGIVITIS

C HIV GINGIVITIS LINEAR MARGINAL ERYTHEMA

D NUG

E CHRONIC PERIODONTITIS AGGRESSIVE PERIODONTITIS

F NUP

Anterior gingiva is most commonly affected, and no periodontal pockets are observed.

E Periodontal LOA in HIV-positive patients with uninflamed or inflamed gingiva suggests chronic periodontitis or aggressive periodontitis, changes that are indistinguishable from those affecting noninfected patients. Changes in the clinical characteristics of the gingiva may appear depending on the progression of the disease (inflammation severity) and quality of the gingiva (fibrous/edematous). Periodontal pockets of widely varying depths are present. Spontaneous bleeding may occur, especially during exacerbation of the problems associated with acquired immunodeficiency syndrome (AIDS).

F LOA with or without pocket formation, accompanied by gingival redness, necrosis, ulceration, profuse bleeding, and pain, are diagnostic for NUP, which probably represents an advanced stage of NUG. Progression is rapid, with gingival and bone destruction, leading in some instances to great LOA, tooth mobility, and severe bony lesions. Deep pockets are rarely seen when gingival and bone necrosis occur simultaneously (Figure 32-2).

Intense pain and fetor oris are important clinical symptoms caused by soft-tissue ulceration and necrosis. Deep pain in the jawbones is common and may be an initial clinical marker of the disease. Bone sequestration may be a finding in this condition. The rapid progression, together with extensive destruction, may produce loosening of the affected teeth.

Additional Readings

Armitage GC. Development of a classification system for periodontal diseases and conditions. Ann Periodontol 1999;4:1.

Barr CE. Periodontal problems related to HIV-1 infection. Adv Dent Res 1995;9:147.

Patton LL. Sensitivity, specificity, and positive predictive value of oral opportunistic infections in adults with HIV/AIDS as markers of immune suppression and viral burden. Oral Surg Oral Med Oral Pathol Oral Radiol Endod 2000;90:182.

Robinson PG. Which periodontal changes are associated with HIV infection? J Clin Periodontol 1998;25:278.

Scheutz F, Matee MI, Andsager L, et al. Is there an association between periodontal condition and HIV infection? J Clin Periodontol 1997;24:580.

33 Diagnosis and Management of Periodontal Diseases Associated with Human Immunodeficiency Virus

Tamer Alpagot

A Periodontal diseases have long been associated with patients who have immune system disorders, such as those who are seropositive for human immunodeficiency virus (HIV), taking immunosuppressive medications (eg, cyclosporine), or have severely uncontrolled diabetes. In HIV-positive patients, the periodontium often exhibits diffuse, marginal erythema, and this is classified as linear gingival erythema (LGE). These lesions are not proportional to the amount of supragingival plaque, and they do not respond well to conventional treatment. Despite the poor response to therapy, LGE must be treated with scaling and root planing, oral hygiene instruction (OHI), and chlorhexidine mouth rinse.

Necrotizing ulcerative gingivitis (NUG) is an acute inflammatory disease of the interdental papillae without loss of attachment (LOA) and covered by a gray pseudomembrane. The other clinical findings include gingival hemorrhage, metallic taste, and fetor oris. NUG may affect the deeper periodontal tissues, becoming a form of necrotizing ulcerative periodontitis (NUP), which is characterized by severe pain, gingival bleeding, extensive soft-tissue necrosis, severe LOA, bone exposure with possible sequestration, deep jaw ache, and fetor oris; the patient is febrile with malaise (Figure 33-1). If untreated, NUP can develop into necrotizing stomatitis (NS), characterized by massively destructive, ulcerative infection extending beyond the mucogingival junction into contiguous palatopharyngeal or mucous tissues. It has been suggested that specific microorganisms such as *Bulleidia extructa, Dialister* spp, *Fusobacterium* spp, *Streptococcus* spp, *Veillonella* spp, as well as certain predisposing factors such as poor oral hygiene and preexisting gingivitis, stress, altered host response, smoking, and socioeconomic status may play a significant role in the pathogenesis of NUG/NUP.

The following laboratory test results assist in the diagnosis and management of HIV-positive patients: peripheral CD4+ lymphocyte count (normal: 544–1663 cells/mm³); CD4+/CD8+ ratio (normal: 0.93–4.5); total and differential white blood cell count (normal: 4,500–10,000 cells/mm³); platelet count (normal: 150,000–400,000 mm³); bleeding time (normal: 2–7 min); and international normalized ratio (INR) test (normal: 2–3). If the platelet count is less than 60,000/mm³, precautions to prevent excessive bleeding are indicated and may necessitate platelet infusions. An INR test score of >3 can also indicate that there may be excessive bleeding with therapy.

B The initial treatment of NUG/NUP in HIV-positive patients consists of scaling and irrigating the affected area with 10% povidone-iodine, followed by systemic use of metronidazole (250 mg four times daily for 5 days) to eliminate anaerobic microorganisms. OHI should be emphasized with the adjunctive use of 3% peroxide diluted 50% with warm water and 0.12% chlorhexidine mouth rinse twice daily. Because the patient may have significant pain, an extensive root planing and scaling is usually not initially feasible. Following resolution of the acute inflammation, meticulous scaling and root planing can be instituted in several visits.

Finally, after therapy is completed, the long-term management of these patients must be considered, including pocket-elimination procedures.

C In immunocompromised HIV patients, preexisting periodontitis may be exacerbated, and thus HIV infection can be considered a modifier of chronic periodontitis. The treatment of chronic periodontitis in HIV-positive patients consists of aggressive scaling and root planing, reevaluation, and pocket-elimination procedures.

Additional Readings

Glick M. Dental management of patients with HIV. Chicago: Quintessence Publishing; 1994.

Greenspan JS, Greenspan D. Oral manifestations of HIV infection. Chicago: Quintessence Publishing; 1995.

Murray PA. Periodontal disease in patients infected by human immunodeficiency virus. Periodontology 2000. 1994;6:50.

Kinane DF. Periodontitis modified by systemic factors. Ann Periodontol 1999;4:54.

Russell MK, Alpagot T, Boches SK, et al. Bacterial species and phylotypes in necrotizing ulcerative periodontitis, J Dent Res 2001;80: 167 (abstract #1050).

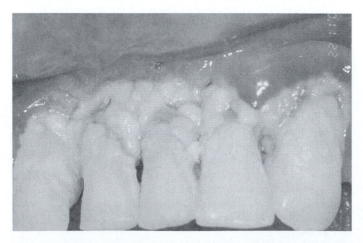

Figure 33-1 Necrotizing ulcerative periodontitis (NUP) associated with HIV infection.

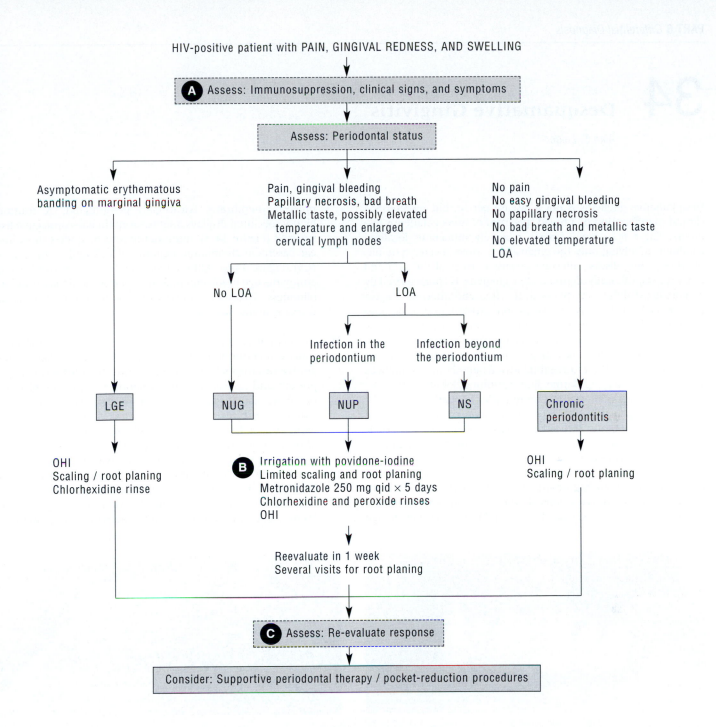

HIV-positive patient with PAIN, GINGIVAL REDNESS, AND SWELLING

A Assess: Immunosuppression, clinical signs, and symptoms

Assess: Periodontal status

Asymptomatic erythematous
banding on marginal gingiva

Pain, gingival bleeding
Papillary necrosis, bad breath
Metallic taste, possibly elevated
temperature and enlarged
cervical lymph nodes

No pain
No easy gingival bleeding
No papillary necrosis
No bad breath and metallic taste
No elevated temperature
LOA

No LOA

LOA

Infection in the
periodontium

Infection beyond
the periodontium

LGE

NUG

NUP

NS

Chronic
periodontitis

OHI
Scaling / root planing
Chlorhexidine rinse

B Irrigation with povidone-iodine
Limited scaling and root planing
Metronidazole 250 mg qid × 5 days
Chlorhexidine and peroxide rinses
OHI

OHI
Scaling / root planing

Reevaluate in 1 week
Several visits for root planing

C Assess: Re-evaluate response

Consider: Supportive periodontal therapy / pocket-reduction procedures

34 Desquamative Gingivitis

Alan S. Leider

Desquamative gingivitis is not a disease per se, but represents a clinical manifestation of a broad spectrum of mucocutaneous disorders. These may range from a relatively innocuous localized condition involving only the gingiva to a more severe, systemic, life-threatening disease affecting extensive areas of the skin and oral mucosa. Clinically, desquamative gingivitis is characterized by a generalized diffuse erythema of the free and attached gingiva (Figure 34-1) with areas of vesiculation, erosion, and/or desquamation. It affects women more often than men; most patients are middle-aged or older. The differential diagnosis includes specific mucocutaneous dermatoses such as benign mucous membrane pemphigoid (BMMP), erosive (bullous) lichen planus, pemphigus vulgaris, erythema multiforme, linear immunoglobulin (Ig) A disease, and a nonspecific group of hormonal or idiopathic origin. Distinction among these entities is based on the presence or absence of eye, skin, or other mucosal lesions, as well as on the histopathologic and immunopathologic findings. A definitive diagnosis requires a biopsy with or without immunofluorescent studies.

A A patient exhibiting desquamative gingivitis with vesiculobullous and erosive lesions of other oral-mucosal tissues and conjunctival eye lesions (Figure 34-2) probably has benign mucous membrane (cicatricial) pemphigoid. A routine biopsy specimen displays a subbasal epithelial–connective tissue split (Figure 34-3). Immunofluorescent studies show linear basement membrane deposits of IgG and complement (C3) (Figure 34-4). Although oral lesions may be painful and annoying, eye involvement is more serious and may result in blindness. Treatment consists of topical and/or short-term use of systemic steroids.

B Desquamative gingivitis in a patient with other oral erosions and peripheral zones of white reticulated striae is suggestive of erosive lichen planus. Cutaneous lesions may be present and appear as scaly keratotic and pruritic plaques on an erythematous base. They are usually observed on the extensor surfaces of the extremities. A biopsy specimen exhibits a subbasal split with a subepithelial, bandlike lymphocytic infiltrate. Globular deposits of C3 and fibrinogen are seen in the basement membrane with immunofluorescent testing of the submitted tissues. Treatment with topical steroids, such as 0.05% fluocinonide in a protective emollient, usually controls the painful erosive and desquamative lesions, but usually will not affect the white components.

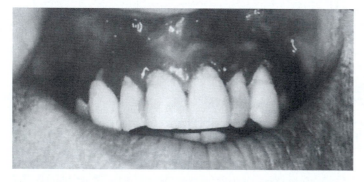

Figure 34-1 Desquamative gingivitis with generalized diffuse erythema of the free and attached gingiva.

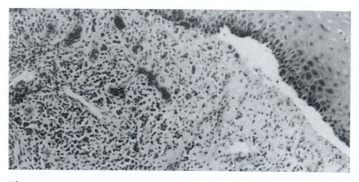

Figure 34-3 Routine histopathologic section of BMMP showing a subbasal epithelial–connective tissue split.

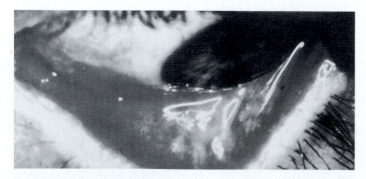

Figure 34-2 BMMP with scarring of the conjunctiva of the eye.

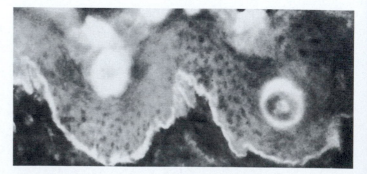

Figure 34-4 Immunofluorescent sections of BMMP with linear basement membrane deposits of IgG and C3.

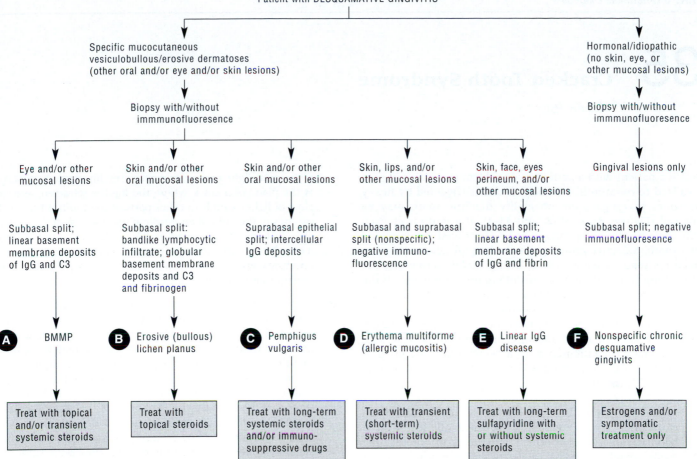

Patient with DESQUAMATIVE GINGIVITIS

Specific mucocutaneous vesiculobullous/erosive dermatoses (other oral and/or eye and/or skin lesions)

Biopsy with/without immmunofluoresence

- **Eye and/or other mucosal lesions**
  - Subbasal split; linear basement membrane deposits of IgG and C3
  - **A** BMMP
  - Treat with topical and/or transient systemic steroids

- **Skin and/or other oral mucosal lesions**
  - Subbasal split: bandlike lymphocytic infiltrate; globular basement membrane deposits and C3 and fibrinogen
  - **B** Erosive (bullous) lichen planus
  - Treat with topical steroids

- **Skin and/or other oral mucosal lesions**
  - Suprabasal epithelial split; intercellular IgG deposits
  - **C** Pemphigus vulgaris
  - Treat with long-term systemic steroids and/or immuno-suppressive drugs

- **Skin, lips, and/or other mucosal lesions**
  - Subbasal and suprabasal split (nonspecific); negative immuno-fluorescence
  - **D** Erythema multiforme (allergic mucositis)
  - Treat with transient (short-term) systemic steroids

- **Skin, face, eyes perineum, and/or other mucosal lesions**
  - Subbasal split; linear basement membrane deposits of IgG and fibrin
  - **E** Linear IgG disease
  - Treat with long-term sulfapyridine with or without systemic steroids

Hormonal/idiopathic (no skin, eye, or other mucosal lesions)

Biopsy with/without immmunofluoresence

- **Gingival lesions only**
  - Subbasal split; negative Immunofluoresence
  - **F** Nonspecific chronic desquamative gingivits
  - Estrogens and/or symptomatic treatment only

C Desquamative gingivitis in a patient with extensive large bullous and erosive lesions throughout the oral mucosa and skin may suggest pemphigus vulgaris. A bullous lesion may be elicited by rubbing uninvolved oral mucosa or skin. This result is referred to as "Nikolsky's sign" and is characteristic for pemphigus, but it may also be observed in all the other desquamative lesions under discussion. A suprabasal epithelial split is seen on a routine biopsy examination, and immunofluorescence exhibits intercellular IgG deposits. Long-term therapy with systemic steroids and/or immuno-suppressive drugs is the treatment of choice. Early diagnosis and initiation of therapy are important in these patients to prevent death from dehydration and septicemia.

D Extensive hemorrhagic-crusted lesions of the lips; erythematous circular iris or target lesions on the skin; a wide variety of intraoral, erythematous, and vesiculoerosive lesions, in conjunction with desquamative gingivitis are highly suggestive of erythema multiforme. When this condition affects the oral mucosa, skin, conjunctiva of the eyes, and external genitalia, it is referred to as "Stevens-Johnson syndrome." A biopsy specimen demonstrates a nonspecific suprabasal and subbasal epithelial split, and immunofluorescent studies are generally negative. Erythema multiforme may represent an allergic mucositis, which is often associated with sulfa drugs, or it may be of idiopathic origin. Treatment consists of short-term (transient) systemic steroids and supportive symptomatic therapy.

E Desquamative gingivitis in a patient with pruritic vesiculobullous skin lesions, ocular lesions, and/or perineal involvement may be indicative of linear IgA disease. This is a chronic autoimmune mucocutaneous disorder seen in mid-

dle age or later with a female predilection. A biopsy specimen shows a subbasal epithelial–connective tissue split. Immunofluorescent studies demonstrate linear deposits of IgA and fibrin in the basement membrane. Patients usually respond to systemic corticosteroids.

F A patient with desquamative gingivitis without any other lesions or systemic symptomology should be suspected of having nonspecific, chronic desquamative gingivitis of hormonal or idiopathic origin. Although in many cases this represents an early stage of BMMP, a biopsy shows a subbasal epithelial–connective tissue split, and immunofluorescence is completely negative. Most of these patients are post-menopausal women, and the treatment of choice is estrogens and/or symptomatic therapy only. Patients should avoid spicy or acidic foods, and a palliative mouthwash with elixir of diphenhydramine hydrochloride and activated attapulgite may alleviate the discomfort.

Additional Readings

Carranza FA Jr, Newman MG. Clinical periodontology. 8th ed. Philadelphia: WB Saunders; 1996. p. 239.

Daniels TE, Quadia-White C. Direct immunofluorescence in oral mucosal disease. Oral Surg 1981;51:38.

Eversole LR. Clinical outline of oral pathology: diagnosis and treatment. 3rd ed. Philadelphia: Lea & Febiger; 1992. Ch. 5.

Porter SR, Bain SE, Scully CM. Linear IgA disease manifesting as recalcitrant desquamative gingivitis. Oral Surg 1992;74:179.

Rogers RS III, Sheridan PJ, Nightingale SH. Desquamative gingivitis: clinical, histopathologic, immunopathologic, and therapeutic observations. J Am Acad Dermatol 1982;7:29.

35 Cracked Tooth Syndrome

Walter B. Hall

When a patient with a periodontal problem complains of pain localized to one tooth, especially if this is triggered by heavy function, investigate the possibility that the tooth may be cracked (Figures 35-1, 35-2, and 35-3). If a tooth is cracked superficially, the symptoms may be controlled by crowning that tooth. Selective grinding may be helpful temporarily, but fractures tend to spread within teeth, making crowning the safest long-term solution to controlling these problems. If the crack is symptomatic, it may be extending to involve the pulp. If the crack is deep already, endodontics may be helpful. If the tooth has been treated endodontically and is now symptomatic, the crack may be affecting the periodontal ligament. When a crack is contiguous with a deep pocket, the prognosis for the tooth is guarded at best, and therapy should be planned with this in mind.

A When a tooth with a periodontal pocket is painful, an endodontic involvement must be ruled out before periodontal surgery is performed. Regardless of whether the tooth is vital or nonvital to electrical pulp testing or to hot and cold, new periapical radiographs should be obtained and evaluated for evidence of periapical radiolucencies. The radiographs should be evaluated visually, and the tooth with

a fiberoptic light source for cracks. The fiberoptic light stops at the plane of a crack where the light is refracted, and no glow of light extends to other parts of the tooth if the crack extends to the pulp. If an intraoral television system is available, this device may visualize the crack even better (Figure 35-4). The tooth should be tapped and pressed in various directions against each cusp to elicit the sharp, brief twinge of pain that is symptomatic of a cracked tooth.

B If a symptomatic tooth tests vital, a radiograph may still suggest an endodontic problem. If no evidence of a crack (visual or symptomatic) can be elicited, use selective grinding to minimize trauma. The tooth should be observed for several months to determine that symptoms have disappeared before any periodontal surgery is undertaken. If evidence of a crack can be elicited, an orthodontic band should be cemented to minimize the likelihood of the crack's spreading. The dentist and patient should decide together to perform endodontic therapy promptly or wait and see whether symptoms subside before undertaking periodontal surgery.

C If a symptomatic tooth tests vital and has no evidence of periapical radiolucency, examine it for cracks or crack symptoms. If no evidence of a crack is elicited, use selective grinding and

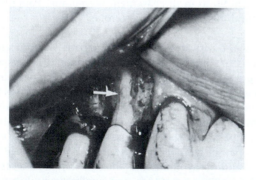

Figure 35-1 An endodontically treated first premolar with a vertical crack and resulting deep periodontal defect.

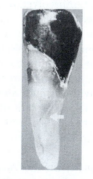

Figure 35-3 A cracked tooth.

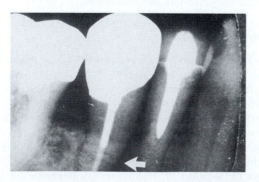

Figure 35-2 A vertical periodontal defect resulting from a cracked tooth.

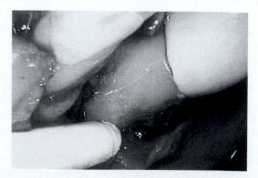

Figure 35-4 Intraoral fiberoptic video picture of a tooth with a clearly visible vertical crack.

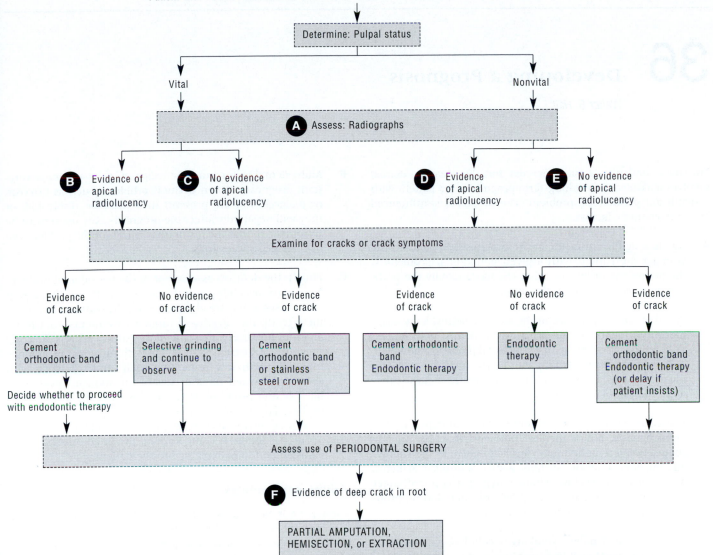

Patient with POCKET DEPTH AND LOCALIZED PAIN OR TWINGES OF PAIN IN A TOOTH

Determine: Pulpal status

Vital — Nonvital

A Assess: Radiographs

B Evidence of apical radiolucency

C No evidence of apical radiolucency

D Evidence of apical radiolucency

E No evidence of apical radiolucency

Examine for cracks or crack symptoms

Evidence of crack

No evidence of crack

Evidence of crack

Evidence of crack

No evidence of crack

Evidence of crack

Cement orthodontic band

Selective grinding and continue to observe

Cement orthodontic band or stainless steel crown

Cement orthodontic band Endodontic therapy

Endodontic therapy

Cement orthodontic band Endodontic therapy (or delay if patient insists)

Decide whether to proceed with endodontic therapy

Assess use of PERIODONTAL SURGERY

F Evidence of deep crack in root

PARTIAL AMPUTATION, HEMISECTION, or EXTRACTION

observation for several months before any periodontal procedures are undertaken. If evidence of a crack can be elicited, cement an orthodontic band or stainless steel crown to minimize fracture spread before periodontal surgery.

D If a symptomatic tooth tests nonvital, this may be confirmed by a radiographic periapical radiolucency. If so, examine the tooth for cracks. If no evidence of a crack can be elicited, complete endodontic treatment promptly before periodontal surgery is undertaken. If evidence of a crack is found, cement an orthodontic band to its crown to minimize fracture spreading. The dentist and patient should agree to initiate endodontic treatment promptly or wait and see. If symptoms do not subside, endodontics should be undertaken before periodontal surgery. If symptoms subside, periodontal surgery can be undertaken with full recognition that an endodontic flare-up could be precipitated, necessitating prompt treatment.

E If a symptomatic tooth tests nonvital and radiographic evidence of a periapical radiolucency is not found, evaluate the tooth for evidence of a crack. If no evidence of a crack can be elicited, the tooth should be treated endodontically before periodontal surgery is performed. If evidence of a crack can be elicited, cement an orthodontic band to the crown and perform endodontic treatment before periodontal surgery is undertaken.

F When periodontal treatment is undertaken in any of these situations, a crack extending down the root where attachment has been lost may become visible. After the area has been débrided, use the fiberoptic light source or intraoral television to search for cracks. If a deep crack is found, the tooth may have to be extracted, one root of a multirooted tooth may be amputated (in maxillary molars), or the tooth may be hemisected (in mandibular molars). If a patient elects not to have such a tooth extracted, the dentist should carefully document the patient's choice and advise that keeping the tooth is risky.

Additional Readings

Cameron CE. The cracked tooth syndrome: additional findings. J Am Dent Assoc 1976;93:971.

Eahle WS, Maxwell EH, Braly BV. Fractures of posterior teeth in adults. J Am Dent Assoc 1986;12:215.

Hiatt WH. Incomplete crown-root fracture. J Periodontol 1973;44:369.

Maxwell EH, Braly BV. Incomplete tooth fracture: prediction and prevention. Calif Dent Assoc 1977;5:51.

Ritchey B, Mendenhall R, Orban B. Pulpitis resulting from incomplete tooth fracture. Oral Surg Oral Med Oral Pathol 1957;10:665.

Turp JC, Gobett JP. The cracked tooth syndrome: an elusive diagnosis. J Am Dent Assoc 1996;127:1502.

36 Developing a Prognosis

Walter B. Hall

The most difficult decision process for the treating dentist involves making a correct long-term prognosis for a patient with a significant periodontal problem. The prognosis is influenced by many complex factors.

A Age is a significant factor in the prognosis. In general, the younger the patient with a given periodontal problem is, the poorer the prognosis. Also, the more rapidly the problem develops, the poorer the prognosis.

B The skills and experience of the treating dentist have a significant influence on the prognosis. A dentist with limited skills *should refer* significant periodontal problems; however, if the patient demands that the dentist treat the problem, the dentist with limited skills must recognize that the prognosis will not be as good.

C The medical status of the patient is of critical importance to the prognosis. Major medical problems that can and do adversely affect periodontal problems include the following: impaired immune system, poorly controlled diabetes, use of medicines that may induce hyperplasia (see Chapter 29), heart or blood pressure problems, and clotting problems or use of anticoagulants (see Chapter 29).

D Poor nutritional habits, smoking, alcohol abuse, and drug abuse have negative effects on the prognosis.

E The ability of the patient to manage stress, follow through with a demanding oral hygiene regimen, and recognize and manage the periodontal problem affect the prognosis—either positively or negatively. Skill in identifying and assessing these nondental factors is a key to the dentist's success as a prognostician.

F Many dental factors must be weighed in developing a long-term prognosis. When occlusal problems such as bruxism or malocclusion are present, they must be resolvable, or they will negatively affect the prognosis. Key teeth must be restorable, so that the restorative aspects of the problem can be managed successfully.

G Finally, the dentist's assessment of the periodontal problem and its manageability is critical to the prognosis. The extent of the disease, its rate of progression, the status of key abutment teeth, the severity of furca involvements, root form, and root proximity are some of the critical aspects affecting prognosis. An extensive problem with rapid loss of support, especially with few remaining solid teeth or teeth with short or crowded roots or severe furcation involvements, has a poorer prognosis than that for a case in which fewer of these factors are negative.

A prognosis is an evolving decision-making process. As additional factors become known, the prognosis should be adjusted and fully explained to the patient.

Additional Readings

Carranza FA Jr, Newman MG. Clinical periodontology. 8th ed. Philadelphia: WB Saunders; 1996. p. 390.

Hirschfeld L, Wasserman B. A long-term study of tooth loss in 600 treated periodontal patients. J Periodontol 1978;49:225.

Ramfjord SP, editor. World workshop in periodontics. Ann Arbor (MI): American Academy of Periodontology; 1966.

Schluger S et al. Periodontal diseases. Philadelphia: Lea & Febiger; 1990. p. 341.

Waerhaug J. The furcation problem: etiology, pathogenesis, diagnosis, therapy, and prognosis. J Clin Periodontol 1980;7:73.

Wilson TG, Kornman KS. Fundamentals of periodontics. Chicago: Quintessence Publishing; 1996. p. 464.

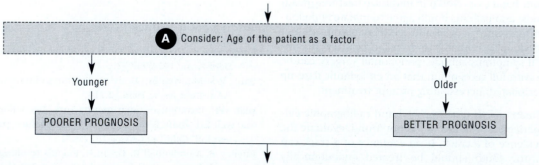

Patient for PROGNOSIS WHOSE DIAGNOSIS AND TREATMENT PLAN ARE COMPLETE

A Consider: Age of the patient as a factor

Younger → POORER PROGNOSIS

Older → BETTER PROGNOSIS

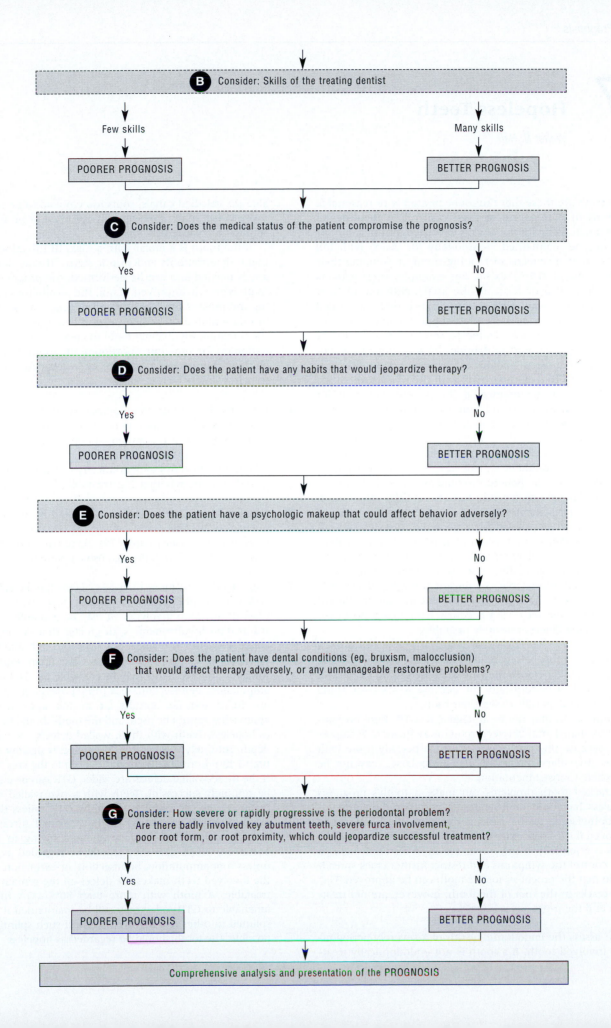

37 Hopeless Teeth

Walter B. Hall

Hopeless teeth are those that cannot be treated with reasonable expectations of eliminating or even controlling their dental problems. Such teeth are not always extracted, but in some situations may be maintained, occasionally for years, with full recognition that no means of treating them or stopping their loss of attachment (LOA) exists. For example, such patients may have lost 50% or more of the attachment on all their remaining teeth. Pocket-elimination surgery might be ruled out on the basis of leaving inadequate support to keep the teeth at all with any reasonable degree of comfort or function. A Widman flap may be used to débride the area once fully, but neither the patient nor the dentist can expect to control the disease process with root planing, even with the use of antibiotics. Such teeth may be maintained, if the patient demands, for some time before abscesses and pain necessitate their removal. Such patients should proceed with full knowledge that their prognosis is hopeless and should be aware of the risks of abscesses and possible danger to general health. The concept of *hopeless,* therefore, should be explained fully when such a prognosis is used so that the patient not only assumes all the attendant risks of keeping such teeth, but also is fully informed in the legal sense (see Chapter 139).

Today, many teeth previously regarded as hopeless are salvageable via guided tissue regeneration (GTR). Badly involved Class II furcation involvements, large three-walled infrabony defects, and osseous craters that were nontreatable have become predictably treatable. Significant numbers of formerly hopeless teeth can be saved by this means today. Recent advances with extensive GTR procedures have made most two-walled infrabony defects routinely treatable.

A Some teeth must be regarded as hopeless because they are not restorable, because they are malposed to an extent not correctable orthodontically, or because vertical or spiral cracks extend apically down their roots.

Some teeth may not be amenable to GTR. Root proximity (less than 1 mm between roots) may make GTR impossible because proximal root surfaces, especially those with furcas (maxillary molars or first premolars), may not be accessible to instrumentation.

Cracked tooth problems can make a tooth's prognosis hopeless. If cracked tooth syndrome exists and the symptoms are bothersome to the patient, the tooth may have to be removed if the crack extends vertically down the root. If the crack is essentially in the crown, placing a restorative crown may control the symptoms and restrict further crack spreading so that the prognosis for the tooth can be improved. Vertical cracks in the root of the tooth, however, are not treatable, and the prognosis is hopeless.

B Next, assess the endodontic health of a severely periodontally involved tooth. If a tooth is not endodontically treatable (ie, calcified canals, roots too crooked to be obturated, severely internally or externally resorbed or perforated), it should be regarded as hopeless.

If the tooth is a molar with a Class III furcation involvement, determine its endodontic status. If endodontic therapy is needed and can be performed, the prognosis for the tooth is greatly improved. If not, the possibilities of improving the molar's prognosis would depend on the possibility of root amputation or hemisection being used to eliminate the furcation involvement and to create a maintainable situation on the remaining portion of the tooth. If this cannot be done (because of root form or fusion), the prognosis is hopeless unless GTR is feasible.

C If the tooth is nonrestorable because of the caries or fracture status of its remaining portion, it should be viewed as hopeless even if it is maintained and the periodontal treatment continues.

If the tooth is not endodontically treatable, the next step is to determine whether it is treatable periodontally.

D Usually, a tooth with less than 50% LOA is treatable by frequent root planing (see Chapter 75) or with mucogingival osseous surgery (see Chapter 79). Teeth with more than 50% LOA usually require more extensive treatment to be saved.

E Some teeth with more than 50% LOA may be salvaged by GTR with highly predictable success. Teeth with Class II or Class III furcation involvement may be treatable. Most Class II furcation involvements with greater than 3 mm of horizontal loss into the furca but not "through-and-through" problems are good candidates for GTR. Teeth with Class III furcation involvements may be treatable by GTR or by root amputation, hemisection, or a tunnel operation. If the roots are fused too far apically or at the apex itself, such approaches cannot be used, and the tooth should be regarded as hopeless. Teeth with three-walled defects, even of severe depth, routinely regenerate if the defect is narrow (no more than 1 mm horizontally from the tooth to the crest of bone). If the three-walled defects are wider, GTR can be expected to be routinely successful. Teeth with a two-walled infrabony crater can be successfully treated by GTR unless their roots are less than 1 mm apart or the proximal furcas are too severely involved to be instrumented owing to restricted access, in which case they should be regarded as hopeless unless root amputation, hemisection, or extraction of one of the involved teeth makes the defect on the remaining tooth treatable. A tooth with more than 50% LOA that is not amenable to GTR today may still be maintained if it can be splinted to other less-involved teeth. If such splinting is not possible, the tooth should be regarded as hopeless.

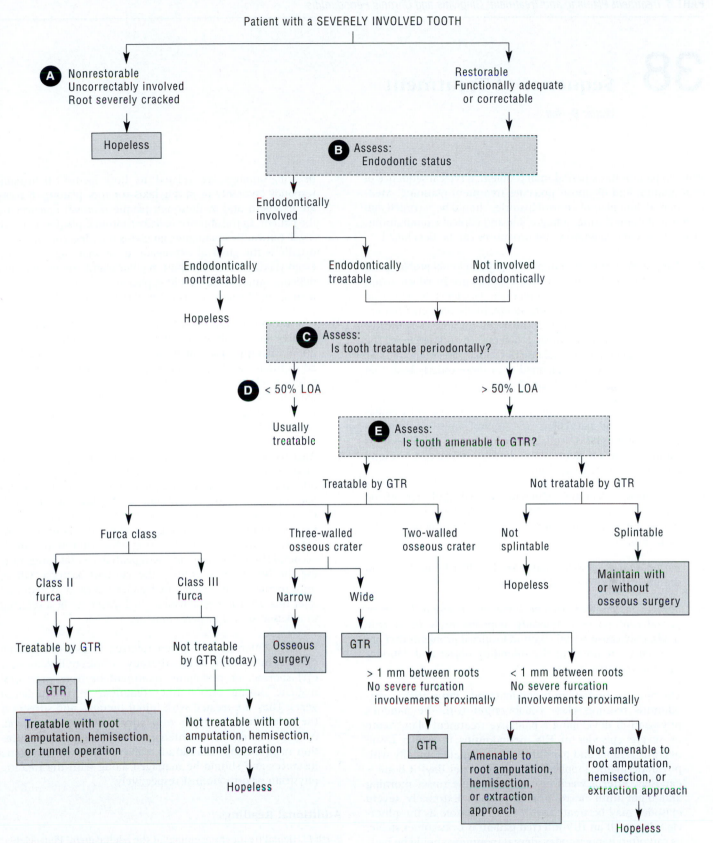

Patient with a SEVERELY INVOLVED TOOTH

A Nonrestorable
Uncorrectably involved
Root severely cracked

Restorable
Functionally adequate
or correctable

Hopeless

B Assess:
Endodontic status

Endodontically
involved

Endodontically
nontreatable

Endodontically
treatable

Not involved
endodontically

Hopeless

C Assess:
Is tooth treatable periodontally?

D < 50% LOA

> 50% LOA

Usually
treatable

E Assess:
Is tooth amenable to GTR?

Treatable by GTR

Not treatable by GTR

Furca class

Three-walled
osseous crater

Two-walled
osseous crater

Not
splintable

Splintable

Class II
furca

Class III
furca

Narrow

Wide

Hopeless

Maintain with
or without
osseous surgery

Treatable by GTR

Not treatable
by GTR (today)

Osseous
surgery

GTR

GTR

Treatable with root
amputation, hemisection,
or tunnel operation

Not treatable with root
amputation, hemisection,
or tunnel operation

> 1 mm between roots
No severe furcation
involvements proximally

< 1 mm between roots
No severe furcation
involvements proximally

Hopeless

GTR

Amenable to
root amputation,
hemisection,
or extraction
approach

Not amenable to
root amputation,
hemisection, or
extraction approach

Hopeless

Additional Readings

Corn H, Marks MA. Strategic extractions in periodontal therapy. Dent Clin North Am 1969;13:817.

Eakle WJ, Maxwell EH, Braly BV. Fractures of posterior teeth in adults. J Am Dent Assoc 1986;12:215.

Everett FG, Stern IB. When is tooth mobility an indication for extraction? Dent Clin North Am 1969;13:791.

Maxwell EH, Braly BV. Incomplete root fracture: predictions and prevention. Cal Dent Assoc J 1977;5:51.

Schluger S et al. Periodontal diseases. 2nd ed. Philadelphia: Lea & Febiger; 1990. p. 341.

38 Sequence of Treatment

Walter B. Hall

When a patient has a periodontal problem, a typical sequence of examination and diagnosis precedes treatment planning. Medical, dental, and plaque-control histories should be recorded and elaborated upon during radiographic and clinical examinations. From these data, diagnoses and prognoses can be developed.

A   For purposes of treatment planning, periodontal problems are divided into acute (symptomatic) problems, in which symptoms are present, and asymptomatic problems, in which no acute problems are present. Symptomatic problems require prompt treatment, usually at the diagnostic visit. Only the five most common symptomatic problems are outlined here. The most common periodontal diseases usually are asymptomatic, and treatment can be planned on a more orderly basis that best fits into the patient's and dentist's schedules.

B   Herpetic gingivostomatitis usually is managed with palliative care (mild painkillers or a topical anesthetic mouthwash), prophylaxis, and instruction about the infectious nature of the problem. Maintain fluid balance in younger children to avoid dehydration.

C   Necrotizing ulcerative gingivitis (NUG) and necrotizing ulcerative periodontitis (NUP) are handled by instrumentation alone or in conjunction with an oral antibiotic, usually penicillin.

D   Periodontal abscesses usually are handled by incision and drainage along with antibiotic therapy.

E   Foreign bodies that become impacted in gingival sulci or periodontal pockets, typically popcorn hulls or sesame seeds, may cause acutely painful localized problems that are relieved by removal of the offending object and débridement of the area.

F   Therapy for human immunodeficiency virus (HIV) periodontitis requires close collaboration with the patient's physician in developing a palliative treatment plan. Acute or severe episodes of HIV periodontitis in which tissue necrosis is rapid and painful should be treated initially with povidone-iodine (applied several times per day) if bone is exposed. After a week, use chlorhexidine rinses morning and night until necrosis is controlled. Extremely severe episodes may be treated with metronidazole as the physician directs. If an HIV-infected patient is or becomes stable, as can often happen today, dental treatment should be handled as with noninfected patients. Even guided tissue regeneration (GTR), using resorbable membranes, has become routine for individuals in stable states.

G   Gingivitis of the typical type probably is the most prevalent disease affecting human beings, and most people experience at least localized inflammations of this type in any given year.

Its subgroupings are related to host factors. It usually responds favorably to prophylaxis (or root planing, if roots are exposed) and to thorough plaque removal practices by the patient. In the absence of daily thorough plaque removal, it will return. Desquamative gingivitis is far less common and usually is the gingival expression of dermatologic diseases. Prophylaxis (or root planing), regular plaque removal (often difficult), and topical steroid applications are common treatments. Oral hygiene instruction (OHI) is essential.

H   Chronic periodontitis is the current name for typical, slowly progressive periodontitis. Its treatment usually consists of initial therapy (root planing, OHI, occasionally occlusal adjustment, and, occasionally, temporary splinting or minor tooth movement). After several weeks or months of patient effort, the response is evaluated and decisions are made regarding the comparative value of surgery or continued maintenance.

I   Aggressive periodontitises include juvenile periodontitis, mixed dentition periodontitis, and rapidly progressive periodontitis; these are discussed elsewhere. Although different bacteria appear to predominate as etiologic agents with these diseases, they are treated in a similar manner. A regimen of tetracycline (250 mg four times daily) or metronidazole is used for 3 weeks, during which all root planing is accomplished. This regimen is repeated several times during the first year to contact the virulent bacteria. Often, only regular maintenance or localized surgery is required after this control is established. Such cases are best referred to a dental school or periodontists.

J   Gingival enlargements (often referred to as hyperplasias) may result from drug therapy (diphenylhydantoin, cyclosporine, or nifedipine treatment or from poor oral hygiene during orthodontic treatment in the pubertal years). They are treated with initial therapy, and surgery if the deformities interfere with adequate plaque removal, occlusion, or regular maintenance. Stopping use of medication or removing orthodontic bands is necessary in some instances and should be managed along with the treating physician or orthodontist respectively.

Additional Readings

Barsh LI. Dental treatment planning for the adult patient. Philadelphia: WB Saunders; 1981. p. 152.

Carranza FA Jr, Newman MG. Clinical periodontology. 8th ed. Philadelphia: WB Saunders; 1996. p. 399.

Genco RJ, Goldman HM, Cohen DW. Contemporary periodontics. St. Louis: Mosby; 1990. p. 359.

Wilson TG, Kornman KS. Fundamentals of periodontics. Chicago: Quintessence Publishing; 1996. p. 307.

Patient with a periodontal problem for TREATMENT PLANNING

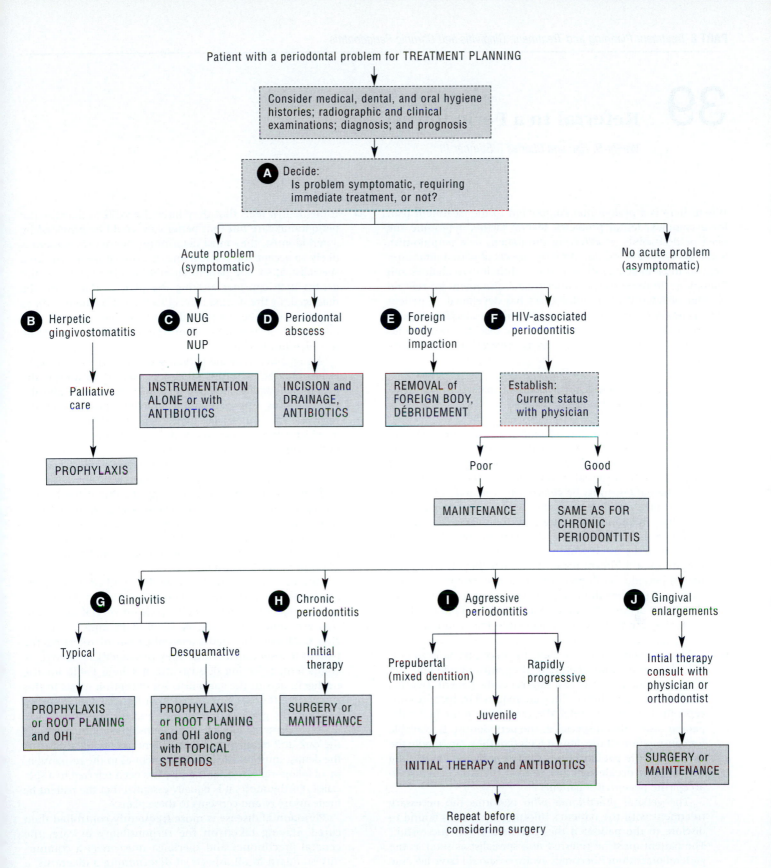

Consider medical, dental, and oral hygiene histories; radiographic and clinical examinations; diagnosis; and prognosis

A Decide: Is problem symptomatic, requiring immediate treatment, or not?

Acute problem (symptomatic)

No acute problem (asymptomatic)

B Herpetic gingivostomatitis

Palliative care

PROPHYLAXIS

C NUG or NUP

INSTRUMENTATION ALONE or with ANTIBIOTICS

D Periodontal abscess

INCISION and DRAINAGE, ANTIBIOTICS

E Foreign body impaction

REMOVAL of FOREIGN BODY, DÉBRIDEMENT

F HIV-associated periodontitis

Establish: Current status with physician

Poor

MAINTENANCE

Good

SAME AS FOR CHRONIC PERIODONTITIS

G Gingivitis

Typical

PROPHYLAXIS or ROOT PLANING and OHI

Desquamative

PROPHYLAXIS or ROOT PLANING and OHI along with TOPICAL STEROIDS

H Chronic periodontitis

Initial therapy

SURGERY or MAINTENANCE

I Aggressive periodontitis

Prepubertal (mixed dentition)

Juvenile

Rapidly progressive

INITIAL THERAPY and ANTIBIOTICS

Repeat before considering surgery

J Gingival enlargements

Intial therapy consult with physician or orthodontist

SURGERY or MAINTENANCE

39 Referral to a Periodontist

Walter B. Hall and Charles F. Sumner III

When there is a periodontal component to the treatment plan for a complex dental problem, several factors determine the need or desirability of referring the patient to a periodontist. Some dentists have mastered many aspects of periodontal care. Dentists must have a realistic concept of their own abilities and limitations. In some states, a quasilegal requirement for referral or offer of referral of complex cases has developed. A patient with a complex problem needs to know that a specialist in periodontics exists and may be consulted. If a case has complexities involving multiple specialized areas, referral is particularly desirable.

A   If there are no significant periodontal aspects in the treatment plan, referral is not necessary.[1]

B   If the treatment plan has a significant periodontal component, dentists must decide whether they have the required skill to treat the periodontal problem or if better care could be provided by a specialist. If the dentist does not have the skill, the patient must be referred to a periodontist or the dentist must refuse to treat the case. General practitioners who have additional training may treat cases that are no longer in the earliest stages. If general dentists decide that the level of disease is within their ability to treat, however, they must still inform patients (1) that they, the patients, have a periodontal disease; (2) about the extent of the disease; and (3) that there are specialists in the treatment of this dental disease. To fail to so inform the patient would be to render care without a complete informed consent.[2,3]

C   If dentists believe that they have the necessary skills to provide the periodontal treatment, they must decide whether referral would be in the best interest of the patient. Dentists must also decide whether they are required by practice concepts in their area to refer the case. They must make the patient aware that a specialist, the periodontist, is available for consultation. If the dentist feels that they can handle the case, and if the patient selects treatment by the dentist, the dentist must decide whether to treat the case or refuse to accept the person as a patient.

The general practitioner who performs the necessary treatment with the patient's informed consent is bound to disclose to the patient if the treatment is not successful.[4] The patient must be referred to a specialist as soon as the general practitioner becomes aware or should have become aware that the therapy initiated is not proving to be as effective as could be expected in the hands of a specialist.

D   If the dentist feels that they have the skills to manage the periodontal care but that better care could be provided by a periodontist, they must determine whether the patient is likely to accept the referral and can afford treatment by a specialist. If so, the patient should be referred. If not, the dentist may consider altering the plan so that it can be managed, or the dentist can refuse to accept the person as a patient. If the patient declines to be referred, the informed consent aspects of the discussion should be recorded in the chart.

A suggestion that the patient seek the care of a specialist is not enough. The practitioner is obliged to inform the patient adequately about the extent of the disease and the consequences if the patient fails to follow through with the referral.[5] The courts have found dentists negligent in cases in which patients have asserted they were not made aware of the consequence of failing to seek care. Thus it would be prudent to follow up on each of the referrals and not simply dismiss the patient who apparently has not taken the advice.

Some courts have held referring dentists liable for not having warned patients of the extent and type of care they would receive from the specialist[6]; however, in most instances, it is the primary obligation of the specialist or a staff member to inform the patient properly and obtain a satisfactory informed consent.[7,8]

Patients are at a disadvantage if they need to rely only on their own resources to choose a specialist. After having informed patients of their needs for special care, dentists are obliged to assist patients in making a prudent choice. Having fulfilled their obligation of referring the patient to a specialist whom they reasonably believe to be competent, referring dentists are not held liable for the negligent acts of the specialist. An exception exists to this rule where there is a partnership or fiduciary relationship between the general practitioner and the specialist.

Having entered into a joint relationship with the patient in the care and treatment of that patient's periodontal disease, the dentist must reach some agreement as to the responsibility of follow-up care after the case has been referred to a specialist. Furthermore, it is equally essential that the patient be made aware of and consents to these plans.

Periodontal disease is more frequently controlled than cured. Having taken on the responsibility of care, the general practitioner and specialist must meet a community standard in all aspects of determining a diagnosis, a treatment plan, and provision of maintenance care. Both parties have a duty to inform the patient of their plans,

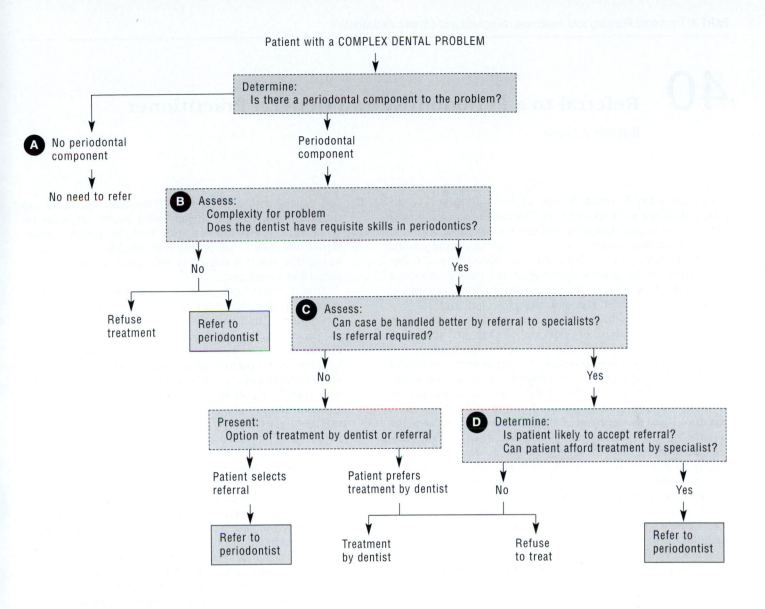

Patient with a COMPLEX DENTAL PROBLEM

Determine:
Is there a periodontal component to the problem?

A No periodontal component

No need to refer

Periodontal component

B Assess:
Complexity for problem
Does the dentist have requisite skills in periodontics?

No

Yes

Refuse treatment

Refer to periodontist

C Assess:
Can case be handled better by referral to specialists?
Is referral required?

No

Yes

Present:
Option of treatment by dentist or referral

D Determine:
Is patient likely to accept referral?
Can patient afford treatment by specialist?

Patient selects referral

Patient prefers treatment by dentist

No

Yes

Refer to periodontist

Treatment by dentist

Refuse to treat

Refer to periodontist

their prognoses, and the consequences of not following the plans. They must also offer the patient an alternative plan, if available, describing its advantages and disadvantages. Only then can the patient make an informed decision and the dentist proceed with an informed consent.

Additional Readings

Grant DA, Stern IB, Listgarten MA. Periodontics. 6th ed. St. Louis: Mosby; 1988. p. 605.

Hall WB. Pure mucogingival problems. Berlin: Quintessence Publishing; 1984. p. 169.

Zinman EJ. Common dental malpractice errors and preventive measures. J West Soc Periodont 1976;23:149.

Legal References

1. Helling v Carey, Wash, 519 P.2d 981 (1974).
2. Canterbury v Spence, 464 F2d 772 (1972).
3. Cobbs v Grant, 104 Cal Rptr 505 (1972).
4. Baldor v Roger, 81 S Rptr 2d 660 (1955).
5. Moore v Preventive Medicine Medical Group, Inc, 178 Cal, App.3d 728;223 Cal Rptr 85 (1986).
6. Llera v Wisner, 557 P.2d 805 (1976).
7. Mustacchio v Parker, 535 So.2d 833, La App.2Cir (1988).
8. Bulman v Myers, DDS, 467 A.2d 1353, Pa.Super. (1983).

40 Referral to a Periodontist by a General Practitioner

Benjamin J. Mandel

Premature referrals result in one of the following: (1) the patient does not see a specialist; (2) the patient sees a specialist but does not accept treatment because the patient is not mentally or financially ready; or (3) the patient leaves the general practitioner because the referral was not successful, and rather than return to the general practitioner, the patient chooses a new dentist. In any event, when premature referrals are made, the general practitioner, specialist, and patient all lose.

The general practitioner should always refer the patient to two specialists. If the patient does not like the first specialist's treatment approach, there is always a second opportunity.

If any problems with compliance develop during treatment by the specialist, the specialist should request the general practitioner's input. The general practitioner must inform the patient of the services provided by a specialist at the onset of treatment and throughout the course of treatment to reinforce the idea that at some point a specialist may be needed. This constant reinforcement throughout the treatment makes the patient more willing to accept the completion of the general practitioner's treatment and the continuation of care at the specialist's office.

Whether the patient accepts or declines the referrals, the patient must be informed in writing of the consequences of failure to obtain treatment. The general practitioner must communicate to the specialist by phone or in writing before the referral is made to familiarize the specialist with all aspects related to this patient. The better the communication, the easier the transition. Communication is the key to this entire process.

A The first step toward a successful referral is a thorough evaluation of the patient by a general practitioner. A complete medical and dental history is reviewed with the patient. Any previous problems with dentists (general practitioners and specialists alike) must be evaluated. Because the patient is to remain with the general practitioner at the beginning and end of treatment, a careful diagnosis, treatment plan, and prognosis must be prepared and understood by the patient before any referrals can be made. The patient and general practitioner must be comfortable with each other as well as with all aspects of the treatment (including emotional and financial). The patient is informed that referrals to specialists in different disciplines may be necessary and that in the end the patient will return to the general practitioner. At this point the goal is to build a level of awareness.

B The second phase is the beginning of treatment. The goals are: (1) to take the patient out of pain and eliminate infection, (2) to begin basic caries control through restorative treatment, and (3) to provide prophylaxis. If no periodontal component is found at the end of this phase, the patient can proceed with advanced treatment (eg, crown and bridge) and then be placed on a 6-month continuing-care program.

C The patient with a periodontal component must undergo thorough root planing therapy with heavy emphasis on home care and follow-up, such that the patient understands the nature of periodontal disease. Oral hygiene instruction (OHI) is offered so that good habits are established and monitored.

If, at the end of this phase, the patient has no periodontal component, the patient is placed on a 3-month continuing-care program, and basic restorative treatment is begun. If the patient has improved somewhat but a few areas of concern remain, those problems are resolved by obtaining written, informed consent of advanced periodontal treatment by the general practitioner or making a referral to the specialist after completing phase two of the basic caries control and simple restorative phase. If the patient refuses a referral to a specialist, the general practitioner should proceed with advanced techniques if comfortable with them. If not comfortable with such techniques, the general practitioner must insist on consultation with a specialist. By this time, the general practitioner has had the opportunity to get to know the patient and can have a thorough discussion about the direction of the treatment, which areas have improved, and which have not improved. If the patient refuses the referral, the general practitioner must inform the patient that if the advanced techniques performed by the general practitioner are not successful, a specialist must be consulted. The above advice must be in writing and must be made part of the written, informed consent of any advanced procedure.

D After advanced techniques are performed, thorough monthly evaluations should be performed and 3-month continuing-care visits should go on as usual. A thorough evaluation, including probing, must be done 6 months after the advanced procedures are performed. As an example, areas that have guided tissue regeneration procedures performed cannot be probed for at least 6 months. If most areas have improved, the patient is maintained on 3-month continuing-care visits, and the patient is offered a referral to a specialist for areas that did not achieve optimal results. It is the general practitioner's responsibility to redo those procedures at no additional cost to the patient.

E This is the most difficult stage because failure to accept referrals to specialists will compromise teeth as well as restorative aspects. Money and fear are important factors, and 3-month continuing-care visits must be continued rather than losing the patient. Perhaps the patient will accept a 1- or 2-month maintenance visit as a compromise. Circumstances may change by keeping the patient in the practice, and the patient might accept a referral sometime in the future. But even if the referral is not accepted, at least the patient is being maintained and home care is being reinforced.

Patient for INITIAL EXAMINATION BY A GENERAL PRACTITIONER

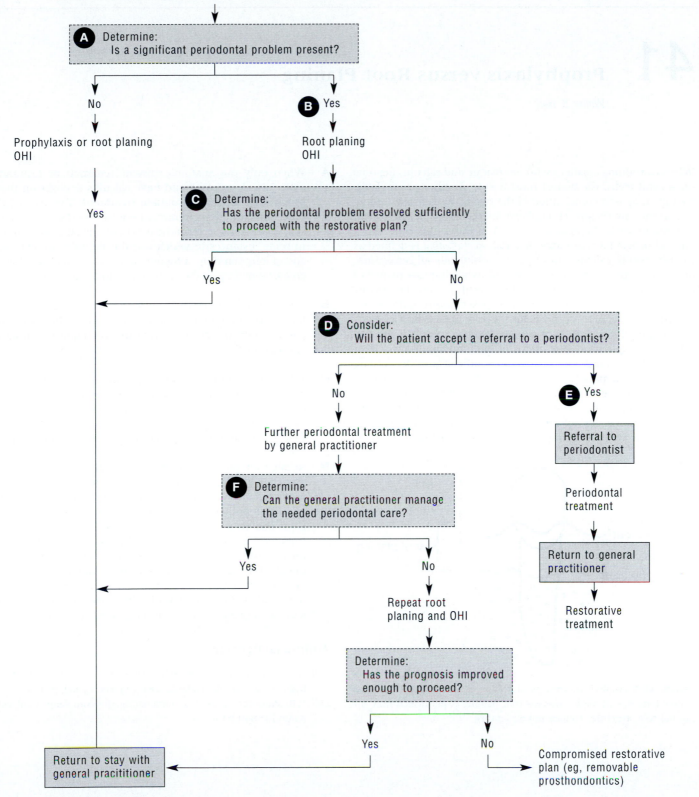

A Determine:
Is a significant periodontal problem present?

No — Prophylaxis or root planing OHI — Yes

B Yes — Root planing OHI

C Determine:
Has the periodontal problem resolved sufficiently to proceed with the restorative plan?

Yes — No

D Consider:
Will the patient accept a referral to a periodontist?

No — Further periodontal treatment by general practitioner

E Yes — Referral to periodontist — Periodontal treatment — Return to general practitioner — Restorative treatment

F Determine:
Can the general practitioner manage the needed periodontal care?

Yes — No — Repeat root planing and OHI

Determine:
Has the prognosis improved enough to proceed?

Yes — No — Compromised restorative plan (eg, removable prosthondontics)

Return to stay with general practitioner

F Successful referral at any stage ends with the patient returning to the general practitioner to complete advanced restorative techniques, with one exception: a referral to a prosthodontist if the general practitioner feels this is in the patient's best interest. In any event, the permanent, continuing-care program must be within the control of the general practitioner.

Additional Readings

Hall WB. Pure mucogingival problems. Berlin: Quintessence Publishing; 1984. p. 169.

41 Prophylaxis versus Root Planing

Walter B. Hall

When examining a patient who has plaque and calculus deposits on several teeth, the dentist must decide whether prophylaxis, root planing, or a combination of the two is the appropriate first step in therapy (Figure 41-1). *Prophylaxis* is defined as the scaling of deposits from the anatomic crown of the tooth, either from enamel or from a restorative material. *Root planing* is defined as the removal of calculus, most plaque, essentially all cementum, and some dentin from the roots of teeth while they are planed to clinical smoothness. The removal of calculus from the crowns (scaling) and the polishing of all exposed tooth surfaces are regarded as part of this process for the sake of ease of documentation and billing. Scaling of the anatomic crowns of teeth is a relatively simple procedure and is of minimal importance. Root planing, however, is one of the most difficult and demanding procedures in dentistry. In planning treatment, the dentist has an obligation to differentiate fairly and correctly between the procedures to charge the patient or a third party properly for the work done. Whenever loss of attachment has occurred and no root restorations are present, root planing must be performed.

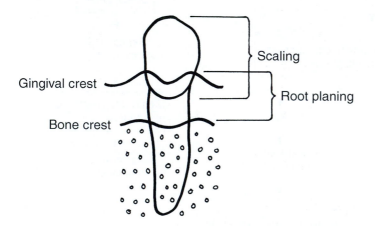

Figure 41-1 Prophylaxis consists of scaling and polishing natural or restored crowns of teeth, whereas root planing is performed only on natural root structures (cementum or dentin).

A When only the anatomic crowns (enamel) or restorative materials are exposed and have calculus deposits on them, prophylaxis is the appropriate treatment. The cost of this procedure usually is minimal because the time, effort, and skill required to perform the procedure usually are minimal. In some instances in which calculus deposits are extensive and of long standing, a higher charge to compensate for the greater time required is justifiable and appropriate.

B When only a few teeth have roots exposed or many teeth have little root exposure, a charge for prophylaxis and perhaps one quadrant or two of root planing would be appropriate.

C When most teeth have root exposure of several millimeters or more, root planing is the appropriate treatment plan. The cost of initial root planing might reasonably be set at four or more times the cost of prophylaxis to reflect the greater time, effort, and skill required to perform this procedure.

D Recall root planing, however, after the roots have been planed by the dentist initially, is a much easier task because many calculi will be relatively new and attached to the previously smoothed dentin much less firmly than the old calculus had been united with cementum. Recall root planing, therefore, makes appropriate a significantly lower fee than for the initial planing, perhaps the same as one quadrant initially for the full mouth on recall. Recall instrumentation of exposed roots should not be termed *prophylaxis*, because only scaling calculus deposits from exposed roots would leave a roughened, irregular, or gouged root surface.

Additional Readings

Hall WB. Clinical practice. In: Steele PF, editor. Dimensions in dental hygiene. 3rd ed. Philadelphia: Lea & Febiger; 1982. p. 143.

Hall WB. Procedure code 452: eliminating the confusion. Calif Dent Assoc J 1983;11:33.

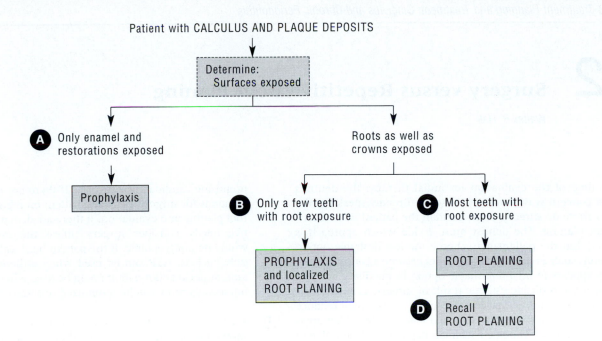

Patient with CALCULUS AND PLAQUE DEPOSITS

Determine:
Surfaces exposed

A Only enamel and
restorations exposed

Prophylaxis

Roots as well as
crowns exposed

B Only a few teeth
with root exposure

PROPHYLAXIS
and localized
ROOT PLANING

C Most teeth with
root exposure

ROOT PLANING

D Recall
ROOT PLANING

42 Surgery versus Repetitive Root Planing

Walter B. Hall

At the time of the evaluation for initial therapy, the dentist's greatest concern is with what to do next. Broadly speaking, the options are to do surgery or to maintain the patient with repetitive root planing. The dentist must decide which approach is indicated, but the patient may choose the less desirable option for reasons such as cost or fear. Esthetics become a concern when surgery appears to be a reasonable option in maxillary anterior regions. If the probable esthetic result of surgery, even if therapeutically successful, is unacceptable to the patient, maintenance is a reasonable alternative. If deep and inaccessible pocket areas remain, the use of a modified Widman flap might be desirable to permit thorough, one-time débridement while minimizing postsurgical exposure. Guided tissue regeneration (GTR) may permit significant restitution of periodontal support on teeth with deep osseous defects, making surgery of this type a most desirable option for a patient with localized severe defects.

A The success of the patient's plaque-control efforts is an important factor in deciding whether a patient "merits" surgery. A patient who has been unable to clean the supragingival portions of the teeth before surgery is not a promising candidate to do well with the more tortuous and minimally accessible areas usually exposed after osseous surgery. A patient who has cleaned these areas well is more likely to be able and willing to clean well after surgery. GTR, if even partially successful, facilitates plaque control.

B A patient who has removed plaque well usually has a good response to initial therapy. Signs of inflammation are diminished or absent, and pocket depth and mobility are likely to have decreased. Occasionally, however, a patient's response is not good, despite efforts at plaque control; surgery for such a patient is less likely to be a good alternative.

C If the patient's response is exceptionally good and there are no requirements that surgery be considered (eg, pure mucogingival problems, inadequate crown exposure), the patient may do well with only repetitive planing rather than surgery. If there are restorative demands for a surgical approach, however, surgery should be considered unless the esthetic results should be unacceptable. If the patient has localized areas that are inaccessible to root planing, consider surgery. When esthetic concerns exist, a modified Widman flap approach would permit a one-time, thorough débridement, which might be advantageous. A patient whose response has been poor despite good plaque control is not a promising candidate for surgery. If there are no restorative demands for surgery, place the patient on regular, repetitive root planing and evaluation. If there are demanding restorative needs, consider surgery unless the esthetic results would be unacceptable. If the patient has localized, inaccessible pockets, GTR can be used when esthetics are important, or pocket elimination might be used when esthetics are not a concern or will be minimized restoratively.

D A patient who has done poorly in plaque control usually shows a poor response to initial therapy; occasionally, however, good responses may occur despite the patient's efforts. For patients with poor oral hygiene who exhibit a good response, surgery may be a practical option if they have restorative needs that surgery would benefit. If a patient has no esthetic concerns, surgery can be done. If the patient has esthetic concerns, maintenance root planing is a better choice. If the patient with good response but poor oral hygiene has no demanding restorative needs, repeat root planing and evaluate again. If the patient has localized, inaccessible pocket areas, GTR is indicated. A patient with poor oral hygiene who has the expected poor response to initial therapy, and no restorative requirements to consider surgery, should be placed on a repetitive root-planing program. If there are restorative requirements, repeat the root planing and evaluate again to determine whether the patient can improve the oral hygiene to a level at which surgery would be reasonable. If the patient has localized, inaccessible pocket areas, a modified Widman flap approach would permit a one-time, thorough débridement. GTR can be considered, despite poor oral hygiene, if a critical tooth can be saved and the patient recognizes the risk of continued poor oral hygiene.

Additional Readings

Carranza FA Jr, Newman MG. Clinical periodontology. 8th ed. Philadelphia: WB Saunders; 1996. p. 565.

Genco RJ, Goldman HM, Cohen DW. Contemporary periodontics. St. Louis: Mosby; 1991. p. 626.

Grant DA, Stern IB, Listgarten MA. Periodontics. St. Louis: Mosby; 1988. p. 602.

Lindhe J. Textbook of clinical periodontology. 2nd ed. Copenhagen: Munksgaard; 1989. p. 328.

Schluger S et al. Periodontal diseases. 2nd ed. Philadelphia: Lea & Febiger; 1990. p. 461.

Periodontitis patient for INITIAL THERAPY EVALUATION

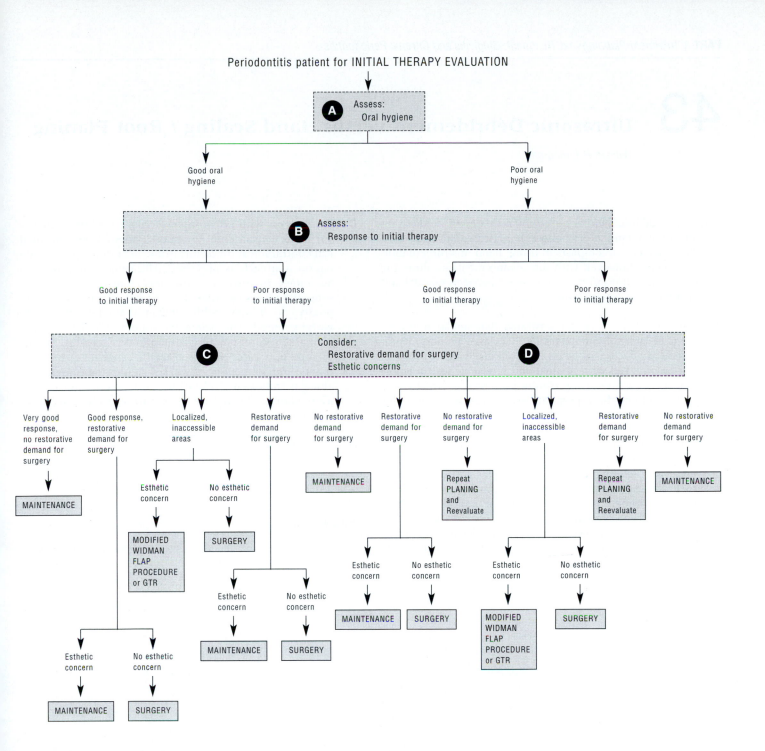

A Assess:
Oral hygiene

Good oral hygiene

Poor oral hygiene

B Assess:
Response to initial therapy

Good response to initial therapy

Poor response to initial therapy

Good response to initial therapy

Poor response to initial therapy

C **D** Consider:
Restorative demand for surgery
Esthetic concerns

Very good response, no restorative demand for surgery

Good response, restorative demand for surgery

Localized, inaccessible areas

Restorative demand for surgery

No restorative demand for surgery

Restorative demand for surgery

No restorative demand for surgery

Localized, inaccessible areas

Restorative demand for surgery

No restorative demand for surgery

MAINTENANCE

Esthetic concern

No esthetic concern

MAINTENANCE

Repeat PLANING and Reevaluate

Repeat PLANING and Reevaluate

MAINTENANCE

MODIFIED WIDMAN FLAP PROCEDURE or GTR

SURGERY

Esthetic concern

No esthetic concern

Esthetic concern

No esthetic concern

Esthetic concern

No esthetic concern

Esthetic concern

No esthetic concern

MAINTENANCE

SURGERY

MAINTENANCE

SURGERY

MODIFIED WIDMAN FLAP PROCEDURE or GTR

SURGERY

Esthetic concern

No esthetic concern

MAINTENANCE

SURGERY

43 Ultrasonic Débridement versus Hand Scaling / Root Planing

William P. Lundergan

Periodontal débridement is an essential treatment modality in the control of inflammatory periodontal disease. This procedure has been largely accomplished using hand instrumentation (curets/scalers); however, with the advancements in ultrasonic technology, the clinician must now select between manual and power-driven instrumentation.

A Clinical studies have demonstrated that similar improvement in clinical parameters (ie, decreased probing depth, increased attachment levels, reduced bleeding on probing) can be achieved with manual and ultrasonic instrumentation. Therefore, patient preference should play a major role in determining the appropriate form of instrumentation for any given patient.

B For patients who strongly prefer ultrasonic over manual instrumentation, the procedure can be completed with ultrasonic débridement alone as long as adequate time is spent to thoroughly débride the exposed root surfaces. Hand instrumentation alone would be indicated if ultrasonic instrumentation is medically contraindicated (ie, owing to a cardiac pacemaker or some infectious diseases). Ultrasonic instrumentation does carry an increased risk for creating contaminated aerosols.

C For patients with no strong preference for ultrasonic versus hand instrumentation (most patients), and no medical contraindication to ultrasonic débridement, a combination approach is preferred. Ultrasonics may offer an advantage in instrumenting deep, narrow pockets and some furcations (ie, Class II and Class III), using contemporary tip designs with smaller diameter and longer working length. Ultrasonic instrumentation does carry an increased risk for creating contaminated aerosols. Manual therapy may offer increased tactile sense for instrumentation and detection of caries. Hand instrumentation alone is indicated if ultrasonic instrumentation is medically contraindicated (ie, owing to a cardiac pacemaker or some infectious diseases).

D For patients who strongly prefer hand instrumentation, ultrasonic therapy should be considered for deep, narrow pockets and Class II / Class III furcation involvements. Hand instrumentation should be used at all other indicated sites.

Additional Reading

Position paper. Sonic and ultrasonic scalers in periodontics. J Periodontol 2000;71:1792.

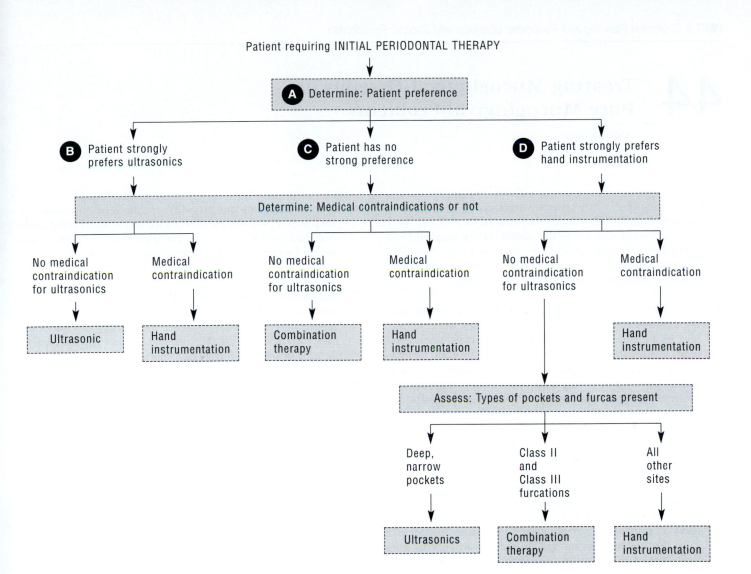

Patient requiring INITIAL PERIODONTAL THERAPY

A Determine: Patient preference

B Patient strongly prefers ultrasonics

C Patient has no strong preference

D Patient strongly prefers hand instrumentation

Determine: Medical contraindications or not

No medical contraindication for ultrasonics → Ultrasonic

Medical contraindication → Hand instrumentation

No medical contraindication for ultrasonics → Combination therapy

Medical contraindication → Hand instrumentation

No medical contraindication for ultrasonics

Medical contraindication → Hand instrumentation

Assess: Types of pockets and furcas present

Deep, narrow pockets → Ultrasonics

Class II and Class III furcations → Combination therapy

All other sites → Hand instrumentation

44 Treating Mucogingival-Osseous or Pure Mucogingival Problems

Walter B. Hall

After determining that periodontal surgery is needed, the dentist or periodontist (to whom the patient may have been referred) first must determine the nature of the surgical problem. Periodontal surgical procedures may be regarded as pure mucogingival procedures or mucogingival-osseous procedures, although the differences are less important today.

A Pure mucogingival procedures include those whose goals are gingival augmentation when inadequate attached gingiva is present. These procedures (from most versatile to least) include the following: connective tissue graft, free gingival graft, and pedicle grafts. Ridge augmentation is a procedure used when no teeth are involved to create a better formed, more esthetic ridge on which to construct a bridge.

The dentist must determine whether recession is active in an area of inadequate gingiva, especially areas with less than 2 mm of attached gingiva. Earlier recordings, photographs, and old study models are more useful than the patient's impressions, although the latter may be all that is available. If recession can be documented as active, gingival augmentation is recommended. If not, the dentist must decide whether proposed orthodontic or restorative treatment requires gingival augmentation. If so, the dentist must discuss the advantages and disadvantages of augmentation with the patient and record the decisions made. If the patient decides not to undergo gingival augmentation or if the orthodontic or restorative treatment does not indicate an immediate need for augmentation, the area may be maintained and a connective tissue graft for root coverage may be used if recession occurs.

B Mucogingival-osseous problems are the result of inflammatory periodontal diseases that cause loss of attachment, bone loss, and pocket formation. These problems demand attention before restoration or orthodontics. Regaining lost attachment is the most desirable goal.

C Guided tissue regeneration (GTR) has been a predictable procedure in the presence of Class II furcation that probe more than 3 mm horizontally between roots (less so for "through-and-through" or Class III furcations), three-walled osseous defects, or osseous craters (two-walled defects).

D When lesions not predictably amenable to new attachment procedures are present, the dentist should consider the desirability of pocket-elimination surgery before restoration or orthodontics—or in some instances (eg, uprighting a tooth), after orthodontics. GTR often is a better alternative. If the problem is relatively minimal and the patient demonstrably motivated, maintenance with frequent root planing alone may be the best option.

Additional Readings

Carranza FA Jr, Newman MG. Clinical periodontology. 8th ed. Philadelphia: WB Saunders; 1996. p. 568.

Hall WB, Lundergan W. Free gingival grafts: current indications and techniques. Dent Clin North Am 1993;37:227.

Schluger S et al. Periodontal diseases. 2nd ed. Philadelphia: Lea & Febiger; 1990. p. 334.

Townsend C, Ammons WF, van-Bellen G. A longitudinal study comparing apically repositioned flaps with and without osseous surgery. Int J Periodont Res Dent 1985;5:11.

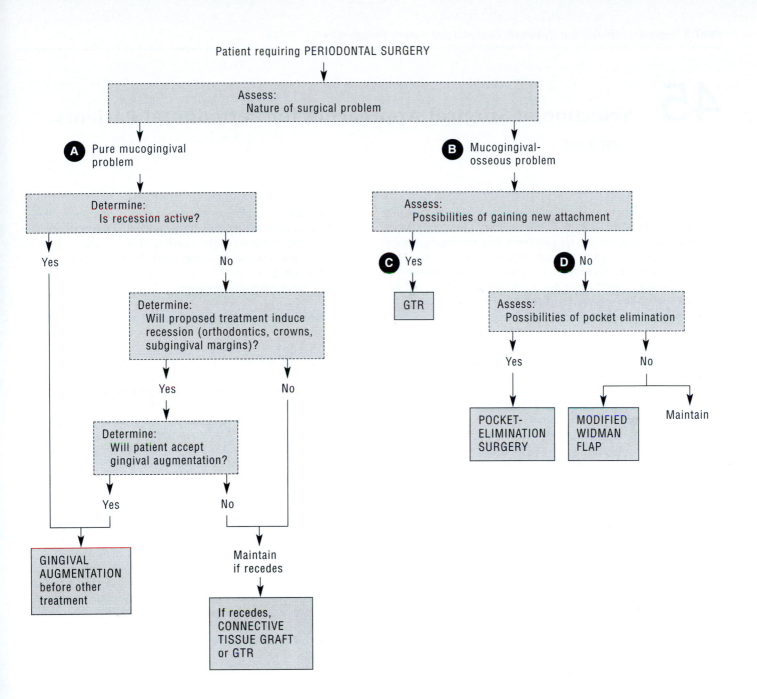

Patient requiring PERIODONTAL SURGERY

Assess:
Nature of surgical problem

A Pure mucogingival problem

B Mucogingival-osseous problem

Determine:
Is recession active?

Yes

No

Determine:
Will proposed treatment induce recession (orthodontics, crowns, subgingival margins)?

Yes

No

Determine:
Will patient accept gingival augmentation?

Yes

No

GINGIVAL AUGMENTATION before other treatment

Maintain if recedes

If recedes, CONNECTIVE TISSUE GRAFT or GTR

Assess:
Possibilities of gaining new attachment

C Yes

D No

GTR

Assess:
Possibilities of pocket elimination

Yes

No

POCKET-ELIMINATION SURGERY

MODIFIED WIDMAN FLAP

Maintain

45 Selection of Surgical Approaches for Periodontal Patients

Walter B. Hall

Discuss with a patient the probability of the need for periodontal surgery if indicated during initial treatment planning. Many patients with complex dental problems require mucogingival-osseous surgery or guided tissue regeneration (GTR). Most patients have been affected by adult (chrome) periodontitis and have a number of teeth with pocket depth, bone loss, and loss of attachment. The character of the bone loss determines the type of surgery indicated.

A   First, the dentist must decide whether the problem involves horizontal bone loss, vertical loss, or mixed loss (some teeth with horizontal bone loss and some with vertical bone loss). If the patient has only horizontal bone loss, the severity of loss and number of severely involved teeth are the factors that determine the treatment plan. If many teeth are severely affected, mucogingival-osseous surgery is contraindicated; however, GTR occurring when several adjacent teeth are involved with vertical bone loss is a promising means of dealing with severe problems. The restorative plan is worked out determining which, if any, teeth can be used. If the horizontal bone loss is not severe or generalized, pocket-elimination surgery performed with osteoplasty to create the most readily maintainable contours may be best. Otherwise, maintenance or extraction should be considered.

B   If vertical bone loss is involved, the types of osseous defects present determine the type of surgery indicated. Shallow one-walled defects should be managed with pocket-elimination surgery and osseous resection (ostec-

tomy and osteoplasty). If a one-walled defect is moderate to deep, consider the value of the individual tooth to the overall treatment plan. If the tooth is of little value, extraction is the best approach. If the tooth is critical to the overall treatment plan, use GTR or GTR with concomitant or second-stage osseous resection.

C   If two-walled defects are present, the surgical approach depends on whether the defects are craters (defects between adjacent teeth where facial and lingual cortical plates remain) of the less common type that affects only one tooth in which a facial or lingual cortical plate and a wall against the adjacent tooth remain. If a crater is present and is a shallow defect, pocket-elimination surgery with osseous resection is best (Figure 45-1). If the crater is moderate to deep, use GTR (Figure 45-2). If the two-walled defect affects only a single tooth, its value to the overall treatment plan determines whether GTR or extraction is best.

D   If a three-walled defect is present, its depth and horizontal width from the root to osseous crest determine the surgical approach. A narrow defect (less than 1 mm horizontal from the root to osseous crest) is amenable to a Prichard fill technique, wherein total débridement is followed by bone fill and new attachment on a predictable basis. If the defect is wide (more than 1 mm horizontal from the root to osseous crest) and moderate to deep, GTR is a predictable means of gaining new attachment. If the defect is wide and shallow, pocket elimination with osseous resection is best.

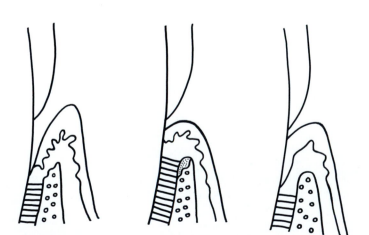

Figure 45-1 A shallow, two-walled infrabony crater is treated by osseous resection.

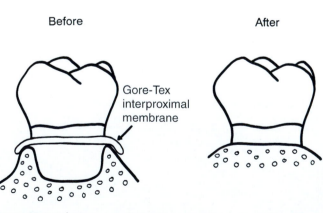

Figure 45-2 A deep, two-walled infrabony crater is treated by GTR.

---

*New World Health Organization terminology.

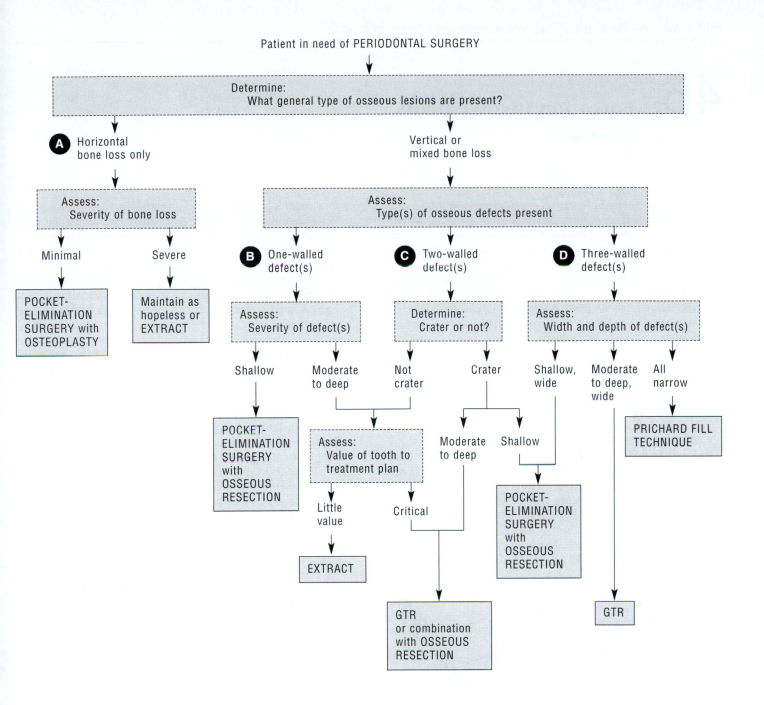

Patient in need of PERIODONTAL SURGERY

Determine:
What general type of osseous lesions are present?

A Horizontal bone loss only

Vertical or mixed bone loss

Assess:
Severity of bone loss

Minimal

Severe

POCKET-ELIMINATION SURGERY with OSTEOPLASTY

Maintain as hopeless or EXTRACT

Assess:
Type(s) of osseous defects present

B One-walled defect(s)

C Two-walled defect(s)

D Three-walled defect(s)

Assess:
Severity of defect(s)

Determine:
Crater or not?

Assess:
Width and depth of defect(s)

Shallow

Moderate to deep

Not crater

Crater

Shallow, wide

Moderate to deep, wide

All narrow

POCKET-ELIMINATION SURGERY with OSSEOUS RESECTION

Assess:
Value of tooth to treatment plan

Moderate to deep

Shallow

PRICHARD FILL TECHNIQUE

Little value

Critical

POCKET-ELIMINATION SURGERY with OSSEOUS RESECTION

EXTRACT

GTR or combination with OSSEOUS RESECTION

GTR

Additional Readings

Carranza FA Jr, Newman MG. Clinical periodontology. 8th ed. Philadelphia: WB Saunders; 1996. p. 566.

Knowles JW. Results of periodontal treatment related to pocket depth and attachment level: eight years. J Periodontol 1979;50:225.

Nevins M, Mellonig JT. Peridontal therapy: clinical approaches and evidence of success. Chicago: Quintessence Publishing; 1998. p. 174, 249.

Pihlstrom BL, McHugh RB, Oliphant TH et al. Comparison of surgical and non-surgical treatment of periodontal disease. A review of current studies and additional results after 6$^{1}/_{2}$ years. J Clin Periodontol 1983;10:524.

Pihlstrom BL, Ortiz Campos C, McHugh RB. A randomized four year study of periodontal therapy. J Periodontol 1981;52:227.

Sato N. Periodontal surgery: a clinical atlas. Tokyo: Quintessence Publishing; 2000. p. 23.

46 Furcation Involvements

Walter B. Hall

The type and severity of furcation involvements on molar teeth represent a critical concern in treatment planning, particularly when surgery is being considered. Furcation involvements are categorized as follows: Class I, incipient; Class II, definite; or Class III, "through and through" (Figure 46-1).

Each furcation should be explored with a pigtail type of explorer, or furca-finder. Insert the instrument into the furcation and move it laterally and coronally to determine whether the instrument can slip out. The type of furcation involvement is recorded on the chart, and the options for treatment are then considered.

A An incipient (Class I) furcation exists when the instrument slips out of the furcation when moved anteriorly, posteriorly, or coronally or in proximal furcations when moved facially, lingually, and coronally. This furcation is recorded with the symbol △ placed appropriately on the tooth diagram. Such furcations are unlikely to influence the treatment plan but should be documented. If the incipient involvement is deep and does not produce a definite catch because adjacent roots are fused, guided tissue regeneration (GTR) (see Chapter 79) should be considered.

B A definite (Class II) furcation exists when a definite catch prevents removal of the furca-finder coronally or laterally but definitely stops before going through and through to another furcation opening. This furcation is recorded with the symbol △ placed in the appropriate furcation area on the tooth diagram. The severity of the involvement horizontally determines the best treatment option. If the furca-finder can be advanced less than 3 mm horizontally into the defect, osseous resection and pocket elimination represent a good treatment option. If the furca-finder can be advanced 3 mm or more into the defect, GTR is a predictable approach for regaining lost attachment and creating a maintainable situation. Often, the horizontal measurement is recorded in millimeters apical to the symbol of the chart.

C A "through-and-through" (Class III) furcation exists when the furca-finder is inserted and appears to connect directly with one or more other furcations. This furcation is recorded by placing the symbol ▲ in each of the appropriate furcation areas on the tooth diagram; therefore, more than one ▲ symbol must be used on a tooth to document a Class III situation. If a tooth with a Class III furcation is not critical to the overall treatment plan, it should be extracted. If its retention does not jeopardize the overall treatment plan, it may be maintained. GTR has become a predictable treatment for such teeth only recently. If the tooth is critical and its retention in a maintainable and useful manner can be achieved by hemisection or root amputation, such an approach, although expensive, often can significantly improve the overall treatment plan for a complex situation.

Additional Readings

Carranza FA Jr, Newman MG. Clinical periodontology. 8th ed. Philadelphia: WB Saunders; 1996. p 640.

Genco RJ, Goldman HM, Cohen DW. Contemporary periodontics. St. Louis: Mosby; 1990. p. 344, 354, 409.

Hemp SE, Nyman S, Lindhe J. Treatment of multi-rooted teeth: results after 5 years. J Clin Periodontol 1975;2:126.

Lindhe J. Textbook of clinical periodontology. 2nd ed, Copenhagen: Munksgaard; 1989. p. 515.

Schluger S et al. Periodontal diseases. 2nd ed, Philadelphia: Lea & Febiger; 1990. p. 541.

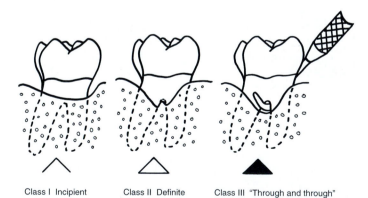

Class I Incipient   Class II Definite   Class III "Through and through"

Figure 46-1 Classes and appearance of furcation involvements, and their respective symbol.

Patient with a COMPLEX DENTAL PROBLEM AND A MOLAR WITH A FURCATION INVOLVEMENT

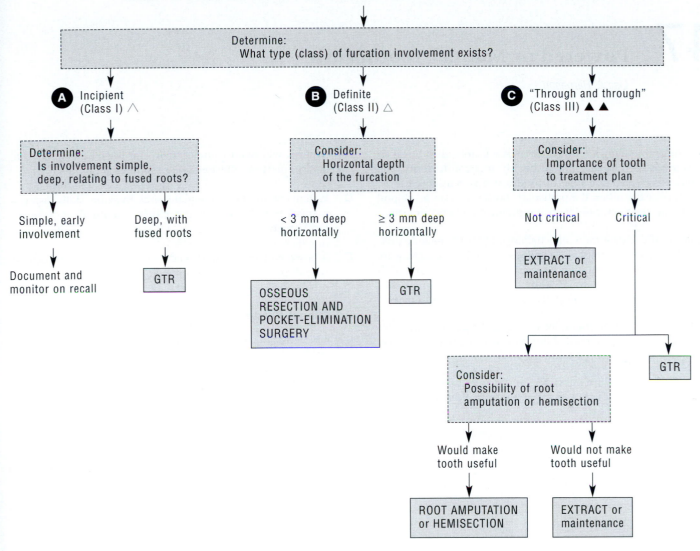

Determine:
What type (class) of furcation involvement exists?

A Incipient
(Class I) △

Determine:
Is involvement simple,
deep, relating to fused roots?

Simple, early
involvement

Deep, with
fused roots

Document and
monitor on recall

GTR

B Definite
(Class II) △

Consider:
Horizontal depth
of the furcation

< 3 mm deep
horizontally

≥ 3 mm deep
horizontally

OSSEOUS
RESECTION AND
POCKET-ELIMINATION
SURGERY

GTR

C "Through and through"
(Class III) ▲ ▲

Consider:
Importance of tooth
to treatment plan

Not critical

Critical

EXTRACT or
maintenance

GTR

Consider:
Possibility of root
amputation or hemisection

Would make
tooth useful

Would not make
tooth useful

ROOT AMPUTATION
or HEMISECTION

EXTRACT or
maintenance

47

Powered or Manual Toothbrush

Lisa A. Harpenau

When recommending a toothbrush, many factors must be taken into account such as periodontal health, manual dexterity, and patient interest. No one type of toothbrush is considered to be superior over the other. If a particular toothbrush can be helpful to a patient, then it should be recommended and encouraged.

A Physically and/or mentally challenged patients include individuals with a variety of disabilities. Within this category are persons with debilitating diseases (such as arthritis) and ill patients under the supervision of a caregiver. Young children who lack brushing skills should also be considered.

B Physically and/or mentally challenged patients and children with compromised ability to use a manual toothbrush should use a powered toothbrush.

C Individuals who are physically and/or mentally challenged but are able to use a manual toothbrush and all other

patients will need to have their oral hygiene evaluated to determine their effectiveness in removing plaque.

D Patients who have adequate oral hygiene skills using a manual toothbrush can use either a manual or powered toothbrush.

E A powered toothbrush should be recommended for patients who display poor plaque removal.

Additional Readings

Hall WB. Decision making in periodontology. 3rd ed. St. Louis: Mosby; 1998. p. 92.

Newman MG, Takei H, Carranza FA Jr. Clinical periodontology. 9th ed. Philadelphia: WB Saunders; 2002. p. 652.

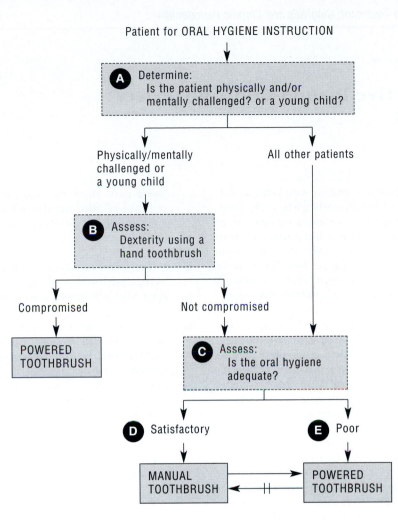

Patient for ORAL HYGIENE INSTRUCTION

A Determine:
Is the patient physically and/or
mentally challenged? or a young child?

Physically/mentally
challenged or
a young child

All other patients

B Assess:
Dexterity using a
hand toothbrush

Compromised

Not compromised

POWERED
TOOTHBRUSH

C Assess:
Is the oral hygiene
adequate?

D Satisfactory

E Poor

MANUAL
TOOTHBRUSH

POWERED
TOOTHBRUSH

48 Adjunctive Plaque-Control Devices

Walter B. Hall

All patients should use a toothbrush, usually employing a sulcular brushing technique. Mechanical toothbrushes (eg, Sonicare, Oral B/Braun) may be more effective for many patients. In addition, adjunctive devices can help clean interproximal areas. Ideally, all patients should also use floss daily; however, some groups of patients are unable to manipulate floss but may be able to use devices that require less dexterity. When disease is advanced, interproximal brushes are more effective than floss.

A Patients with a variety of handicaps are unable to use floss, usually because of compromised dexterity. Physical handicaps that restrict arm and hand movement may be of long-term or short-term duration. Arthritis often creates problems with finger movement. Many older patients lose dexterity. Many mentally handicapped people, however, can be taught to use floss, although the learning process may be long and tedious. For the handicapped who cannot use handheld floss, a floss holder may permit its use. Thin birchwood sticks shaped to fit interproximal spaces are easily manipulated and require little dexterity. In northern Europe, these sticks often are used instead of floss and achieve good removal of interproximal plaque. Stimudents are less satisfactory because of their much larger dimensions. Interproximal brushes, especially those with short handles, are excellent devices for the removal of interproximal plaque. They are particularly appropriate for patients with loss of attachment and/or poor dexterity.

B Not all patients who are able to use floss are willing to do so regularly. Also, some localized situations are better managed with adjunctive devices (Figures 48-1 and 48-2).

C Where roots are close together, certain devices cannot be inserted into the available space. Where space is adequate, interproximal brushes, especially those with short handles, are most effective and easy to use. The Perio Aide (a round toothpick-holding device) may be quite effective; however, it is difficult to use and can cause damage if it is pressed into pockets or is broken off. Superfloss (dental tape with thickened areas at regular intervals) may be effective where plain floss is not; however, it must be used with a shoeshine approach, which can produce "floss cuts" and tooth abrasion. For situations in which root proximity makes these devices

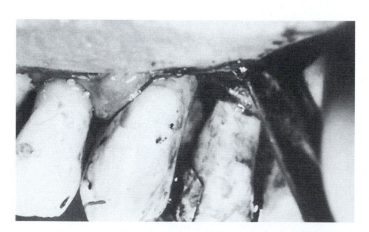

Figure 48-1 A deep fluting in the root structure of a maxillary first molar that cannot be cleaned by flossing.

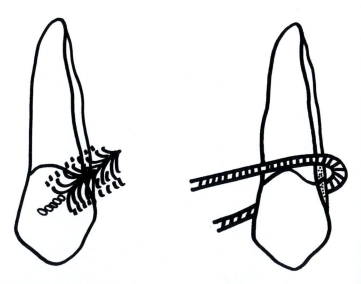

Figure 48-2 Various adjunctive devices may be used to clean hard-to-reach areas.

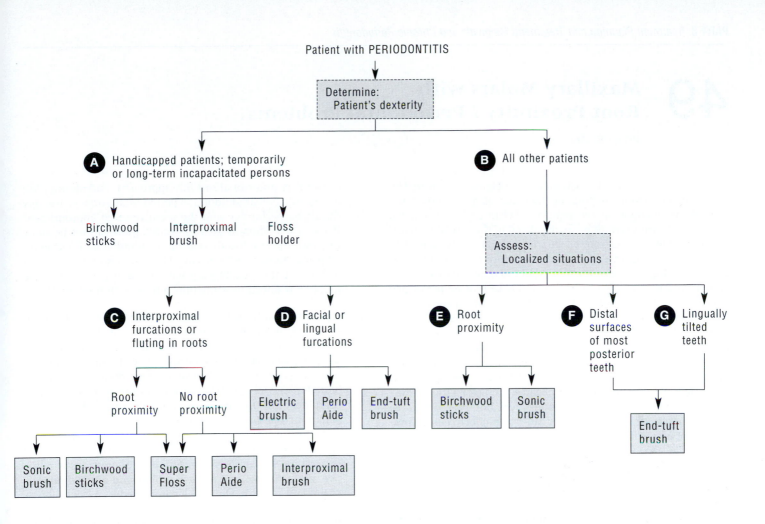

Patient with PERIODONTITIS

Determine: Patient's dexterity

A Handicapped patients; temporarily or long-term incapacitated persons

- Birchwood sticks
- Interproximal brush
- Floss holder

B All other patients

Assess: Localized situations

C Interproximal furcations or fluting in roots

- Root proximity
  - Sonic brush
  - Birchwood sticks
  - Super Floss
- No root proximity
  - Super Floss
  - Perio Aide
  - Interproximal brush

D Facial or lingual furcations

- Electric brush
- Perio Aide
- End-tuft brush

E Root proximity

- Birchwood sticks
- Sonic brush

F Distal surfaces of most posterior teeth

- End-tuft brush

G Lingually tilted teeth

- End-tuft brush

---

unusable or dangerous, the thin, birchwood sticks may be effective if furcations are not too badly involved.

D The Sonicare brush, a mechanical brush that moves at sonic vibration speed, has proven especially effective; the Braun brush is equally effective. The end-tuft brush is a single-tufted brush designed to clean anatomically difficult areas such as the distal surfaces of the most distal teeth or isolated teeth serving as removable partial abutments.

E Where roots are close together or irregularly aligned, the thin birchwood sticks are most effective and easily used. They are readily available in northern Europe but difficult to obtain in North America or elsewhere.

F An end-tuft toothbrush may be purchased for the distal surfaces of the most posterior teeth, or such a toothbrush can be made easily with an old brush. All the tufts are cut off close to the handle, except for the last few nearest the end of the handle. After these tufts are cut off, the remaining ones can be applied to the distal surface of the most

posterior teeth without the missing tufts pushing against the occlusal surface and restricting contact on the distal surface.

G Many patients have difficulty removing plaque from the lingual surfaces of lingually tilted teeth for much the same reason that the distal surfaces of the most posterior teeth are difficult to clean. The end-tuft brush may also be used quite effectively in these situations.

Additional Readings

Carranza FA Jr, Newman MG. Clinical periodontology. 8th ed. Philadelphia: WB Saunders; 1996. p. 551.

Gjermo P, Flotra L. The effect of different methods of interdental cleaning. J Periodont Res 1970;5:230.

Gjermo P, Flotra L. The plaque-removing effect of dental floss and toothpicks: a group comparison study. J Periodont Res 1969;4:170.

Lindhe J. Textbook of clinical periodontology. 2nd ed. Copenhagen: Munksgaard; 1989. p. 346.

Schluger S et al. Periodontal diseases. 2nd ed. Philadelphia: Lea & Febiger; 1990. p. 362.

49 Maxillary Molars with Root Proximity / Periodontal Problems

Walter B. Hall

Maxillary molar teeth with periodontal problems complicated by root proximity (roots so close together that plaque removal and root planing cannot be accomplished because plaque-removal devices and curets cannot be manipulated in the available space) are a commonly encountered puzzle that has to be solved in planning the treatment. A surgical procedure that would eliminate pocketing but leave an area where plaque removal by the patient and root planing by the therapist cannot be performed effectively is not a wise choice for therapy. Extraction or root amputation on one or both of the molars can create a sound, maintainable, functional unit, but this does involve extensive treatment including endodontics and/or prosthodontics as well as periodontal treatment. Such treatment is expensive and must be within the patient's means. Guided tissue regeneration (GTR) is not feasible if root proximity negates the possibility of thorough débridement of the periodontal defect; however, if the area can be thoroughly débrided, GTR can be an effective and comparatively inexpensive approach (Figure 49-1).

A   If the defect between the two molars can be thoroughly débrided with a curet or new thin ultrasonic tip after flap displacement, GTR is the best option.

B   If GTR is not feasible, the endodontic status of the two molars should be determined next. If no pulpal problem exists, a determination should be made whether root canal therapy and a room amputation can be done. If so, the restorability of the teeth and their value to the overall treatment plan should be assessed. If restoration is feasible and useful, and the periodontal problem can be resolved by root amputation on either or both of the molars (and the patient

consents to and can afford this approach), endodontics followed by root amputation / periodontal surgical therapy should be performed and the teeth restored appropriately. If root canal therapy or root amputation cannot be done (eg, root tips are fused) or if the restorative and periodontal problems cannot be resolved by root amputation, either or both of the molars may have to be extracted and the problem resolved prosthodontically or with implants.

C   If either or both of the molars also have endodontic problems, the possibility of performing successful root canal therapy should be evaluated first. If they can be treated, the sequence of decision making would be the same as in "B," namely: (1) Can a root amputation be done? (2) Can the periodontal problem be resolved and the teeth restored to usefulness in the overall treatment plan? (3) Can the patient accept and afford this approach?

If the answer to each question is positive, proceed with endodontics, root amputation / periodontal surgery, and restoration. If the answer to any of the questions is negative, extraction of one or both molars and a prosthodontic or implant solution should be considered.

D   If one or both of the molars have existing endodontics, the adequacy of the existing endodontics (including "cracked tooth" signs or symptoms) should be evaluated first. If the endodontics are satisfactory, and no vertical root fractures can be detected, the sequence of decision making would be the same as in "C." If the answer to each question is positive and no endodontic treatment is needed, root amputation and elimination of the periodontal defects should be performed and followed by appropriate restoration. If the answer to each question is positive and the existing endodontics is unsatisfactory, but it can be redone successfully or the problem is around the root to be amputated, necessary endodontic retreatment followed by root amputation / periodontal surgery and restoration should be planned. If any answers are negative, extraction and a prosthodontic or implant alternative should be used.

Additional Readings

Carranza FA Jr, Newman MG. Clinical periodontology. 8th ed. Philadelphia: WB Saunders; 1996. p. 732.

Genco RJ, Goldman HM, Cohen DW. Contemporary periodontics. St. Louis: Mosby; 1990. p. 582, 589.

Hall WB. Periodontal preparation of the mouth for restoration. Dent Clin North Am 1980;24:197.

Hall WB. Removal of third molars: a periodontal viewpoint. In: McDonald RE et al, editors. Current therapy in dentistry. St. Louis: Mosby; 1980. p. 228.

Nevins M, Mellonig JT. Periodontal therapy: clinical approaches and evidence of success. Tokyo: Quintessence Publishing; 1998. p. 221.

Schluger S et al. Periodontal diseases. 2nd ed. Philadelphia: Lea & Febiger; 1990. p. 102, 343, 511.

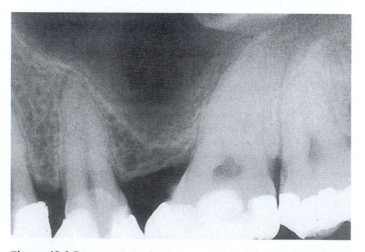

Figure 49-1 Root proximity between second and third molars appears to jeopardize access to treat or maintain the distal furcation involvement successfully on the second molar. Reproduced with permission from Hall WB, Roberts WE, LaBarre EE. Decision making in dental treatment planning, St. Louis: Mosby; 1994.

Patient with MAXILLARY MOLARS WITH ROOT PROXIMITY/PERIODONTAL PROBLEMS

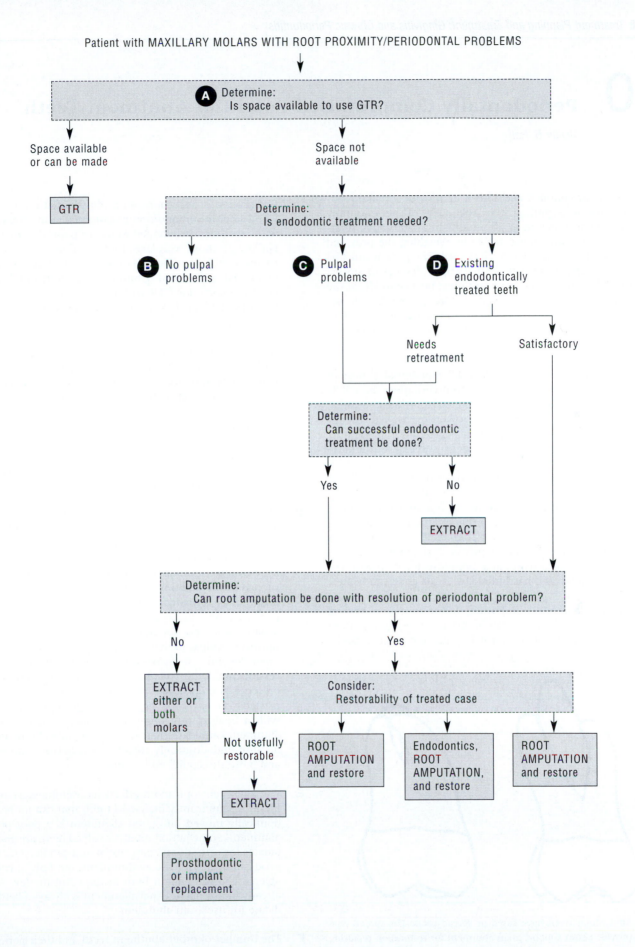

50 Periodontally Compromised Potential Abutment Teeth

Walter B. Hall

One of the most complex decisions a dentist must make regularly involves determining the adequacy of periodontally involved teeth to function as abutments in a restorative treatment plan. The dentist must decide by weighing the pros and cons of each of the many factors involved. The patient must be informed of and able to cope with various degrees of uncertainty in such complex decisions and must be able to afford the cost of the whole treatment plan before proceeding. If the patient elects not to proceed, the dentist must advise the patient of the probable consequences of this decision. Such complex situations require careful documentation.

A The status of the attachment of the potential abutment tooth is extremely important. A tooth with more than 50% loss of attachment (LOA) is a poor risk as an abutment; however, if that tooth has a narrow, three-walled osseous defect, it is a candidate for a bone regeneration procedure. There is a reasonable likelihood of success sufficient to change the prognosis for the tooth. In situations in which guided tissue regeneration (GTR) has a strong probability of success (see Chapters 78 and 79), a tooth that would be a poor abutment can be converted to one that may make a good-to-excellent abutment. If this situation does not exist, and the tooth has lost more than half its support, it is unlikely to be a good abutment risk. If the tooth has moderate LOA, it has a reasonable prognosis for successful use as an abutment. If it has little LOA, it is a good candidate.

B Root form is another important factor to assess. Several radiographs of the tooth can be used to give an important conceptualization of the form for the root (Figure 50-1).

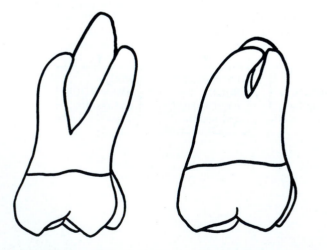

Figure 50-1 Molar teeth have fused or spread roots. The spread type usually provide better support as an abutment for restoration replacing a missing tooth.

Exploration of furcations on a multirooted tooth can provide useful information on its potential cleansability. Teeth with small or cone-shaped roots are poor abutments compared with those with large roots (or flared roots on multirooted teeth). If a molar has a Class II furcation involvement that is involved 3 mm or more horizontally, it is a good candidate for GTR with eventual use as an abutment (see Chapter 88). If a molar has a "through-and-through" involvement, GTR may be used or root amputation or hemisection may make its remaining parts useful as an abutment if the patient can afford that approach (see Chapter 72). A molar with minimal furcation involvement and flared roots, however, is a good abutment candidate, even where pocket- elimination surgery is used.

C The status of the crown of the potential abutment area is important. If it is badly broken down, it is a poorer candidate than if it can be restored readily. Crown lengthening can improve the potential restorability of some poorer candidates (see Chapter 149).

D The pulpal status affects the potential of a tooth to be used as an abutment. If the tooth has been endodontically treated but either requires further treatment (ie, apicoectomy) or retreatment or appears to have a cracked root, its usefulness as an abutment depends on the likelihood of success of the additional treatment. If its root is cracked or it cannot be retreated, it is not a potential abutment. If the earlier endodontic procedure appears satisfactory, the tooth usually is a good potential abutment. If the tooth has an untreated pulpal problem, its potential for use as an abutment depends on factors affecting the probability for successful endodontic treatment (ie, accessibility of root canals, presence of pulp stones, internal resorption). If the tooth is treatable, it has good potential as an abutment. A tooth with a healthy pulp, however, is almost always a better abutment candidate than is an endodontically treated one because endodontically treated teeth become more brittle and more susceptible to fractures.

E The alignment of a tooth affects its usefulness as an abutment. A significantly malposed tooth that cannot be orthodontically moved into good alignment is a poor potential abutment. Some periodontally involved teeth are good candidates for orthodontic movement and can become fair-to-good candidates for use as abutments, but only at considerable cost to the patient both in time and money. A tooth already in normal or usual alignment is always a better candidate for use as an abutment.

F The number of other abutment teeth and their periodontal statuses affect the potential usability of the tooth in question

Patient with a PERIODONTALLY COMPROMISED POTENTIAL ABUTMENT TOOTH

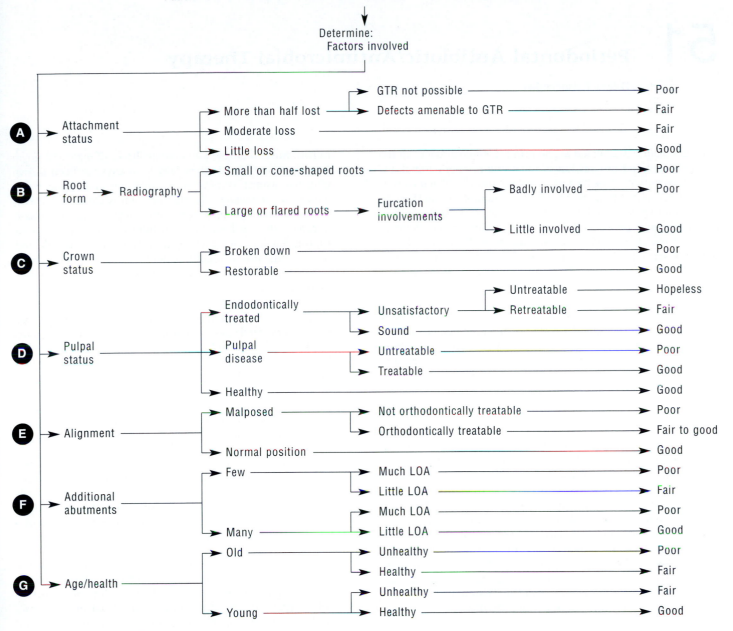

as an abutment. If few other potential abutments are present and they have much LOA, the tooth in question is a poorer candidate for use as an abutment because more will be demanded of it. If the other potential abutments, although few, have little LOA, the tooth in question is a better candidate. If there are many additional potential abutment teeth, but all or most have significant LOA, the potential use of the tooth in question is less. If the other potential abutments have lost little attachment, the tooth in question has better possibilities for use as an abutment.

G   Other factors (such as plaque-removal skills of the patient and regularity of dental care) must be weighed by the dentist and patient in deciding the potential for a periodontally involved tooth to be used as an abutment. Age and health are two essential factors, however. In one sense, older patients have poorer prognoses than younger patients

because their healing capabilities may be lower. In another sense, older patients have better prognoses in that their teeth and dental work will not have to last as long on the average. A potential abutment tooth that is periodontally compromised in an otherwise healthy patient has a better prognosis in general than does such a tooth in an unhealthy mouth.

Additional Readings

Grant DA, Stern IB, Listgarten MA. Periodontics. 6th ed. St. Louis: Mosby; 1988. p. 982.

Hall WB. Periodontal preparation of the mouth for restoration. Dent Clin North Am 1980;24:195.

Schluger S et al. Periodontal diseases. 2nd ed. Philadelphia: Lea & Febiger; 1990. p. 341.

51

Periodontal Antibiotic/Antimicrobial Therapy

William P. Lundergan

Bacterial plaque is accepted as the primary etiologic agent in the establishment and progression of inflammatory periodontal disease. Recognition of the bacterial etiology has stimulated considerable interest in antimicrobial agents as adjuncts to mechanical periodontal therapy. Today, antibiotics and antimicrobial rinses have a role in periodontal therapy as an adjunct to débridement, but their use should not be indiscriminate and it is not without potential hazards. The clinician should be thoroughly familiar with all of the potentially adverse reactions before prescribing or recommending any chemotherapeutic agent.

A Patients treated with antibiotic therapy should be closely monitored for therapeutic response and potential side effects. Patients who fail to respond to therapy may require a culture of the subgingival flora with evaluation of antibiotic sensitivity. Pretreatment and post-treatment microbiologic analysis may prove useful in monitoring therapeutic success.

B Periodontal abscess, periocoronitis, and necrotizing ulcerative gingivitis (NUG) are acute diseases often requiring emergency treatment. Treatment of the acute signs and symptoms is generally best accomplished with local débridement. Antibiotics are usually unnecessary, unless the patient is febrile, exhibits lymphadenopathy, is in danger of developing cellulitis, or does not respond to local débridement within 24 hours. If an antibiotic is indicated, amoxicillin or penicillin is the drug of choice. Cephalexin or clindamycin can be used if the infection is not responding in 24 to 48 hours. If the patient is allergic to penicillin, azithromycin or clindamycin are good alternatives. Metronidazole has been used in the treatment of NUG and necrotizing ulcerative periodontitis (NUP).

C Antibiotics generally offer no advantage over conventional periodontal therapy (ie, mechanical plaque control, root planing, elimination of secondary local factors, periodontal surgery, and maintenance) in the treatment of chronic periodontitis. Consider using local controlled delivery products (Actisite [tetracycline fibers], Arestin [minocycline microspheres], and Atridox [doxycycline gel]) as an adjunct to débridement in treating recurrent disease.

D Antibiotics can be useful adjuncts to conventional therapy in the treatment of aggressive and refractory periodontitis. Collection of subgingival microbial samples with antibiotic sensitivity testing should be considered. Tetracycline hydrochloride, doxycycline, metronidazole, clindamycin, ciprofloxacin, amoxicillin/clavulanic acid, metronidazole in combination with amoxicillin, and metronidazole in combination with ciprofloxacin have all been used. Although systemic antibiotics have been shown to be an effective adjunctive therapy in treating aggressive and refractory forms of periodontitis, optimal dosing regimens have not been deter-

mined. Metronidazole and amoxicillin (250 mg each) given in combination three times daily for 8 days has been shown effective against *Porphyremonas gingivalis* and *Actinobacillus actinomycetemcomitans*. Augmentin (amoxicillin and clavulanic acid) may be preferred to amoxicillin because it incorporates the β-lactamase inhibitor clavulanic acid. Ciprofloxacin is useful when enteric organisms are cultured, but it should not be used in patients who are under 18 years of age. Ciprofloxacin can also be given in combination with metronidazole (500 mg each) taken twice daily for 8 days. Clindamycin should be used with caution because of its association with pseudomembranous colitis, which can prove to be fatal. Locally controlled delivery of antibiotics can be considered for localized aggressive or refractory sites; however, few data are available for controlled delivery products in treating these forms of periodontal disease. Actisite (tetracycline fibers), Arestin (minocycline microspheres), and Atridox (doxycycline gel) are commercially available in the United States. PerioChip is another locally controlled delivery product that delivers the antiseptic chlorhexidine.

E NUP occurs as a more acute periodontal lesion characterized by tissue necrosis and sequestration. Treatment of such acute conditions can be augmented with metronidazole (250–500 mg) given three to four times daily for 7 days. The patient's physician should be consulted before antibiotic therapy is prescribed.

F Chemical plaque control represents an attractive adjunct to mechanical plaque control; thus several products are now being marketed as chemical plaque inhibitors. Current information suggests that some commercial mouth rinses and toothpastes can reduce plaque and decrease gingival inflammation. Supragingival and subgingival irrigation has been evaluated as an alternative mode of delivery for some of these mouth rinses. Irrigation has an apparent advantage over rinsing in that it increases the ability of the product to reach the subgingival flora. Compliance and the requirement for some level of patient dexterity are problems commonly associated with irrigation. Although these products can reduce gingival inflammation, little information is available regarding the use of these products as rinses or irrigants in preventing and treating periodontitis. Only Peridex (chlorhexidine gluconate) and Listerine (and generic formulations of Listerine), mouth rinses, and Total toothpaste (triclosan) have been accepted by the American Dental Association's Council on Dental Therapeutics as antiplaque/antigingivitis agents.

G Numerous studies have demonstrated the safety and effectiveness of chlorhexidine when used in the control of supragingival plaque and gingivitis. The most appropriate use of chlorhexidine seems to be as a short-term adjunct to

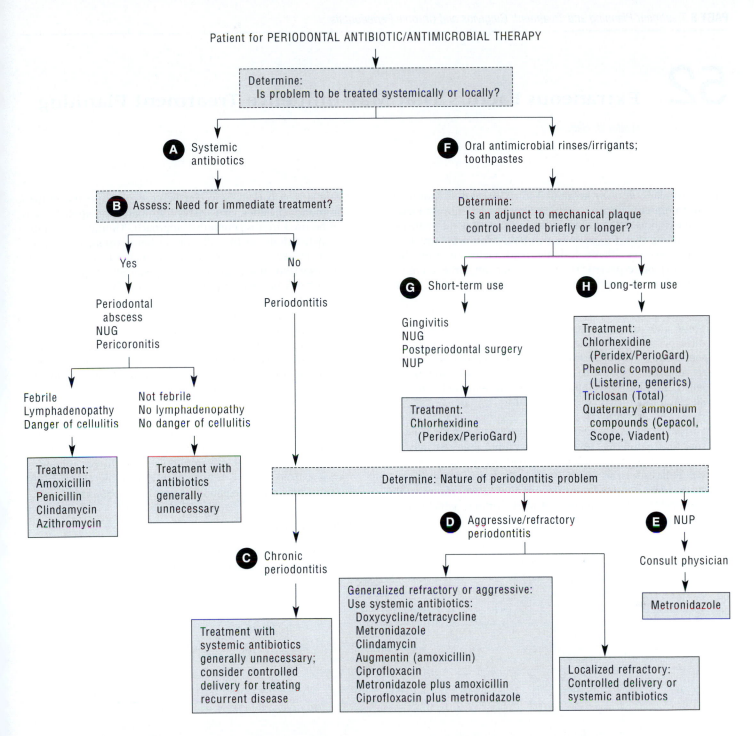

Patient for PERIODONTAL ANTIBIOTIC/ANTIMICROBIAL THERAPY

Determine:
Is problem to be treated systemically or locally?

A Systemic antibiotics

F Oral antimicrobial rinses/irrigants; toothpastes

B Assess: Need for immediate treatment?

Determine:
Is an adjunct to mechanical plaque control needed briefly or longer?

Yes

No

G Short-term use

H Long-term use

Periodontal abscess
NUG
Pericoronitis

Periodontitis

Gingivitis
NUG
Postperiodontal surgery
NUP

Treatment:
Chlorhexidine
(Peridex/PerioGard)
Phenolic compound
(Listerine, generics)
Triclosan (Total)
Quaternary ammonium
compounds (Cepacol,
Scope, Viadent)

Febrile
Lymphadenopathy
Danger of cellulitis

Not febrile
No lymphadenopathy
No danger of cellulitis

Treatment:
Chlorhexidine
(Peridex/PerioGard)

Treatment:
Amoxicillin
Penicillin
Clindamycin
Azithromycin

Treatment with
antibiotics
generally
unnecessary

Determine: Nature of periodontitis problem

D Aggressive/refractory periodontitis

E NUP

Consult physician

C Chronic periodontitis

Generalized refractory or aggressive:
Use systemic antibiotics:
Doxycycline/tetracycline
Metronidazole
Clindamycin
Augmentin (amoxicillin)
Ciprofloxacin
Metronidazole plus amoxicillin
Ciprofloxacin plus metronidazole

Metronidazole

Treatment with
systemic antibiotics
generally unnecessary;
consider controlled
delivery for treating
recurrent disease

Localized refractory:
Controlled delivery or
systemic antibiotics

mechanical plaque control. Short-term use of chlorhexidine during the initial healing phase after periodontal surgery may represent one useful application; gingival and dentinal sensitivity often hamper mechanical plaque-control efforts postsurgically. Treatment of NUG and NUP requires professional débridement followed by proper home care. Initially, because of gingival discomfort, proper mechanical plaque control is difficult for these patients to achieve. Short-term use of chlorhexidine during the treatment of NUG or NUP can represent another useful application.

H The clinician should evaluate carefully the risk-to-benefit ratio before recommending long-term use of Peridex or PerioGard (0.12% chlorhexidine). Stain, altered taste, and increased supragingival calculus can be expected. Stain is

especially a problem around composite restorations. Several other over-the-counter antimicrobial rinses are available, and they have shown some efficacy in reducing plaque and gingivitis. Most of these agents are also associated with varying degrees of tooth discoloration, and some cause a temporary burning sensation. Total toothpaste (triclosan) should also be considered for long-term use.

Additional Readings

Systemic antibiotics in periodontics. J Periodontal 1996;67:831.
Ciancio SG. Antiseptics and antibiotics as chemotherapeutic agents for periodontitis management. Compendium 2000;21:59.
The role of controlled drug delivery for periodontitis. J Periodontol 2000;71:125.

52 Extraneous Factors That May Influence Treatment Planning

Walter B. Hall

Treatment planning may be altered for nonscientific, nonmedical, and nondental reasons, which may not be entirely logical to the practitioner. When these issues surface, they may rule out the treatment that the practitioner feels would be the most effective; however, these strongly held views of individual patients must be respected. The practitioner can agree to choose a less promising approach or refer the patient to another practitioner.

A Some patients may reject a proposed regenerative procedure because it includes the use of bovine xenographic material (see Chapter 95). Such a consideration may relate to religious beliefs (in the case of persons of the Hindu faith). An alternative approach, human allographic material could be utilized (see Chapter 96).

B Various fears may prevent some patients from agreeing to specific treatments. Bovine xenographic material may be rejected by a patient who fears "mad cow disease." No scientific basis for this fear exists; however, the patient's concerns may necessitate using an alternative regenerative approach. Little is understood about prions, which cause mad cow disease.

C Similarly, a patient may fear being exposed to the human immunodeficiency virus (HIV) if human allographic bone is to be used in a regenerative approach. Though all credible evidence indicates that allographic bone supplied by various agencies (eg, Red Cross) is safe, the patient's wishes should be respected, and an alternative regenerative approach (perhaps a bovine xenographic material) could be considered.

D Some patients' fears may be such that they cannot consider any surgical approach. This fear is the most common one the practitioner may face. Maintenance therapy, regular supportive periodontal therapy visits may be the only viable option. Documenting the "informed consent" for this decision is very important.

E Whenever any of these extraneous factors leads to a decision to choose an alternative to the approach that the practitioner believes would be most effective, the practitioner must decide whether he or she is willing to proceed as the patient wishes or not. If he or she is unwilling to change his approach, the dentist may refer the patient to another practitioner.

Additional Reading

Ramfjord SP et al. Four modalities of periodontal treatment compared over 5 years. J Clin Periodontal 1987;14:445.

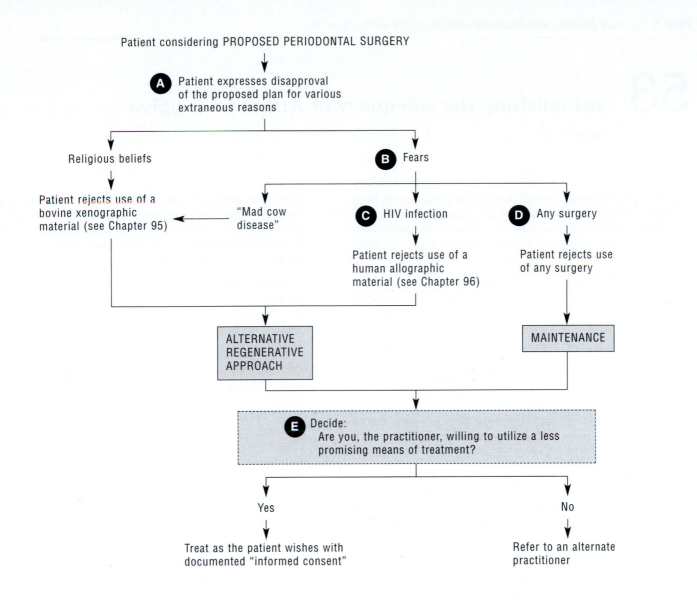

Patient considering PROPOSED PERIODONTAL SURGERY

A Patient expresses disapproval of the proposed plan for various extraneous reasons

Religious beliefs

B Fears

Patient rejects use of a bovine xenographic material (see Chapter 95)

"Mad cow disease"

C HIV infection

D Any surgery

Patient rejects use of a human allographic material (see Chapter 96)

Patient rejects use of any surgery

ALTERNATIVE REGENERATIVE APPROACH

MAINTENANCE

E Decide:
Are you, the practitioner, willing to utilize a less promising means of treatment?

Yes

No

Treat as the patient wishes with documented "informed consent"

Refer to an alternate practitioner

53 Establishing the Adequacy of Attached Gingiva

Walter B. Hall

A tooth with a minimal amount of attached gingiva on its facial or lingual surface should be indicated as a potential pure mucogingival problem. The term *inadequate attached gingiva* was coined during the 1960s and has been defined loosely by many investigators. Rather than being a fixed number of millimeters of attached gingiva, this term refers to a clinical estimate by the treating dentist of the adequacy of the attached gingiva on an individual tooth to remain stable and healthy under conditions imposed by any planned dental treatment or in the absence of any dental treatment involving the tooth (Figure 53-1). Hall (1984) defined *attached gingiva* as "that gingiva extending from the free margin of the gingiva to the mucogingival line minus the pocket or sulcus depth measured with a thin probe in the absence of inflammation." That the gingiva is "inadequate" in an individual case is a clinical decision made by the treating dentist based on a judgment of the tooth's needs in the patient's overall treatment plan. The decision on the need to treat is made with the concurrence of the informed patient (or parent).

A   A simple guideline for determining whether a pure mucogingival problem exists is to record all areas with less than 2 mm of total gingiva as being potential problems because they will have 1 mm or less attached gingiva when the crevice depth is subtracted from the total gingiva. This does not mean that all such cases require grafting. Conversely, although a tooth may have more than 2 mm of total gingiva, it may still have 1 mm or less of attached gingiva when the crevice depth is subtracted from the total

gingiva. In such an instance, the need for grafting would be treated similarly to any situation with 1 mm or less of attached gingiva. Grafting may still be required if the tooth functions as an abutment for a rest-proximal plate-I (RPI) bar-type removable partial denture or an overdenture.

B   For teeth with less than 1 mm of attached gingiva, the patient's age must be considered. Younger children are more likely than older patients to require treatment because of the longer time they can (as a group) expect to keep their teeth.

C   If a young patient has less than 1 mm of attached gingiva on a tooth and is having active recession (ie, any root exposure at this age), consider using a graft on a periosteal bed, which has a high predictability of success. This is preferable to using a graft that depends on new attachment to an exposed root. If the young patient has no recession but restorative procedures (such as Class V restoration) or orthodontic treatment is planned, observe the area for change at all future visits rather than grafting at this time. If the patient is older, has less than 1 mm of attached gingiva on a tooth, and has active recession, consider augmentation. If the situation appears stable (with or without root exposure), the need to treat depends on restorative or orthodontic plans. If crowns, bridges, RPI partials, or overdentures are planned involving this tooth or if orthodontic work is planned, consider augmentation; if not, observe the area for evidence of recession at later dates.

D   If the patient has 2 mm or more of attached gingiva on a tooth that will not serve as an abutment for an RPI removable partial or an overdenture, grafting does not need to be considered. If such a restoration is planned, however, the tooth may require grafting to create at least 3 mm of attached gingiva over which the RPI clasp would be positioned or to support the movement resulting from an overdenture. If the tooth has 3 mm or more of attached gingiva, grafting is not likely to be needed.

Additional Readings

American Academy of Periodontology. World Workshop in Clinical Periodontics. Nevins M, Becker N, Kornman K eds. Chicago: 1989. p. VII–10.

Hall WB. Present status of soft tissue grafting. J Periodontol 1977;48:587.

Hall WB. Pure mucogingival problems. Berlin: Quintessence Publishing; 1984. p. 61.

Lang NP, Loe H. The relationship between the width of the attached gingiva and gingival health. J Periodontol 1972;43:623.

Lindhe J. Textbook of clinical periodontology. 2nd ed. Copenhagen: Munksgaard; 1989. p. 422.

Maynard JG, Wilson RDK. Physiologic dimensions of the periodontium significant to the restorative dentist. J Periodontol 1979;50:170.

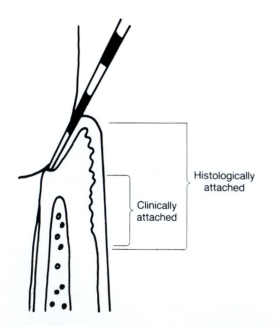

Figure 53-1 A probe in the sulcus illustrating the difference between clinically and histologically attached gingiva.

Patient with INADEQUATE ATTACHED GINGIVA

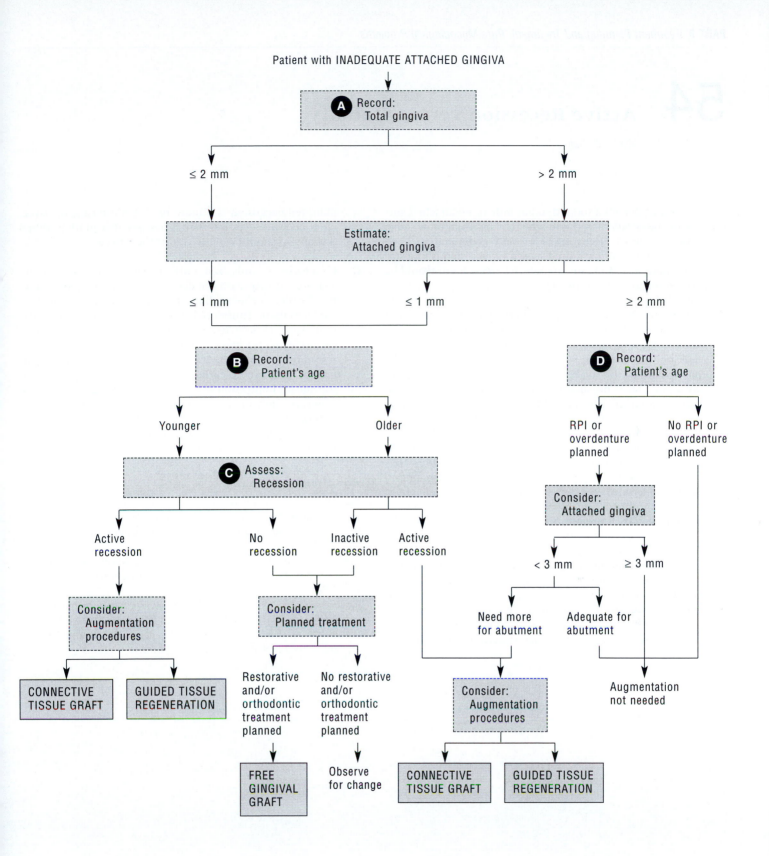

107

54 Active Recession versus Stability

Walter B. Hall

When a dentist detects a tooth that has little or no attached gingiva, he or she should determine whether the situation is stable or active recession is occurring before any additional attached gingiva is created. If a tooth predisposed to recession is in a stable state, there is no impetus to graft; whereas, there would be if active recession were occurring.

A When a tooth that is predisposed to recession because of lack of adequate attached gingiva has no root exposure, the situation is stable. If restorative or orthodontic treatment plans indicate that recession could be precipitated on the predisposed tooth by this treatment, consider prophylactic free gingival grafting. If no such treatment is planned, inform the patient about the problem and evaluate the tooth regularly for indications of change. The dentist and patient together may decide to proceed with restorative work or orthodontics without grafting prophylactically. If recession occurs or progresses, a connective tissue graft (CTG) (see Chapter 109) usually would be the treatment of choice in attempting to repair the receded area; however, guided tissue regeneration (GTR) is another option, especially if no adequate fatty donor site for the CTG is present.

B If root exposure is present, earlier records are helpful in determining whether recession is active or the condition is stable. If such records exist and indicate that the situation is stable, continue to observe the area unless restorative or orthodontic plans indicate the need to create more gingiva before proceeding. If comparison with earlier records demonstrates that recession has occurred, CT grafting is

indicated because it is a more predictable means of covering roots with recession than is free gingival grafting. When this option is not possible, GTR is the choice.

C If no earlier records exist, only the patient's impressions are available to help with the decision whether to graft or not. If the patient believes that recession is occurring actively, a CTG should be considered. If the patient believes that the root exposure occurred earlier and is stable now, document the problem area and observe it regularly for change unless restorative or orthodontic plans indicate a need to graft now. If there are no earlier records, and the patient cannot provide an impression as to the stability of the area of root exposure, document and observe the area regularly for change unless other treatment, which is planned, indicates a need to graft now. If treatment is needed now or in the future, CTG or GTR would be the options.

Additional Readings

Gartrell JR, Mathews DP. Gingival recession: the condition, process and treatment. Dent Clin North Am 1976;20:199.

Hall WB. Pure mucogingival problems. Berlin: Quintessence Publishing; 1984. p. 178.

Nevins M, Mellonig JT. Periodontal therapy: clinical approaches and evidence of success. Chicago: Quintessence Publishing; 1998. p. 279, 293.

Rateitschak KH, Egli V, Fingeli G. Recession: a four-year longitudinal study after free gingival grafts. J Clin Periodontol 1979;6:158.

Wilson RD. Marginal tissue recession in general practice: a preliminary study. Int J Periodontol Res Dent 1983;3:41.

Patient with a TOOTH PREDISPOSED TO RECESSION

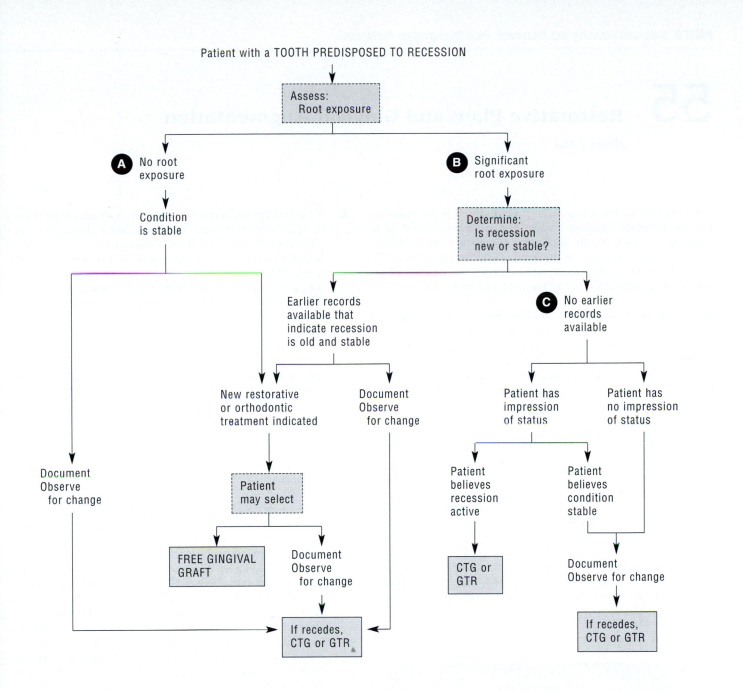

Assess:
Root exposure

A No root exposure

B Significant root exposure

Condition is stable

Determine:
Is recession new or stable?

Earlier records available that indicate recession is old and stable

C No earlier records available

New restorative or orthodontic treatment indicated

Document Observe for change

Patient has impression of status

Patient has no impression of status

Document Observe for change

Patient may select

Patient believes recession active

Patient believes condition stable

FREE GINGIVAL GRAFT

Document Observe for change

CTG or GTR

Document Observe for change

If recedes, CTG or GTR

If recedes, CTG or GTR

55 Restorative Plans and Gingival Augmentation

Walter B. Hall

On determining that a tooth that is predisposed to recession by lack of adequate attached gingiva has restorative needs or is going to be used as an abutment, the dentist must decide whether grafting to increase the band of attached gingiva is indicated. The patient who elects not to proceed with a graft when indicated must be informed of the potential problems.

A   If the predisposed tooth requires restoration, the type of restoration and its locale are most important. If the restoration is a Class V but is to be supragingival, there is no need to graft. If the Class V restoration is to be close to the gingival margin or subgingival, consider a graft. If the restoration is to be of any other class, grafting does not need to be considered.

B   If the predisposed tooth requires a crown, and the crown margins are to be supragingival, there is no need to graft. However, if the crown margin is to be placed at the gingival margin or subgingivally, grafting is indicated because the diamond bur will cut soft tissue as well as tooth structure when carried subgingivally and will induce recession as a consequence of the soft-tissue curettage. If the entire crown of the tooth is to be visible and recession would expose a chamfer or shoulder, the patient must be aware that not grafting is likely to result in a visible gold margin apical to the porcelain. Grafting beforehand is strongly encouraged, because the successful covering of such an exposed chamfer or shoulder surgically after crown placement is exceedingly unlikely (Figure 55-1).

C   If the predisposed tooth is to become an abutment for a fixed bridge, consider grafting whether or not a subgingival margin will be placed in the area of inadequate attached gingiva because cleaning under the pontic or between it and the tooth is likely to produce recession. If a three-quarter crown design is to be used, grafting should be considered, but is not as essential as when a full-crown restoration is to be placed.

D   If the predisposed tooth will serve as an abutment for a rest-proximal plate-I (RPI) bar-type removable partial denture, a graft should be placed sufficiently large enough that the entire I-bar is over the gingiva. If this is not done, the patient who removes the partial denture by placing a fingernail under the apical end of the I-bar is likely to cause wounding and induce recession (see Figure 55-1). A graft usually cannot be placed under an existing I-bar, because the space is inadequate for a graft of sufficient thickness to be placed; therefore, a new partial denture would have to be constructed after grafting.

E   If the predisposed tooth is to be used as an abutment for an overdenture, much the same situation applies. If recession occurs, which is likely when a full denture is placed in the area, the denture could be relieved and a graft placed, or the denture could be left out while the graft heals. In either situation, the graft is likely to be moved about—and to fail. Instead, a large flange of acrylic must be cut away, the graft placed, and the overdenture rebased after healing is completed. The more advisable course is to graft on any predisposed tooth before the overdenture treatment begins. If a graft is to be placed for restorative reasons, the type to be used involves considering the options among free gingival grafts, pedicle grafts, or connective tissue grafts (see Chapter 112).

Additional Readings

American Academy of Periodontology. World Workshop in Clinical Periodontics. Chicago: The Academy; 1989. p. VII–16.

Genco EJ, Goldman HM, Cohen DW. Contemporary periodontics. St. Louis: Mosby; 1990. p. 621.

Hall WB. Periodontal preparation of the mouth for restoration. Dent Clin North Am 1980;24:195.

Hall WB. Pure mucogingival problems. Berlin: Quintessence Publishing; 1984. p. 41.

Maynard JG, Wilson RD. Physiologic dimensions of the periodontium significant to the restorative dentist. J Periodontol 1979;50:170.

Nevins M, Mellonig JT. Periodontal therapy: clinical approaches and evidence of success. Chicago: Quintessence Publishing; 1998. p. 286, 291.

Sato N. Periodontal surgery: a clinical atlas. Tokyo: Quintessence Publishing; 2000. p. 81.

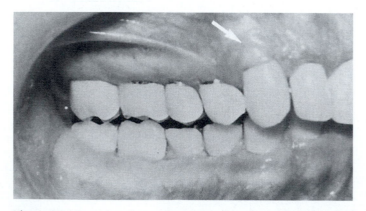

Figure 55-1 Recession of 3 mm has occurred on the canine (which had inadequate attached gingiva) after crown placement.

Patient has tooth with ATTACHED GINGIVA INADEQUATE FOR RESTORATION

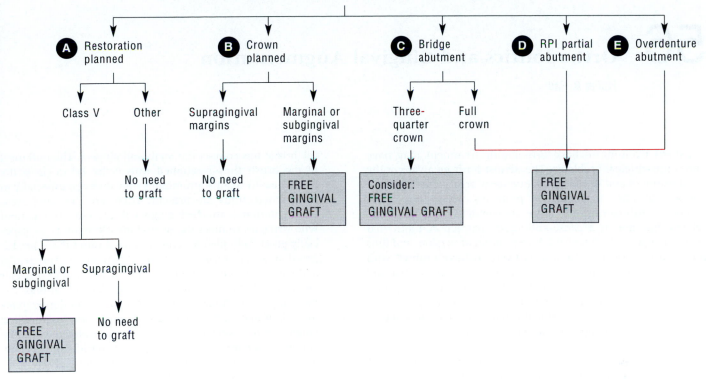

A Restoration planned

Class V

Other → No need to graft

Marginal or subgingival → FREE GINGIVAL GRAFT

Supragingival → No need to graft

B Crown planned

Supragingival margins → No need to graft

Marginal or subgingival margins → FREE GINGIVAL GRAFT

C Bridge abutment

Three-quarter crown → Consider: FREE GINGIVAL GRAFT

Full crown

D RPI partial abutment → FREE GINGIVAL GRAFT

E Overdenture abutment

56 Orthodontics and Gingival Augmentation

Walter B. Hall

A patient planning to have orthodontic treatment may have pure mucogingival problems. The dentist must be aware of the relationship of and the correct sequence of treatment for orthodontic and pure mucogingival problems when they occur together. Orthodontic and pure mucogingival problems are related, but not in a cause-and-effect manner. A tooth that erupts in a position in which it is in prominent version, and thus prone to occlusal trauma, also is likely to have erupted with minimal attached gingiva. The two problems are related and occur together frequently, but (to repeat) not in a cause-and-effect relationship. Both relate to the prominent eruptive position of the tooth. Understanding this relationship is most important in planning therapy for these cases.

A   The age of the patient is important in deciding the way to sequence treatment of combined pure mucogingival and orthodontic problems.

B   If the patient is young and has an overbite/overjet discrepancy that prohibits free gingival grafting on mandibular incisors before some orthodontic movement, proceed with some orthodontic treatment in the maxillary arch before grafting, so that the graft will not be disturbed directly when the patient closes in centric relation. Adult patients in good periodontal health should be treated similarly.

C   If the young patient does not have an overbite/overjet problem but has pure mucogingival problems, consider grafting before beginning orthodontic treatment, because the placement of a vestibular arch wire will alter the approach to brushing. After the arch wire is placed, the brush must be positioned apically to it and turned so that

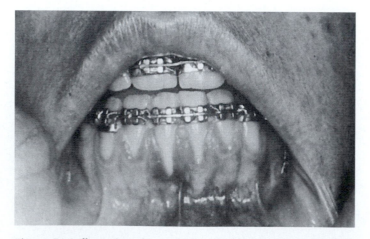

Figure 56-1 Illustration of a recession that a patient with inadequate attached gingiva experienced after the start of orthodontic treatment.

the bristle tips contact the teeth and gingiva. The bulkiness of the brush thus positioned causes the lip to press the brush heavily against prominent root surfaces, especially in areas where frena are present. These are the same areas where minimal attached gingiva is present. The patient who struggles to meet the orthodontist's requests for especially good daily plaque removal may wound these predisposed areas, producing recession (Figure 56-1). The dentist and patient, and parent when appropriate, should consider gingival grafting of mandibular incisors and all canines that have pure mucogingival problems before orthodontic treatment is initiated. The option of waiting and augmenting gingiva if recession occurs must be considered with the patient, and parent, as well. The same considerations apply for patients who have completed correction of overbite/overjet discrepancy problems.

D   With predisposed first premolars, another aspect of orthodontic therapy must be considered. In many orthodontic situations, four first premolars or two first premolars are extracted to create space for realignment of the remaining teeth. If a first premolar has minimal attached gingiva and is going to be extracted, there is no pure mucogingival concern. If the predisposed tooth is to be retained, however, the need to consider grafting before orthodontic treatment is most important.

E   If periodontitis is present in the adult patient, the status of potential anchor teeth must be considered first. A molar with a definite furcation involvement or worse is not a good candidate to serve as an anchor tooth without prior successful guided tissue regeneration (GTR). Some teeth with deep pockets may have to be extracted; others may be moved into or out of periodontal defects after inflammation is controlled and prognoses have improved. If mucogingival-osseous and pure mucogingival problems exist, their surgical treatment usually is accomplished at the same time. In adult orthodontic cases for which one objective is to move a periodontally involved tooth into or out of an osseous defect prior to surgery, the pure mucogingival grafting procedure may be delayed until after the orthodontic goal has been achieved. Then the mucogingival-osseous and pure mucogingival problems can be treated together surgically, if indicated. If there are no periodontitis problems requiring uprighting, and no orthodontic movement into defects is being considered, mucogingival-osseous surgery may be used to correct pocketing and pure mucogingival problems via an apically positioned flap (see Chapter 90). If problems amenable to GTR exist (see Chapter 85), that approach should be used before or after orthodontic treatment as a means of regaining lost attachment and creating a greater band of attached gingiva.

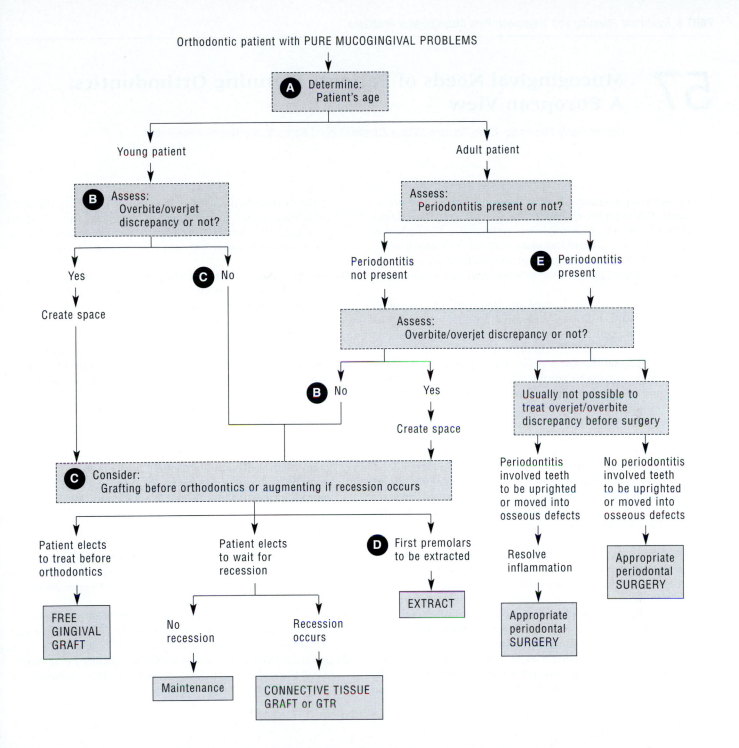

Orthodontic patient with PURE MUCOGINGIVAL PROBLEMS

A Determine: Patient's age

Young patient

B Assess: Overbite/overjet discrepancy or not?

Yes

C No

Create space

Adult patient

Assess: Periodontitis present or not?

Periodontitis not present

E Periodontitis present

Assess: Overbite/overjet discrepancy or not?

B No

Yes

Create space

Usually not possible to treat overjet/overbite discrepancy before surgery

Periodontitis involved teeth to be uprighted or moved into osseous defects

No periodontitis involved teeth to be uprighted or moved into osseous defects

Resolve inflammation

Appropriate periodontal SURGERY

Appropriate periodontal SURGERY

C Consider: Grafting before orthodontics or augmenting if recession occurs

Patient elects to treat before orthodontics

Patient elects to wait for recession

D First premolars to be extracted

FREE GINGIVAL GRAFT

No recession

Recession occurs

EXTRACT

Maintenance

CONNECTIVE TISSUE GRAFT or GTR

Additional Readings

American Academy of Periodontology. World Workshop in Clinical Periodontics. Chicago: The Academy; 1989. p. VII–2.

Boyd RL. Mucogingival considerations and their relationship to orthodontics. J Periodontol 1978;49:67.

Coatoam GW, Behrents RG, Bissada NF. The width of traumatized gingiva during orthodontic treatment. J Periodontol 1981;52:307.

Dorfman HS. Mucogingival changes resulting from mandibular incisor tooth movement. Am J Orthod 1978;74:286.

Hall WB. Can attached gingiva be increased non-surgically? Quint Int 1982;13:455.

Hall WB. Pure mucogingival problems. Berlin: Quintessence Publishing; 1984. p. 44.

Nevins M, Mellonig JT. Periodontal therapy: clinical approaches and evidence of success. Chicago: Quintessence Publishing; 1998. p. 158, 294.

57 Mucogingival Needs of Patients Planning Orthodontics: A European View

Giovan Paolo Pini-Prato, Carlo Clauser, Giliana Zuccati, Tiziano Baccetti, and Roberto Rotundo

A Proper plaque control is crucial during orthodontic treatment. Orthodontic appliances are a factor in plaque retention, which can cause gingivitis. Additionally, the patient is required to use a more traumatic method of toothbrushing. Traumatic toothbrushing and plaque accumulation are the main etiologic factors in the development of recession.

B Local plaque removal may be impaired by anatomic mucogingival conditions, such as inadequate attached gingiva, shallow vestibule, and pulling frena. These conditions should be corrected before orthodontic treatment.

Buccolingual thickness rather than apicocoronal extent of the gingiva may be considered as a *locus minoris resistentiae* for the development of recession in relation to the direction of planned orthodontic movement. An orthodontic movement that tends to position the tooth within the alveolar bone (generally a lingual movement) is considered a favorable one. On the contrary, a movement that tends to position the tooth outside of the alveolar bone (generally a buccal movement) is considered an unfavorable one. When an unfavorable orthodontic movement is planned, and the gingiva is thin, an augmentation procedure to increase the gingival thickness should be considered.

C When an unfavorable orthodontic movement is scheduled on a tooth with existing gingival recession, treatment of the recession should be performed prior to orthodontic therapy. On the contrary, favorable orthodontic movement, in the presence of adequate plaque control, may result in a reduction of the gingival recession; therefore, appropriate monitoring of the patient should be carried out. Due to esthetic requirements of the patient at the end of the orthodontic treatment, root coverage procedures may be needed. Despite favorable orthodontic movement, gingival recession in patients who do not exhibit good plaque control in the areas of recession may require mucogingival procedures, such as free gingival graft (FGG), guided tissue regeneration (GTR), or apically positioned flap (APF), often for root coverage.

D Ectopic tooth eruption may lead to mucogingival problems. The ectopic tooth may be completely unerupted, in either a submucosal position or a deep infraosseous location. In a case of superficial impaction, an APF can be performed. In case of infraosseous impaction, orthodontic treatment is aimed to guide the tooth to the center of the alveolar ridge. Each of these therapeutic approaches may be considered as preventive procedures to maintain a physiologic amount of gingiva.

Buccally erupting teeth can entrap and destroy the gingiva between the erupting cusp and the deciduous tooth. This entrapped tissue can be saved and used as donor material to create a satisfactory width of gingiva for the permanent tooth. Different interceptive mucogingival procedures may be performed depending upon the distance from the erupting cusp to the mucogingival junction (MGJ).

Additional Readings

Pini-Prato GP, Baccetti T, Magnani C, Agudio G, Cortellini P. Mucogingival interceptive surgery of bucally erupted premolars in patients scheduled for orthodontic treatment. I. A 7-year longitudinal study. J Periodontol 2000;71:172.

Wennstrom JL, Lindhe J, Sinclair P, Thilander B. Some periodontal tissue reactions to orthodontic tooth movement in monkeys. J Clin Periodontol 1987;14:121.

Zachrisson BU. Orthodontics and periodontics. In: Lindhe J et al, editors. Clinical periodontology and implant dentistry. Copenhagen: Munksgaard; 1997.

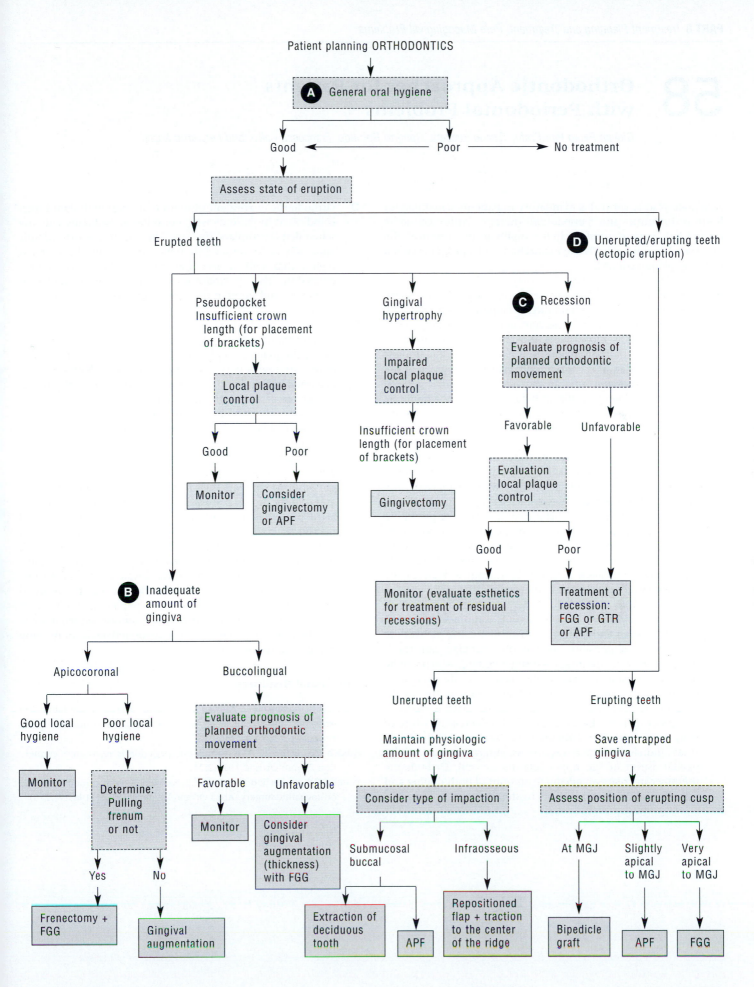

Patient planning ORTHODONTICS

A General oral hygiene

Good ←————— Poor ————→ No treatment

Assess state of eruption

Erupted teeth

D Unerupted/erupting teeth (ectopic eruption)

Pseudopocket Insufficient crown length (for placement of brackets)

Local plaque control

Good → Monitor

Poor → Consider gingivectomy or APF

Gingival hypertrophy

Impaired local plaque control

Insufficient crown length (for placement of brackets)

Gingivectomy

C Recession

Evaluate prognosis of planned orthodontic movement

Favorable

Unfavorable

Evaluation local plaque control

Good

Poor

Monitor (evaluate esthetics for treatment of residual recessions)

Treatment of recession: FGG or GTR or APF

B Inadequate amount of gingiva

Apicocoronal

Buccolingual

Good local hygiene → Monitor

Poor local hygiene → Determine: Pulling frenum or not

Yes → Frenectomy + FGG

No → Gingival augmentation

Evaluate prognosis of planned orthodontic movement

Favorable → Monitor

Unfavorable → Consider gingival augmentation (thickness) with FGG

Unerupted teeth

Maintain physiologic amount of gingiva

Consider type of impaction

Submucosal buccal

Infraosseous

Extraction of deciduous tooth

APF

Repositioned flap + traction to the center of the ridge

Erupting teeth

Save entrapped gingiva

Assess position of erupting cusp

At MGJ → Bipedicle graft

Slightly apical to MGJ → APF

Very apical to MGJ → FGG

58 Orthodontic Approaches for Patients with Periodontal Problems

Giovan Paolo Pini-Prato, Tiziano Baccetti, Roberto Rotundo, Francesco Cairo, and Leonardo Muzzi

Adequate plaque control is mandatory in patients scheduled for both orthodontic and periodontal therapy. Although some orthodontic measures may help to simplify plaque removal, the keystone for oral health is the maintenance of a proper regimen of home plaque control.

A   The relationship between malpositioning of the teeth, crowding in particular, and the development of periodontal diseases is controversial. The determining factor for gingival inflammation is more likely the amount of accumulated local plaque than the malposition itself. When the amount of bacterial plaque is considerably greater in regions of the dentition showing severe crowding than the general amount of plaque in the individual patient, orthodontic correction of the dental disharmony can be beneficial for more effective local oral hygiene.

B   Restorative dentistry in patients with insufficient tooth crown height must be performed after procedures that allow for the establishment of physiologic biologic width. Otherwise, the periodontal tissues may develop increased probing depth and limitations with respect to plaque control. When a procedure for crown lengthening is scheduled, the amount of bone support must be assessed. If bone support is adequate, resective surgery is indicated; if not, orthodontic extrusion of the tooth, with or without fiberotomy, can be helpful to increase the supragingival crown length of the tooth.

C   Some malocclusions result in chronic traumatic contact of gingival tissues and teeth due to mismatching of overbite and overjet dimensions. Periodontal damage can result from the gingival trauma. Excessive overbite, which can be observed in patients with angle Class II division 2 malocclusion, may lead to typical gingival lesions on the buccal aspect of the lower incisors and/or on the palatal aspect of the upper incisors. Elective therapy for decreasing overbite is by tooth intrusion. Patients with excessive overjet angle (Class II division 1) may experience gingival trauma on the palatal aspect of the upper incisors as well. Orthodontic therapy can create an adequate amount of both tipping and intrusion of the lower incisors to stop damage.

D   Orthodontic movement of tooth extrusion with light forces is indicated in patients with periodontal problems who are scheduled for implant therapy. The aim of the orthodontic approach is to reestablish bone support in the alveolar region that will receive the implant. After orthodontic extrusion the periodontally compromised tooth is extracted, and implant therapy is performed.

E   The presence of a papilla between the maxillary incisors is an important esthetic requirement of many patients. In some, the papilla is either reduced or absent. Some orthodontic strategies may assist in creating an adequate interproximal space for the residual papilla. Both alignment and shape of the teeth play a relevant role with regard to this type of orthodontic approach. The first example relates to the presence of diverging roots of the maxillary incisors. In these patients, the aim is to restore the physiologic alignment of both crowns and roots. After orthodontic therapy, an asymmetrical profile of the incisal margin (due to uneven incisal wear) may become apparent and require incisal restoration. A second clinical condition is the presence of space above the interproximal contact of maxillary incisors in association with abnormal tooth shape. In these patients, the crowns of the incisors are much wider at the incisal edge than in the cervical part. The interproximal surfaces of the incisors may have to be recontoured before orthodontic closure of the residual embrasures. Similarly, when the papilla is reduced in presence of a diastema, orthodontic therapy aimed at closing the interproximal space can be beneficial in improving papillary esthetics.

Additional Readings

Ingervall B, Jacobsson U, Nyman S. A clinical study of the relationship between crowding of teeth, plaque and gingival condition. J Clin Periodontol 1976;4:214.

Kokich VG. Esthetics: the orthodontic-periodontic restorative connection. Semin Orthod 1996;2:21.

Poulton DR. Correction of extreme deep overbite with orthodontics and orthognathic surgery. Am J Orthod Dentofac Orthop 1989;96:275.

ORTHODONTIC APPROACHES FOR A PATIENT WITH PERIODONTAL PROBLEMS

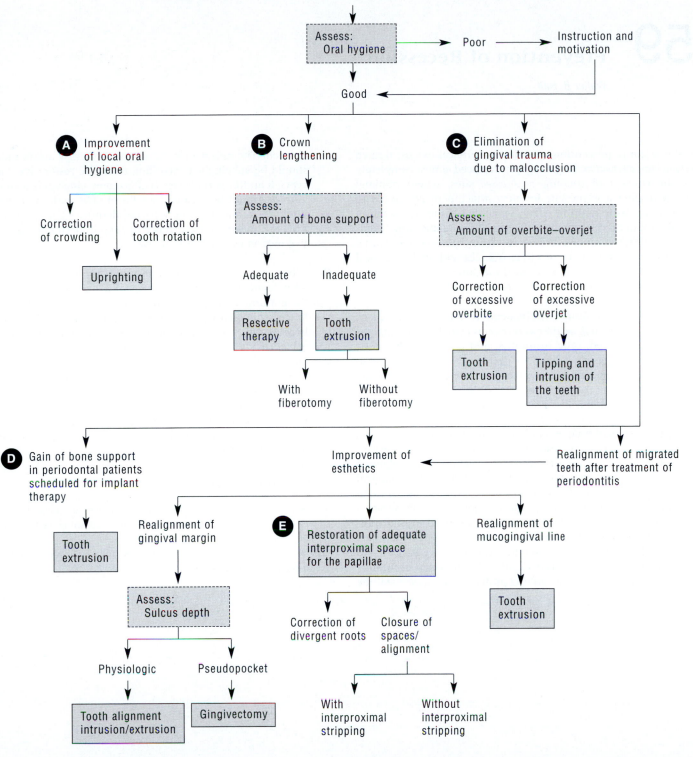

59 Prevention of Recession

Walter B. Hall

The concept of preventing recession by surgical means, termed *prophylactic gingival grafting,* has been replaced almost completely by the concept of treating *predisposed* sites, where minimal attached gingiva is present for new attachment by means of connective tissue grafting (CTG) or guided tissue regeneration (GTR), should recession occur. The need for augmenting "inadequate" attached gingiva before recession has occurred can be justified in a limited set of circumstances, although the legal aspects of "informed consent" in these situations are still in a state of flux in some American states.

A If a patient has a site with inadequate attached gingiva (see Chapter 53), and neither is recession activity occurring nor has it occurred, only restorative and possibly orthodontic plans need be considered in deciding whether to graft to prevent recession. If recession has occurred or is actively occurring, the treatment would be therapeutic rather than preventive (and is discussed in Chapter 60).

B In a site where "inadequate" attachment gingiva is noted and a crown, a Class V restoration, or a rest-proximal plate-I (RPI) style clasp for a removable partial denture is planned involving that site, the use of a prophylactic free gingival graft (FGG) or a CTG to prevent recession relating to tooth preparation or clasp design must be considered. If the site is one with esthetic concerns as well, the need to graft pre-emptively is greatest, because the position of the free margin of new gingiva—created by a therapeutic CTG GTR—in relation to crown margins cannot be predicted accurately enough to assure that gold chamfers or shoulders will be covered. The apical margins of metal Class V restorations should be subgingival according to classic restorative concepts. If an RPI partial clasp is affected by gingival recession, gingiva cannot be created by CTG or GTR without a commitment to making a new partial denture. A prophylactic FGG can make the occurrence of such undesirable restorative outcomes much less likely.

C When orthodontic treatment involving teeth with sites with "inadequate" attached gingiva is planned, prophylactic grafting before proceeding with orthodontics is no longer a mandatory consideration (see Chapter 56). This is because root coverage with new attachment can be achieved, should recession occur, utilizing CTG or GTR surgical procedures. However, a discussion of the complex issues with the patient and/or parents in order to achieve "informed consent" (see Chapter 139) before proceeding with orthodontics can prevent misunderstandings should recession occur during orthodontic treatment.

Careful sucular soft-tissue brushing remains the best means of preventing recession.

Additional Readings

Nevins M, Mellonig JT. Periodontal therapy: clinical approaches and evidence of success. Chicago: Quintessence Publishing; 1998. p. 279–288, 291–300.

Sato N. Periodontal surgery: a clinical atlas. Tokyo: Quintessence Publishing; 2000. p. 82–3.

Patient with a site with INADEQUATE ATTACHED GINGIVA

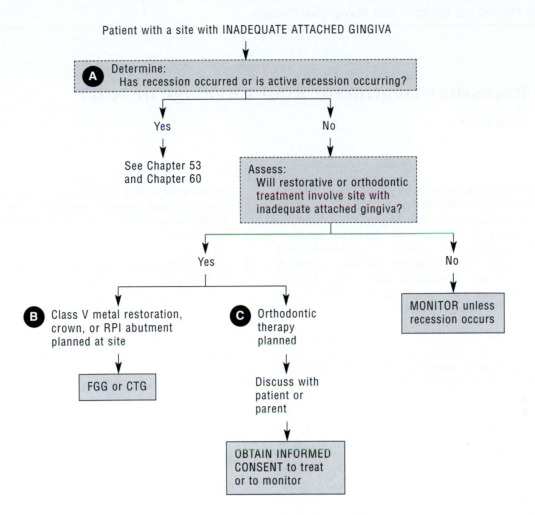

A Determine:
Has recession occurred or is active recession occurring?

Yes

No

See Chapter 53
and Chapter 60

Assess:
Will restorative or orthodontic
treatment involve site with
inadequate attached gingiva?

Yes

No

B Class V metal restoration,
crown, or RPI abutment
planned at site

C Orthodontic
therapy
planned

MONITOR unless
recession occurs

FGG or CTG

Discuss with
patient or
parent

OBTAIN INFORMED
CONSENT to treat
or to monitor

60 Recession Treatment: Root Coverage or Not?

Walter B. Hall

If a patient has a root or roots exposed by recession, esthetic and restorative needs influence the need for grafting in an inter-related manner. If the band of attached gingiva is adequate, but recession has occurred, surgery may be performed to cover exposed roots if an esthetic need exists. If no esthetic need exists, and no restoration affecting the gingival margin is planned, maintenance care alone should suffice. If the band of attached gingiva is "inadequate" in the dentist's opinion, the need to consider gingival augmentation is greater.

A   Decide on the "adequacy" of the existing band of attached gingiva and assess the patient's overall dental needs. An adequate band of attached gingiva is one that is sufficient to prevent initial or continued recession. The patient's age, other dental needs, oral hygiene status, caries activity, and esthetic needs are some factors influencing a decision regarding whether treatment is needed if the band of attached gingiva is judged inadequate to prevent initial or continued recession.

B   If the patient has an adequate band of attached gingiva, and no cosmetic or esthetic need to attempt root coverage exists, dental health should be maintainable with regular oral hygiene efforts, prophylaxis, or root planing. If a Class V restoration or crown is to be placed, the apical margin of the restoration may be placed within the gingi-val crevice without strong likelihood of inducing recession or placed supragingivally if root sensitivity, caries activity, or other restorative requirements (eg, crown length) are not involved. Maintenance care should suffice to preserve dental health.

C   If root coverage is necessary to meet esthetic (or cosmetic) goals, and the band of attached gingiva on the tooth or teeth with recession is adequate, a coronally positioned pedicle graft or flap (see Chapters 110 and 111) is one pos-sible treatment; however, a connective tissue graft (CTG) or guided tissue regeneration (GTR) should be considered (see Chapter 109).

D   If an inadequate band of attached gingiva is present and esthetic, cosmetic, or restorative goals indicate the need for root coverage, a CTG is most appropriate, particularly if sev-eral teeth are involved. If an adequate donor site for such a graft is not available (ie, the donor site in the rugae area is insufficiently thick), GTR is the choice for augmentation (see Chapter 109).

E   If the patient has inadequate attached gingiva to meet dental needs without initiating recession or further recession, and no cosmetic or esthetic concern exists, a free gingival graft (FGG) without root coverage may be performed for stabilization.

Additional Readings

Allen EP, Miller PD. Coronal positioning of existing gingiva: short-term results in the treatment of shallow marginal tissue recession. J Peri-odontol 1989;60:316.

American Academy of Periodontology. World Workshop in Clinical Periodontics. Chicago: The Academy; 1989. p. VII–1.

Hall WB. Pure mucogingival problems. Berlin: Quintessence Publishing; 1984. p. 61.

Langer B, Langer L. Subepithelial connective tissue graft technique for root coverage. J Periodontol 1985;56:715.

Matter J. Free gingival grafts for the treatment of gingival recession—a review of some techniques. J Clin Periodontol 1980;9:103.

Nevins M, Mellonig JT. Periodontal therapy: clinical approaches and evidence of success. Chicago: Quintessence Publishing; 1998. p. 339.

Sato N. Periodontal surgery: a clinical atlas. Tokyo: Quintessence Pub-lishing; 2000. p. 335.

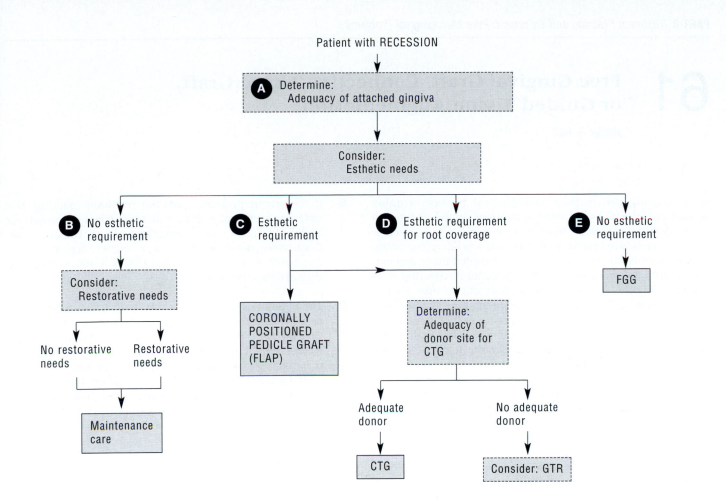

61 Free Gingival Graft, Connective Tissue Graft, or Guided Tissue Augmentation

Walter B. Hall

After deciding that a pure mucogingival problem requires surgery to create a broader band of attached gingiva, the dentist must select the technique most likely to achieve root coverage to minimize future recession. Esthetics is a primary consideration. Connective tissue grafts (CTG) and guided tissue regeneration (GTR) are more likely to be successful in covering roots and matching the appearance of adjacent gingiva than are free gingival grafts (FGG). Connective tissue grafting is more successful than GTR in the author's experience; therefore, if root coverage is a goal, the CTG is preferable to other graft procedures unless an adequately thick donor site for a CTG is not available (see Chapter 109).

A If no esthetic concern exists, as in most mandibular and maxillary molar areas, a free gingival graft is one option. If no existing recession requiring root coverage is present, a free gingival graft is an acceptable choice and is the easiest to perform.

Free gingival grafts for covering roots have long been desired goals of those practicing pure mucogingival surgery. The predictability of success with a FGG is not great, although claims for improved success through root treatment either with citric acid or complicated suturing have been made. The FGG usually is taken from the palate, which may be of a markedly different color than the gingiva adjacent to the area to be grafted. If the donor gingiva is such a poor color match that it would create a greater esthetic problem if successful than that created by root exposure, free gingival grafting for root coverage should not be attempted.

B If no esthetic problem exists but recession requiring root coverage is present or if an esthetic problem is present, use a CTG or GTR for root coverage and a better esthetic result. Connective tissue grafts have a higher degree of predictability of success in the author's experience; therefore, they are the first choice.

C The optimal donor site for a CTG is in the anterior palatal area beneath the rugae, where the submucosa is fatty (see Chapter 109). If finger pressure suggests that little spongy-feeling submucosa is present, GTR as a means of augmentation and root coverage is the alternative choice.

If the area of recession is so great—more than 6 to 8 mm from the cementoenamel junction to the bony crest—that excision of a donor specimen would extend close to the anterior palatine artery, GTR is a safer approach.

Additional Readings

American Academy of Periodontology. World Workshop in Clinical Periodontics. Chicago: The Academy; 1989. p. VII–1.

Carranza FA Jr, Newman MG. Clinical periodontology. 8th ed. Philadelphia: WB Saunders; 1996. p. 651.

Hall WB. Pure mucogingival problems. Berlin: Quintessence Publishing; 1984. p. 129.

Langer B, Langer L. Subepithelial connective tissue graft technique for root coverage. J Periodontol 1983;56:175.

Nevins M, Mellonig JT. Periodontal therapy: clinical approaches and evidence of success. Chicago: Quintessence Publishing; 1998. p. 355, 365.

Sato N. Periodontal surgery: a clinical atlas. Tokyo: Quintessence Publishing; 2000. p. 359.

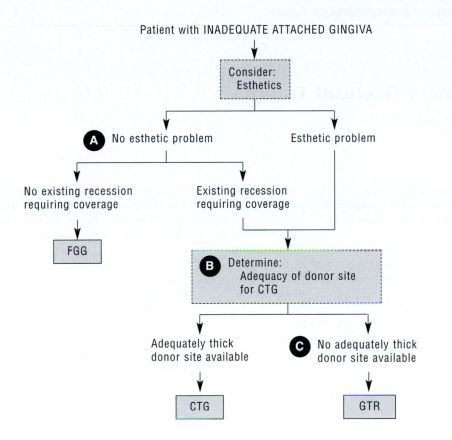

Patient with INADEQUATE ATTACHED GINGIVA

Consider:
Esthetics

A No esthetic problem

Esthetic problem

No existing recession
requiring coverage

Existing recession
requiring coverage

FGG

B Determine:
Adequacy of donor site
for CTG

Adequately thick
donor site available

C No adequately thick
donor site available

CTG

GTR

62 Primary Occlusal Trauma

Walter B. Hall

Primary occlusal trauma occurs when a tooth with normal support is overloaded and as a result is wounded. The problem may be localized or generalized in several teeth.

A Localized, primary occlusal trauma most typically is related to a "high" restoration, a common sequela of the placement of a new restoration in an individual tooth that has been extensively instrumented. An anesthetized patient whose mouth has been opened wide for some time often is unable to detect such an early contact. Selective grinding usually is all that is required to correct the problem; however, severe discrepancies may best be resolved by replacing the restoration.

B Malaligned teeth also may be subjected to primary occlusal trauma, especially when they are locked in facial or lingual version. Selective grinding may resolve minor malalignments. Orthodontic movement is often the best treatment choice. In severe crowding, however, selective extraction of teeth may be a simple and satisfactory solution.

C Generalized, primary occlusal trauma usually is of a different origin. Clenching and grinding habits including bruxism (night grinding) are the most common causes. Occlusal adjustment or (occasionally) selective grinding of a high "trigger" tooth may resolve some problems; however, the psychologic component of clenching and grinding habits, especially bruxism, may improve with counseling to control the patient's psychic disturbances. Because such problems are difficult to resolve, a bite guard (night guard) often is used to control the damage caused by grinding, especially bruxism. The skill of the dentist in managing such problems, which often have complex psychologic overtones, often is sorely tried.

D Another less common etiology is "occupational" bruxism, wherein certain occupations cause patients to grind their teeth. Jobs that involve riding a tractor, hauling nets on rocking fishing boats, using a jackhammer, and driving a taxi with bad springs have been implicated. Changing jobs may not be an option open to the patient; however, a bite guard often can be worn during work hours in such occupations.

E *Recreational bruxism* is a term used to describe the extreme gnashing of teeth that accompanies the use of some "recreational" drugs. The best solution to such problems is to discontinue the use of the drugs. Counseling may be helpful in correcting such habits. Occasionally, a bite guard may be helpful if the patient cannot stop using the drug.

F Postorthodontic clenching may occur when a major occlusal discrepancy occurs after orthodontic therapy. A so-called double bite may be created if the patient has a maximal occlusal position a half tooth or more forward of a centric relation occlusion. As the patient rocks between these two positions, severe trauma usually occurs. If it is detected before periodontitis is present, occlusal adjustment may be somewhat helpful; however, the discrepancies often are too great to be ground out. Further orthodontic treatment, even orthognathic surgery, should be undertaken with patient consent. A bite guard may be useful in controlling damage; however, a lifetime of wearing such a device is rarely a palatable alternative. Full-mouth reconstruction to establish a stable, centric relation occlusion is an expensive but reasonable alternative.

Additional Readings

Carranza FA Jr, Newman MG. Clinical periodontology. 8th ed. Philadelphia: WB Saunders; 1996. p. 314.

Genco RJ, Goldman HM, Cohen DW. Contemporary periodontics. St. Louis: Mosby; 1990. p. 493.

Prichard JF. Advanced periodontal disease. 2nd ed. Philadelphia: WB Saunders; 1992. p. 823.

Schluger S et al. Periodontal diseases. 2nd ed. Philadelphia: Lea & Febiger; 1990. p. 388.

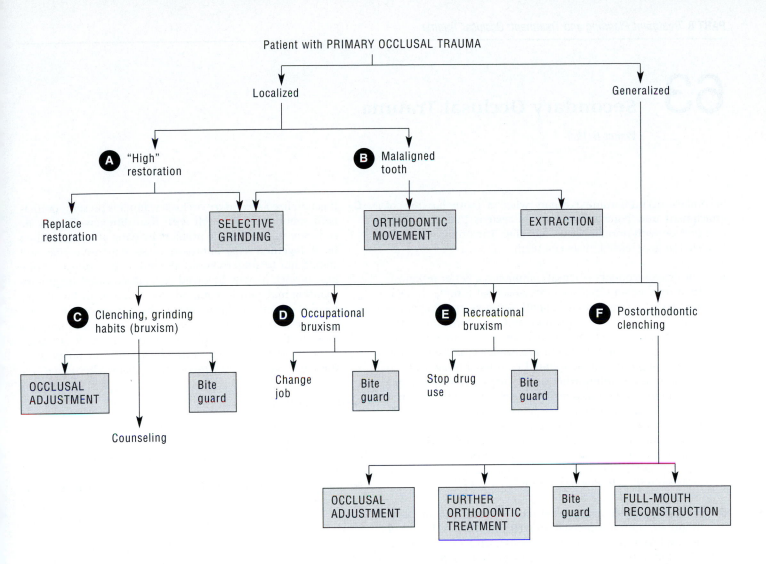

63 Secondary Occlusal Trauma

Walter B. Hall

Secondary occlusal trauma occurs when a tooth has loss of attachment and bone support to the extent that wounding occurs even with normal occlusal loading. The problem may be localized or generalized in several teeth.

A Localized secondary occlusal trauma has a better prognosis than does generalized secondary occlusal trauma. If adjacent teeth have adequate support, selective grinding of the tooth that has lost support may minimize function on the tooth by placing most function on the teeth with good support. If good abutment teeth are available, the tooth that has lost support may be splinted with fixed bridgework to the abutments, minimizing heavy function on the weakened tooth. The more remaining teeth with sufficient support to act as abutments or otherwise assist the compromised tooth, the better the prognosis. If the compromised tooth is amenable to guided tissue regeneration (GTR) (see Chapters 79 and 80), it may be treated, obviating the need for splinting; otherwise, it should be extracted and replaced with a bridge or implant.

B If no good adjacent abutment teeth remain, but the compromised tooth is amenable to GTR, that approach cannot be employed; the tooth should be extracted or maintained with full recognition that its prognosis is hopeless (see Chapter 37).

C If generalized secondary occlusal trauma is present, permanent splinting of all teeth with fixed bridgework may be sufficient to stabilize the problem by tying all compromised teeth together. This approach is an expensive one and should not be undertaken if all teeth have extensive bone loss. In such heavily involved generalized cases, temporary splinting may permit maintenance of the teeth for shorter periods. Another alternative is the placement of a bite guard, especially if the patient grinds the teeth at night. If most teeth have lost substantial support, GTR on large numbers of teeth is not currently practical or predictable; therefore, extraction is the only reasonable alternative.

Additional Readings

Carranza FA Jr, Newman MG. Clinical periodontology. 8th ed. Philadelphia: WB Saunders; 1996. p. 315.

Genco RJ, Goldman HM, Cohen DW. Contemporary periodontics. St. Louis: Mosby; 1980. p. 493.

Schluger S et al. Periodontal diseases. 2nd ed. Philadelphia: Lea & Febiger; 1990. p. 405.

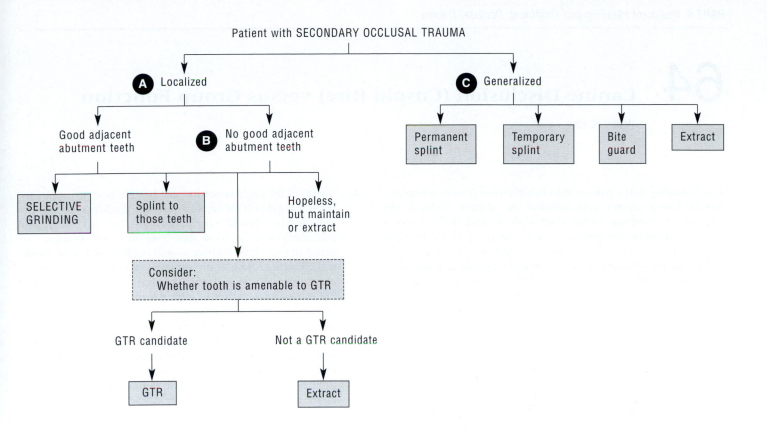

64 Canine Disclusion (Cuspid Rise) versus Group Function

Walter B. Hall

After deciding that a patient may benefit from selective grinding during treatment for periodontitis, the dentist must decide whether establishing canine disclusion (cuspid rise) or group function in lateral movements is best (Figure 64-1). Canine disclusion may provide a "cuspid-protected" occlusion in parafunctional lateral movements that may be beneficial if posterior teeth have significant bone loss, considerable occlusal wear, or a number of cracks, and if the patient clenches or grinds the teeth. Canine disclusion is preferable to group function of weakened posterior teeth, but if canine disclusion cannot be employed, group function is used.

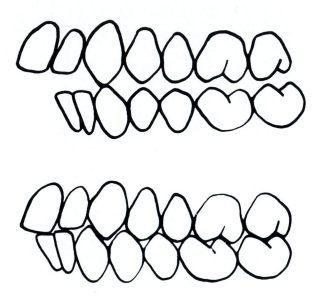

Figure 64-1 Working side contacts in canine disclusion or group function situations.

A If both of the canines on one side have little or no bone loss, the first condition for the use of canine disclusion is met. The radiographs should show normal-sized maxillary and mandibular canine roots that have little radiographic evidence of bone loss. Probing should confirm that little attachment has been lost. If the canines occlude in lateral movement toward the side in which these teeth are present, canine rise is a logical objective of selective grinding. If sound maxillary and mandibular canines do not occlude in lateral movement, canine disclusion cannot be attained. If the posterior teeth have little or no bone loss, group function is the objective. If the posterior teeth have moderate-to-severe bone loss and the canines are essentially sound, however, either the canines may be restored to create canine disclusion, or orthodontic positioning of the canines can be used to permit it.

B If one or both canines on one side have moderate-to-severe bone loss and guided tissue regeneration is not feasible, canine disclusion should be discarded as an objective. If the adjacent posterior teeth have little or no bone loss, group function is the logical objective. If the adjacent posterior teeth have moderate-to-severe bone loss, as do the canines, splinting to distribute the loading more evenly is necessary, especially if the teeth are very mobile. If mobility is minimal, selective grinding to "smooth out" the group function may suffice.

Additional Readings

D'Amico A. The canine teeth: normal functional relation of the natural teeth of man. Calif Dent Assoc J 1958;26:6.

Grant DA, Stern JB, Listgarten MA. Periodontics. 6th ed. St. Louis: Mosby; 1988. p. 986.

Ramfjord S, Ash MM. Occlusion. 3rd ed. Philadelphia: WB Saunders; 1983. p. 370.

Schluger S et al. Periodontal diseases. 2nd ed. Philadelphia: Lea & Febiger; 1990. p. 392.

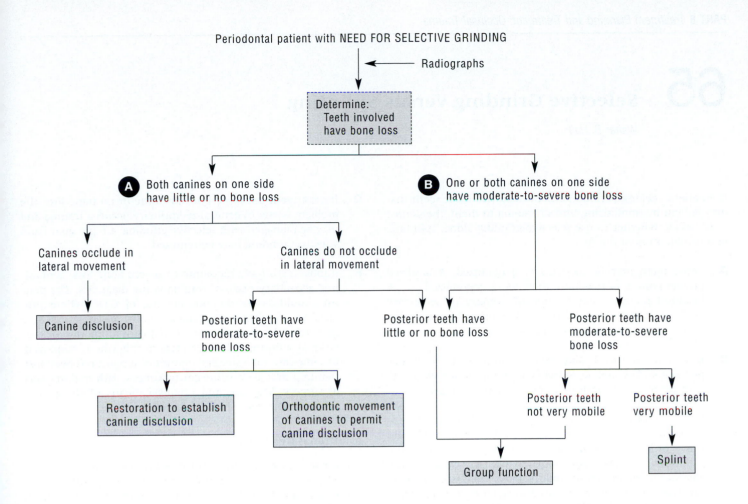

Periodontal patient with NEED FOR SELECTIVE GRINDING

← Radiographs

Determine:
Teeth involved
have bone loss

A Both canines on one side
have little or no bone loss

B One or both canines on one side
have moderate-to-severe bone loss

Canines occlude in
lateral movement

Canines do not occlude
in lateral movement

Canine disclusion

Posterior teeth have
moderate-to-severe
bone loss

Posterior teeth have
little or no bone loss

Posterior teeth have
moderate-to-severe
bone loss

Restoration to establish
canine disclusion

Orthodontic movement
of canines to permit
canine disclusion

Posterior teeth
not very mobile

Posterior teeth
very mobile

Group function

Splint

65 Selective Grinding versus Splinting

Walter B. Hall

If a patient seeking periodontal treatment has loose teeth that may benefit by minimizing further trauma to them, the dentist must decide whether to use selective grinding alone, splinting, or a combination of the two.

A Loose teeth may be localized or generalized. A localized problem offers more options than does a generalized one. A localized problem may be one of primary or secondary occlusal trauma. A generalized problem may be one mostly of primary or secondary occlusal trauma.

B Localized loose teeth may have lost little or no bone support but still be mobile. Selective grinding should eliminate such problems of localized primary occlusal trauma.

C Localized loose teeth, however, may have lost a moderate-to-severe amount of bone. If most other teeth are sound (have little bone loss), selective grinding may reduce the loading to the loose teeth enough to minimize trauma. If the adjacent teeth are sound, and the loose tooth is moderately involved, splinting may be used to stabilize it. If the loose tooth has lost substantial support, guided tissue regeneration (GTR) may be considered. If GTR is a predictable procedure for the severely involved tooth, it should be used (see Chapter 79). If GTR is not possible or acceptable to the patient and the adjacent abutments are adequate, the compromised tooth should be extracted and replaced with a bridge rather than jeopardizing sound abutment teeth to maintain a tooth with a guarded-to-hopeless prognosis.

D If most teeth are loose but have little or no bone loss, the problem is one of generalized primary occlusal trauma and may be managed with selective grinding; a night guard and selective grinding may be required.

E If most teeth have moderate-to-severe bone loss, generalized secondary occlusal trauma is the diagnosis. The dentist should assess the possible use of GTR, where predictable, to change individual tooth prognosis. Where practical, GTR should be employed with temporary or provisional splinting before permanent splinting is employed. In some cases, if a smaller amount of support has been lost, splinting may be a sufficient treatment with maintenance of surgery. The age and financial means of the patient influence the decision.

Additional Readings

Newman MG, Takei HH, Carranza FM Jr. Carranza's clinical periodontology. 9th ed. Philadelphia: WB Saunders; 2002. p. 101–2.

Nyman S, Lindhe J, Lundgren D. The role of occlusion for the stability of fixed bridges in patients with reduced periodontal support. J Clin Periodontol 1975;22:53.

Ramfjord S, Ash MM. 3rd ed. Philadelphia: WB Saunders; 1983. p. 384.

Ringli HH. Splinting of teeth: an objective assessment. Helv Odontol Acta 1971;15:129.

A periodontal patient with LOOSE TEETH

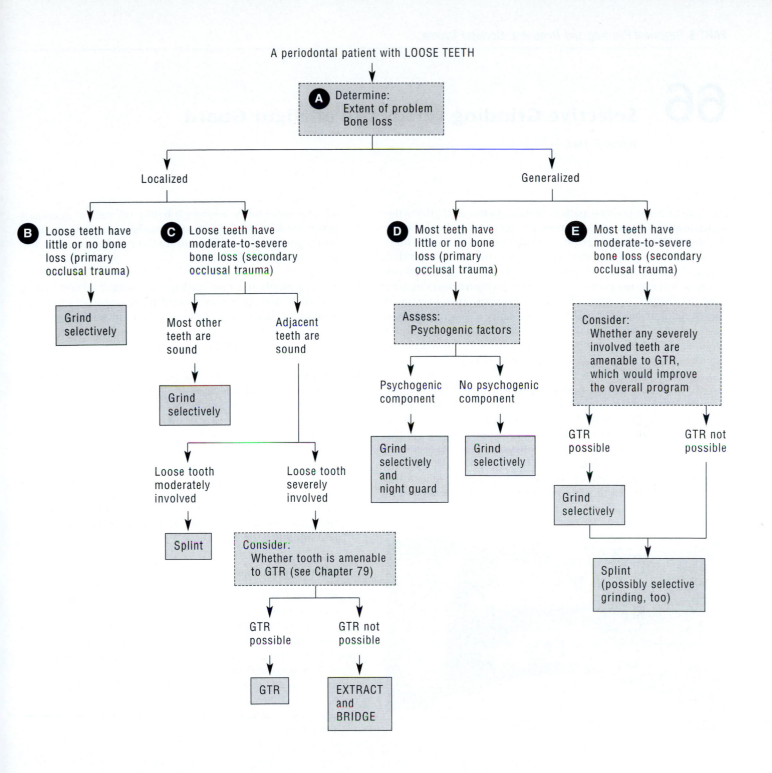

66 Selective Grinding versus Use of Night Guard

Walter B. Hall

In treating a periodontal patient who clenches and grinds the teeth and has loose or symptomatic teeth, the dentist must decide whether selective grinding or night guard therapy is indicated. Selective grinding may smooth out the occlusion so that "trigger" discrepancies are eliminated or may better distribute forces so less trauma occurs. A night guard (Figure 66-1) may be used to control trauma relating to bruxism (parafunctional clenching or grinding at night). Occasionally a patient also may be able to wear such a guard for periods during the day. If the problems are of psychologic origin, selective grinding may be of little help in stopping the clenching and grinding.

A   If the patient has an essentially satisfactory occlusion, but still has loose or symptomatic teeth, only a night guard is indicated. The guard does not prevent the patient from clenching and grinding, but it does minimize trauma to the teeth while it is worn. Such patients usually have a psychogenic need to clench and grind. Not all such patients will wear a night guard. The dentist should explain to the patient the need to wear one in bed and the tendency to

salivate more while wearing it before the patient decides to have one fabricated. Some patients become so accustomed to a night guard that they cannot sleep if they lose it or forget to bring it with them.

B   Some patients have an inadequate number of teeth or an occlusion that cannot be treated by selective grinding. If a restorative plan to provide a better, less traumatogenic occlusion cannot be financed by the patient, a night guard may be used to minimize the trauma.

C   In some cases in which the patient has loose or symptomatic teeth, and selective grinding is both indicated and feasible, the patient may reject selective grinding. If so, a night guard may be a helpful alternative. If the patient agrees to selective grinding, and the dentist can determine a psychogenic component to the etiology of the clenching and grinding, both selective grinding and a night guard should be used. If psychogenic factors are minimal or absent, and the dentist can detect "trigger tooth" disharmony, selective grinding alone may be sufficient to control the clenching and grinding, improve the firmness of teeth, and minimize the symptoms.

Additional Readings

Glickman I et al. When and to what extent do you adjust the occlusion during periodontal therapy? J Periodontol 1970;41:536.

Muhlemann HR, Herzog H, Rateitschak KH. Qualitative evaluation of the therapeutic effect of selective grinding. J Periodontol 1957;28:11.

Possellt V, Wolff IB. Treatment of bruxism by bite guards and bite plates. Calif Dent Assoc J 1963;29:773.

Ramfjord S, Ash MM. Occlusion. 3rd ed. Philadelphia: WB Saunders; 1983. p. 365.

Schluger S et al. Periodontal diseases. 2nd ed. Philadelphia: Lea & Febiger; 1989. p. 405.

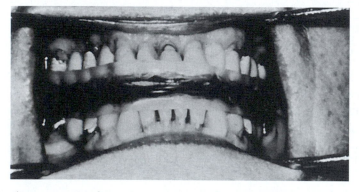

Figure 66-1 Paired maxillary and mandibular night guards.

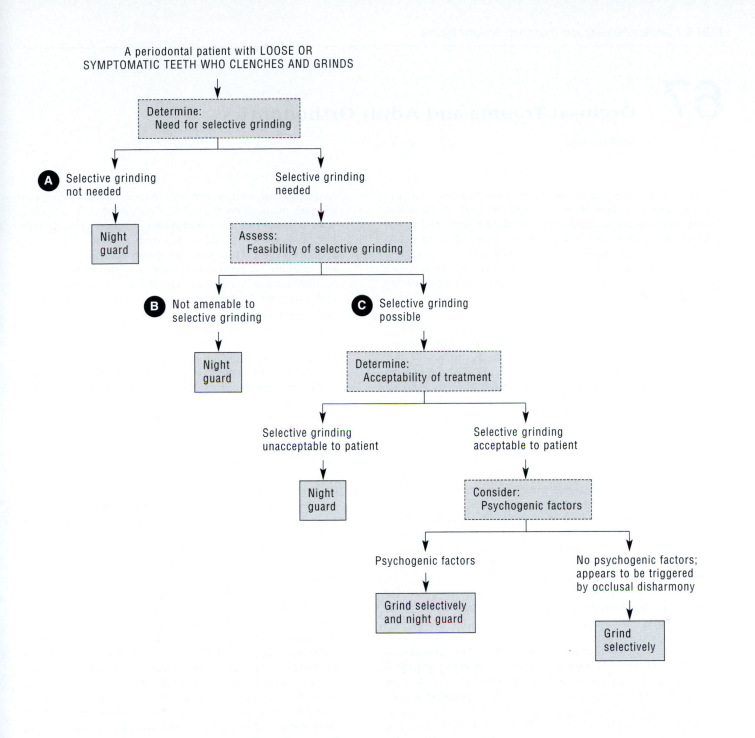

A periodontal patient with LOOSE OR
SYMPTOMATIC TEETH WHO CLENCHES AND GRINDS

Determine:
Need for selective grinding

A Selective grinding
not needed

Night
guard

Selective grinding
needed

Assess:
Feasibility of selective grinding

B Not amenable to
selective grinding

Night
guard

C Selective grinding
possible

Determine:
Acceptability of treatment

Selective grinding
unacceptable to patient

Night
guard

Selective grinding
acceptable to patient

Consider:
Psychogenic factors

Psychogenic factors

Grind selectively
and night guard

No psychogenic factors;
appears to be triggered
by occlusal disharmony

Grind
selectively

67 Occlusal Trauma and Adult Orthodontics

Vicki Vlaskalic

Orthodontic therapy can be an efficient way to treat and prevent occlusal traumatic lesions caused by tooth malposition. Adults experiencing such trauma may present signs and symptoms including increased tooth mobility, localized worn dentitions, pain on mastication, temporomandibular joint pain, and periodontal disease. Many of these conditions may be reversed with orthodontic tooth movement, in patients without existing inflammatory disease.

A   The diagnosis of occlusal trauma is not typically made based on a single examination due to the necessarily progressive nature of the injury. Once a diagnosis of primary or secondary occlusal trauma is made, the cause of the trauma must be assessed. Orthodontic correction of tooth malposition will not necessarily address trauma due to ill-designed partial dentures, poor restorations, or habits. In cases where tooth malposition is the prime cause of the trauma, we need to determine the teeth involved and whether moving these teeth is a reasonable course of action. Orthodontic tooth movement may augment periodontal therapy in many situations including functional anterior crossbite causing jiggling trauma, tipped teeth with periodontal pocketing, and the extrusion or intrusion of teeth with compromised bone morphology. In these situations, pocket depth and bone morphology may be reduced and normalized if root surfaces remain débrided and free of plaque. Additional factors such as the morphology and prognosis of the teeth involved, and the direction and magnitude of movement required will influence the decision of whether or not orthodontic tooth movement is indicated.

B   Treatment decisions involving orthodontic mechanotherapy will largely depend on the assessment of the entire periodontal health status of the patient. The three broad categories that patients will fall into will be those with no periodontal concerns, those with previous periodontal disease but no inflammatory conditions present, and those with active lesions. The patients displaying total periodontal health are candidates for orthodontic evaluation, whereas those with either previous periodontal conditions or active lesions should be treated and/or assigned a periodontal maintenance regimen. Once the periodontal health of the patient becomes stable, and all inflammatory conditions are controlled, the patient can then be assessed for orthodontic treatment. If, however, the periodontal health of the patient is not well controlled, and inflammatory disease does not subside, orthodontic tooth movement is contraindicated due to the increased risk of further, rapid periodontal deterioration.

C   Before any attempt at tooth movement is made, a diagnosis of the entire occlusion is necessary. This is to ensure that the patient does not undergo treatment aimed at only a symptom of a broader problem. Occlusal trauma may be a localized tooth malposition problem, or more usually a symptom of tooth malposition related to a comprehensive malocclusion. Occlusal factors such as posterior interdigitation, overbite, and overjet should be assessed, as well as transverse relations such as crossbites. Significant deviations from centric relation to centric occlusion are also important, as occlusal trauma is often associated with mandibular shifts, either as a predisposing factor or secondarily as an avoidance mechanism. If a comprehensive malocclusion exists, it is standard of care to inform the patient that the ideal corrective treatment would likely include treatment of two full arches. It is not uncommon for patients to refuse full treatment due to the esthetic objection to most fixed appliances, and to opt for an approach limited to treating only the teeth directly involved in traumatic occlusion. This may be an acceptable compromise only if the patient has been fully informed of the larger problem with the occlusion and attempts are made, such as retention of the occlusion, to prevent further relapse and/or physiologic tooth movement.

D   Patients experiencing occlusal trauma who have been assessed to this point require orthodontic diagnosis and treatment planning with the correction of the traumatic tooth position as only one occlusal goal of many. The process of orthodontic treatment planning involves collection and evaluation of records including full mouth radiographs, lateral cephalometric film, intra- and extraoral photographs, and study cases. Those patients who have had compromised periodontal health would also require a periodontal evaluation indicating the absence of active disease. A problem list including extraoral esthetic evaluation, as well as intraoral soft-tissue, skeletal, and dental evaluation is compiled, headed by the patient's chief complaint. A treatment plan is devised that best addresses as many of these problems as possible. It is prudent to consider the correction of the whole malocclusion at this stage, rather than focus specifically on the trauma, as if an ideal occlusion situation is created for the patient, this will correct the trauma most of the time. The treatment plan should make provision for the type of long-term retention that would best suit the patient's needs concerning the prevention of a recurrence of the trauma and periodontal needs.

E   Fixed appliance therapy is the traditional modality used in the treatment of malocclusions requiring three-dimensional correction. These appliances provide maximum control over root position. The disadvantage is that they are often unesthetic and may obstruct periodontal maintenance and routine oral hygiene procedures. Recently, an alternative appliance system known as the Invisalign System of tooth movement has become popular among esthetically minded adult patients due to the removable nature of these sequentially worn, clear, overlay appliances. This system may be

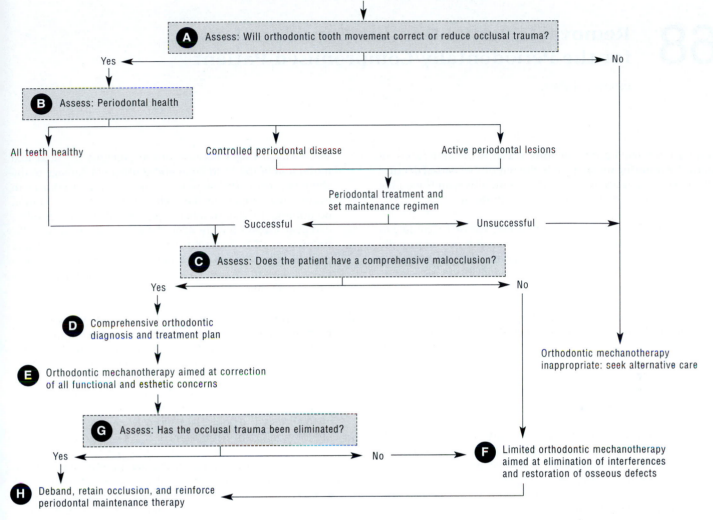

Adult Patient with OCCLUSAL TRAUMA AND ORTHODONTICS

A Assess: Will orthodontic tooth movement correct or reduce occlusal trauma?

Yes — No

B Assess: Periodontal health

All teeth healthy — Controlled periodontal disease — Active periodontal lesions

Periodontal treatment and set maintenance regimen

Successful — Unsuccessful

C Assess: Does the patient have a comprehensive malocclusion?

Yes — No

D Comprehensive orthodontic diagnosis and treatment plan

E Orthodontic mechanotherapy aimed at correction of all functional and esthetic concerns

Orthodontic mechanotherapy inappropriate: seek alternative care

G Assess: Has the occlusal trauma been eliminated?

Yes — No

F Limited orthodontic mechanotherapy aimed at elimination of interferences and restoration of osseous defects

H Deband, retain occlusion, and reinforce periodontal maintenance therapy

---

specifically indicated for adult patients with periodontal compromise, as routine oral hygiene procedure are not obstructed. During treatment, patients should be screened for signs of periodontal disease and root resorption at intervals related to the risk profile of the patient.

F Limited orthodontic mechanotherapy assumes that either the traumatic lesion is the only evidence of a malocclusion or that patients have been informed of and rejected treatment aimed at comprehensive treatment of their malocclusion. They still require an adequate record base for diagnosis; however, the treatment plan is restricted in its goal to elimination of the occlusal trauma. Typically, the treatment will take less time to accomplish and will require only partial application of fixed appliances or the use of removable appliances.

G Before orthodontic appliances are removed, the clinician should ensure that occlusal interferences are eliminated. This assessment should be made both in static occlusion and in functional excursions. Investigations that may aid this decision may include visual inspection using articulation paper, shoulder of occlusion, mobility assessment, radiographs, feedback from the patient, and, lately, the use of computer-aided occlusal evaluation systems. Study models will also be beneficial in assessing arch coordination and

posterior cusp relations. Specific attention should be paid to low lingual cusp position of maxillary molars.

H Once traumatic occlusion has been eliminated via tooth movement (perhaps supplemented with minor occlusal equilibration), and other treatment goals are obtained, the patient may be debanded and the retention phase started. Retention should be custom-designed for each patient taking into account the nature of the initial malocclusion and the periodontal status of the patient. Bonded retainers may not be indicated if they prevent compliance with oral hygiene routine. Settling of the occlusion is common, even during the retention phase. This may necessitate minor equilibration to perfect the static and functional occlusion.

Additional Readings

Boyd RL, Vlaskalic V. Three dimensional diagnosis and orthodontic treatment of complex malocclusions with the Invisalign appliance. Semin Orthod 2001;7:232.

Melsen B. Tissue reaction following application of extrusive and intrusive forces to teeth in adult monkeys. Am J Orthod 1986;89:469.

Ramfjord SP, Ash MM Jr. Significance of occlusion in the etiology and treatment of early, moderate and advanced periodontitis. J Periodontol 1981;52:511.

68 Removable Partial Denture Considerations for the Periodontally Compromised Patient

Eugene E. LaBarre

Although the fixed partial denture (FPD) is the restoration of choice for restoring missing teeth, the removable partial denture (RPD) becomes necessary when the edentulous span is too long or when there is no end tooth (distal extension).

A The need for tooth replacement is first assessed according to the patient's esthetic or functional disability. Not all partially edentulous patients require restoration; when all molars are missing, a well-integrated second premolar occlusion is satisfactory for many people.

B When an RPD is fabricated for a periodontally compromised patient, the prosthesis should fit well, be rigid, and result in minimal coverage of marginal gingiva by the metallic portion. Open major connector designs placed at least 3 mm apically to marginal tissue in the mandible (6 mm in the maxilla) are preferred over plated designs, which cover the lingual surfaces of multiple teeth.

C Edentulous areas that are capable of supporting occlusal loads are covered fully, particularly in distal extension situations. The altered cast impression technique provides soft tissue contact simultaneously with seating the rests, minimizing rocking of the restoration in function. A variety of mechanical clasping systems have been described to reduce functional leverage-type forces on distal extension RPD abutments (Figure 68-1). If precision attachments are desirable esthetically, resilient designs that permit tissue-ward movement and rotation are necessary for periodontally compromised abutments.

D Splinting is required to reinforce mobile RPD abutments and is strongly recommended for free-standing premolar pier abutments. Double abutting also may be necessary for non-mobile abutments adjacent to severely resorbed distal exten-

sion residual ridges because of the potential for increased movement of the restoration and consequent damage to the abutment teeth. The presence of six or fewer anterior teeth as the only support in the arch for an RPD is a common occurrence. In this situation, splinting all the teeth offers excellent support for the RPD. Highly mobile teeth have little value as RPD abutments and should be extracted. There must be at least two strategic nonmobile abutments or abutment groups to support an RPD; otherwise, a complete denture is indicated.

E The optimal occlusion for the reduced support RPD involves uniform posterior centric contacts without significant laterally displacing forces. Natural tooth guidance, if it exists and is nondestructive, should be maintained. Prosthetic tooth materials should have wear properties compatible with those of opposing dentition to preserve occlusal contact patterns: acrylic opposite acrylic; metal opposite enamel, metal, or porcelain fused to metal; and porcelain opposite porcelain denture teeth.

The success of any restoration in a compromised oral scheme depends on effective home care and regular recall. Removable restorations should be kept scrupulously clean and should be removed from the mouth for a minimum of 8 hours each day.

Additional Readings

Carranza FA. Glickman's clinical periodontology. 7th ed. Philadelphia: WB Saunders; 1990. p. 945.

Gomes BC, Renner RP. Periodontal considerations of the removable partial overdenture. Dent Clin North Am 1990;34:653.

Renner RP, Boucher IJ. Removable partial dentures. Chicago: Quintessence Publishing; 1987. p. 53.

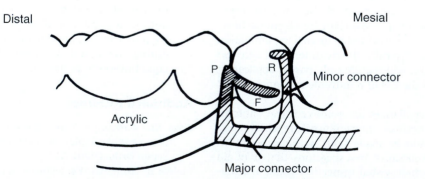

Figure 68-1 Illustration of a stress-releasing clasp. The minor connector provides bracing action and is designed to cover the soft tissue minimally. The major connector is placed apically to the free gingival margin. F = circumferential clasp placed at or gingival to the tooth height of contour; P = distal plane; R = mesial rest.

Patient who is PARTIALLY EDENTULOUS WITH REDUCED PERIODONTAL SUPPORT

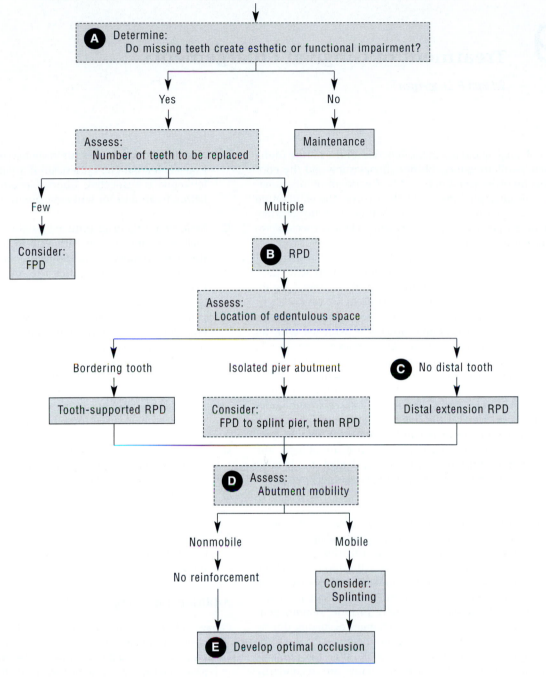

69 Treatment of Gingival Enlargements

William P. Lundergan

Treatment of gingival enlargement depends on the nature of the enlargement—inflammatory, fibrotic, neoplastic—and the etiologic factors involved (see Chapter 29). Treatment of inflammatory or fibrotic enlargements generally involves the elimination of local factors, followed by surgical treatment of any residual enlargement. Suspected neoplasms require a biopsy specimen to establish or confirm a diagnosis.

A   During the treatment of a gingival abscess or an acute periodontal abscess, the dentist gives a local anesthetic, establishes drainage, and débrides the lesion. In the case of a gingival abscess, blade incision is used to establish drainage. Drainage for the periodontal abscess is achieved with an external incision or by curette via the pocket. Care should be taken not to overinstrument the root surface, because this decreases the prospects for reattachment. After drainage is established, irrigate the lesion with warm saline solution or water. For a periodontal abscess, antibiotics should be prescribed if the patient is experiencing malaise or lymphadenopathy or is febrile. Analgesics may be prescribed for pain. After treatment of an acute abscess, the patient should return the next day. The dentist should evaluate the area for further treatment (eg, surgery) after the acute symptoms have resolved.

B   Treatment of chronic inflammatory gingival enlargements requires a heavy emphasis on proper daily plaque control, elimination of other local irritants (ie, calculus, poor dental restorations, caries, open contacts with food impaction, mouth breathing, orthodontic braces, and poorly fitted removable appliances), and identification of potential systemic factors. Systemic factors may include vitamin deficiency, leukemia, and hormonal changes occurring during pregnancy or puberty or in association with oral contraceptives. Some enlargements may resolve after the etiologic factors are eliminated; however, many are secondarily fibrotic and require surgical treatment. Evaluate the need for surgery (gingivectomy or flap procedure) after sufficient time has been allowed for response to the initial therapy. Consult the patient's physician if a vitamin C deficiency or leukemia is suspected. Check bleeding and clotting times before treatment for leukemic gingival enlargement.

C   Treatment of a drug-induced gingival enlargement should include a consultation with a physician regarding alternative drug therapy. Drug-induced enlargement may regress or completely resolve after the medication is discontinued. In most cases, however, an alternative drug therapy is not practical. Treatment then involves meticulous plaque control and removal of local irritants. If the enlargement interferes with esthetics or mastication or presents a significant plaque-control problem, gingivectomy or flap surgery may be performed. Recurrence is a problem, but it can be minimized with proper attention to daily plaque control and regular professional cleanings. Some clinicians use positive-pressure appliances after surgery to help discourage recurrence.

D   Hereditary gingival fibromatosis is treated surgically (gingivectomy or flap procedure) if it interferes with esthetics or mastication or becomes a significant plaque-control problem. The condition may recur despite meticulous oral hygiene, and it often regresses after tooth extraction.

E   Suspected neoplasms require a biopsy specimen to establish or confirm a diagnosis. Treatment depends on the nature of the neoplasm, and referral to a specialist is often indicated.

Additional Readings

Carranza FA Jr, Newman MG. Clinical periodontology. 8th ed. Philadelphia: WB Saunders; 1996. p. 672.

Lundergan WP. Drug-induced gingival enlargements—dilantin hyperplasia and beyond. J Calif Dent Assoc 1989;17:48.

Newman MG, Takei HH, Carranza FA Jr. Carranza's clinical periodontology. 9th ed. Philadelphia: WB Saunders; 2001. p. 279.

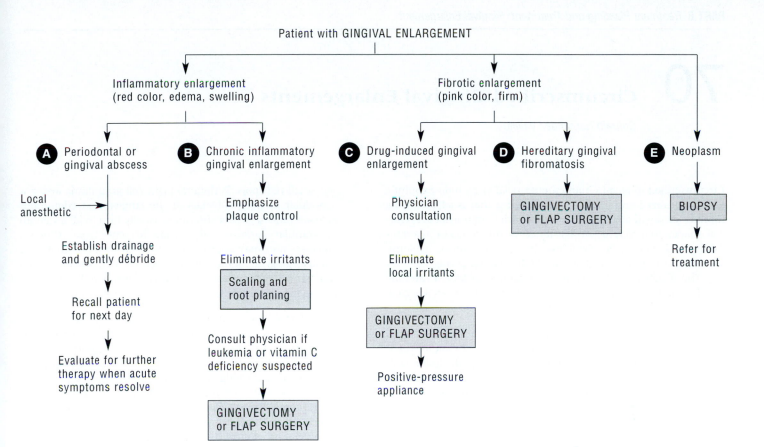

Patient with GINGIVAL ENLARGEMENT

Inflammatory enlargement
(red color, edema, swelling)

Fibrotic enlargement
(pink color, firm)

A Periodontal or gingival abscess

Local anesthetic →

Establish drainage and gently débride

↓

Recall patient for next day

↓

Evaluate for further therapy when acute symptoms resolve

B Chronic inflammatory gingival enlargement

↓

Emphasize plaque control

↓

Eliminate irritants

Scaling and root planing

↓

Consult physician if leukemia or vitamin C deficiency suspected

↓

GINGIVECTOMY or FLAP SURGERY

C Drug-induced gingival enlargement

↓

Physician consultation

↓

Eliminate local irritants

↓

GINGIVECTOMY or FLAP SURGERY

↓

Positive-pressure appliance

D Hereditary gingival fibromatosis

↓

GINGIVECTOMY or FLAP SURGERY

E Neoplasm

↓

BIOPSY

↓

Refer for treatment

70 Circumscribed Gingival Enlargements

Gonzalo Hernández Vallejo

Circumscribed gingival enlargements (CGEs) include exophitic lesions localized and limited to the gingiva that is adjacent to a tooth or group of teeth. CGEs adopt a variety of nonspecific clinical shapes that may be of assistance to the clinician in establishing a diagnosis. Nevertheless, in most instances, a biopsy specimen is required to establish a definitive diagnosis.

The diagnostic sequence for CGE should include a carefully detailed medical and dental history. After a CGE has been detected, the inflammatory appearance of the lesion must be assessed.

A   Inflamed lesions are characterized by redness, edema, and bleeding. They may appear at the attached or marginal papillary gingiva, and the inflammatory origin of the lesion does not necessarily mean that it appears inflamed. Radiographic investigation of the morphology of the lesion and probing the sulcus are important steps in making the diagnosis.

B   Inflamed CGEs located at the attached gingiva may adopt a pedunculated or polypoid shape. Dental pain and negative vitality with the presence of a polypoid lesion near the border between attached gingiva and alveolar mucosa suggest a parulis (a draining chronic alveolar abscess), which can be easily confirmed by studying the radiograph. If the lesion appears in the socket corresponding to a removed tooth, the dentist should suspect an epulis granulomatosa. The presence of partial or complete dentures accompanied by exophitic hyperplastic tissue at the periphery of the prosthesis provides enough information to diagnose an epulis fissurata.

CGEs that display a nodular dome shape with a smooth, shiny surface should be checked for acute infections. Gingival abscess is usually limited to the marginal or interdental gingiva and is clinically characterized by acute pain, redness, and fluctuance with no loss of attachment. Periodontal abscesses, however, show features of periodontal disease and radiographic evidence of bone loss.

C   Inflamed CGEs involving marginal or papillar gingiva are common lesions. Radiography is important in evaluating the involvement of the underlying bone. Red polypoid or nodular masses that bleed easily and are accompanied by bone radiolucency may indicate a central giant cell granuloma.

If no bone involvement is observed, the dentist should review the following conditions. Chronic inflammatory enlargements sometimes appear as painful, red, localized papillar or marginal masses and are associated with local factors such as bacterial plaque and calculus. Pyogenic granuloma is an inflammatory hyperplasia that clinically consists of a red or purple, very soft, friable, nodular or pedunculated mass, frequently with an eroded or ulcerated surface that bleeds under the slightest trauma. Pregnancy tumor occurs in 3 to 5% of pregnancies; it appears as a spherical or flattened mass located in marginal and interdental papilla. The surface of a pregnancy tumor is dusky red or magenta, and it displays numer-

ous small red spots. Peripheral giant cell granuloma arises as a nodular or polypoid mass at the gingiva and edentulous alveolar mucosa; its consistency is usually firm, with a smooth or granular surface, and it may become large. Gingival abscesses also may appear circumscribed to the marginal or papillar gingiva. Some rarities such as hemangiomas and Kaposi's sarcoma in cases of acquired immunodeficiency syndrome may resemble lesions belonging to this group.

D   Noninflamed CGEs include conditions that exhibit clinical characteristics in which inflammation is absent. An evaluation of the color of the lesion is extremely important in this group of entities. White color is a typical feature in papillomas and verruca vulgaris, which usually show a pedunculated shape with a cauliflowerlike appearance. Brown CGEs are rare and are associated with hyperparathyroidism. They appear as multiple tumoral lesions accompanied by bone involvement; clinical history, radiography, and biochemical data support the correct diagnosis. Blue lesions include hemangioma, hematoma, eruption cysts, and, less frequently, the blue variety of peripheral giant cell granuloma. Careful examination can provide information about a history of trauma (hematoma) or reveal the presence of unerupted teeth (eruption cyst). Red or pink CGEs comprise the majority of gingival tumors and tumorlike conditions. Clinical characteristics are of little help in differentiating these entities; therefore, biopsy is the method of choice to confirm the diagnosis. Clinical diagnosis, however, must be focused on the texture and consistency of the CGE.

E   Hard lesions with bonelike consistency must be assessed using radiography. Exostoses are common developmental lesions that can occur in alveolar bone and give a radiopaque image. Radiolucencies accompanied by CGEs are associated with central exophitic lesions.

F   Soft-to-firm (not hard) CGEs may display normal bone or bone changes under radiographic examination. Radiopaque images can be observed in peripheral fibromas with calcification or in peripheral ossifying fibromas. The presence of radiopaque foci within the tumors, together with the feature of separated teeth in this area, may help in the diagnosis. Radiolucencies appear frequently in cases of central giant cell granuloma, malignant central tumors with peripheral invasion, and cysts. Gingival cysts arising from remnants of odontogenic epithelium may cause erosion of the alveolar bone, giving a circumscript radiolucency.

G   Soft-to-firm masses that concur with normal bone include most of the neoplasias. The dentist must evaluate these conditions while paying careful attention to the age of the lesion, rate of growth, external aspect of the lesion (surface), and location. Special care should be taken not to confuse normal anatomic variations such as retromolar papilla

Patient with CIRCUMSCRIBED GINGIVAL ENLARGEMENT

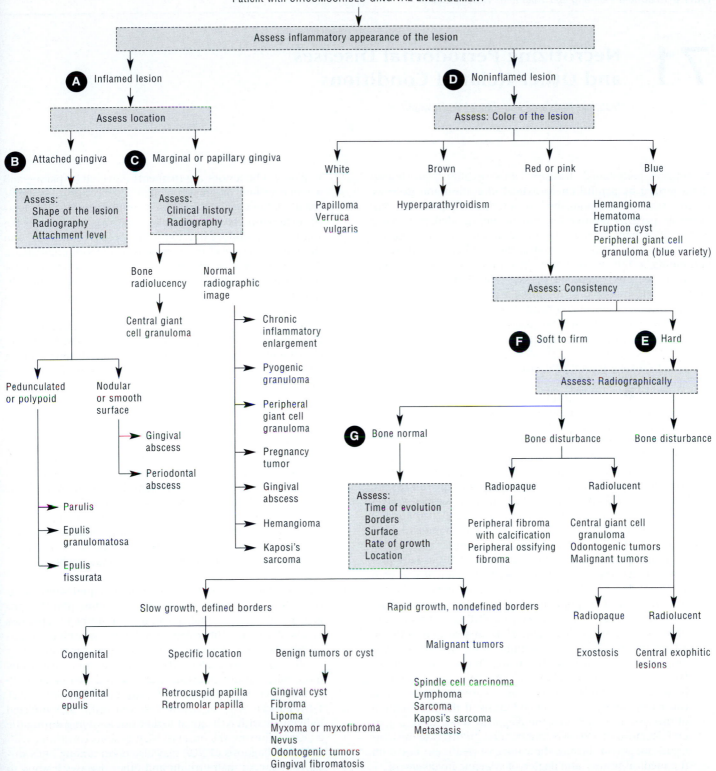

and retrocuspid papilla. Congenital epulis appears at birth as a large polypoid swelling and is easily recognizable. Benign tumors and gingival cysts show slow growth and well-defined borders and include a great number of lesions arising from the gingiva. Gingival fibromatosis may appear as a CGE located in the palatal posterior areas.

CGEs with a rapid rate of growth and nondefined borders should be suspected for malignancies, whether the lesions are growing from gingival tissues, central bone, or metastases from other locations.

Additional Readings

Cawson RA, Binnie WH, Speight PM, et al. Luca's pathology of tumors of the oral tissues. 5th ed. London: Churchill Livingstone; 1998. p. 199.

Lindhe J. Clinical periodontology and implant dentistry. 3rd ed. Copenhagen: Munksgaard; 1998. p. 356.

Wood NK, Goaz PW. Differential diagnosis of oral and maxillofacial lesions. 5th ed. St. Louis: Mosby; 1997. p. 130.

71 Necrotizing Periodontal Diseases and Other Related Conditions

Mauricio Ronderos and Randal W. Rowland

Necrotizing periodontal diseases (NPDs) exhibit acute lesions characterized by painful interproximal ulceration and necrosis. In the severely malnourished or immunocompromised, for example, patients positive for human immunodeficiency virus (HIV), NPDs may extend into the basal bone and mucosa (ie, necrotizing stomatitis) or extend farther to the perioral tissues perforating to the external face (ie, cancrum oris/noma). Cancrum oris is often preceded by systemic viral infections (eg, measles). The presence of interproximal necrosis distinguishes NPD from other painful conditions, for example, herpetic gingivostomatitis (see Chapter 27), mucocutaneous disorders (see Chapter 34), and aphthous ulcers.

A Due to their intraoral pain, patients with an NPD generally seek treatment. The pain is usually localized to a specific area. There are two forms of NPD: necrotizing ulcerative gingivitis (NUG) and necrotizing ulcerative periodontitis (NUP). Both NUG and NUP are characterized by pain, interproximal gingival necrosis, and bleeding that occurs spontaneously or upon minimal manipulation. However, they differ in the extent of periodontal tissue destruction. NUG exhibits necrosis that is generally limited to the soft tissues; whereas NUP features gingival necrosis with a loss of alveolar bone and minimal pocketing. NUG and NUP are also distinct from an epidemiologic perspective. In industrialized countries, NUG is a disease of young adults, whereas, in developing countries, it affects children. NUP usually presents in a severely immunocompromised patient (eg, with HIV) in developed countries, but may present in the non–HIV-infected population especially in developing countries. It has been suggested that NUP is the progression of NUG in a susceptible patient. NPDs appear to result from a bacterial infection in a susceptible host. A possible influence of herpes viruses in the etiology has also been speculated. It may be difficult for clinicians to distinguish between NUP and NUG when there is preexisting bone loss caused by other forms of periodontitis. If the presentation of the lesions is such that the diagnosis is not clear, a general diagnosis of NPD is recommended. In this case the clinician's judgment dictates the course of treatment based on the medical history and degree of systemic involvement.

B NUG (formerly known as ANUG, Vincent's gingivitis, or trench mouth) lesions are characterized by necrosis and ulceration of one or more interdental areas resulting in "punched-out" papillae. NUG lesions often extend to the facial and lingual marginal gingiva and are accompanied by foul odor. The lesions are frequently covered by plaque and a white-yellow or grayish slough due to fibrin. Systemic manifestations may or may not be present and include lymphadenopathy, fever, and malaise. NUG is localized to the soft tissues and does not involve loss of alveolar bone, and the lesions may lead to minimal or no loss of attachment. The distribution of the lesions varies; however, anterior teeth are frequently affected. The lesions appear to be self-limiting in extent and duration and generally resolve rapidly to mechanical débridement. NUG lesions have been associated with the presence of different bacteria including spirochetes, *Fusobacterium* spp, and *Prevotella intermedia*. Under electron microscopy, NUG lesions have four distinct zones: a bacterial zone (outer layer), a neutrophil-rich zone, a necrotic zone, and a spirochetal-infiltrated zone.

The incidence of NUG in industrialized countries has declined during the past decades, and it is now rare. However, the disease is still common in some developing nations. In industrialized countries, NUG mostly affects young adults of low socioeconomic status. Meanwhile, in developing nations, the disease mainly affects children. Historically, persons under psychological stress are more prone to be affected, for example, those in the military and students. Other risk factors include cigarette smoking, poor oral hygiene, malnutrition, and immunosuppression (eg, neutropenia, leukemia, and HIV infection). Risk factors other than poor oral hygiene, however, may not be obvious.

C NUP (formerly know as HIV-associated periodontitis) is characterized by pain and necrosis extending past the gingiva into the periodontal attachment, resulting in rapid loss of alveolar bone. The lesions usually involve the interdental periodontium. Sequestration of bone is common.

NUP generally affects HIV-infected persons, especially those who are not receiving antiretroviral treatment. NUP is associated with severe immunosuppression (eg, CD4+ T-lymphocyte counts below 200 cells/mL). HIV-infected individuals with NUP are at higher risk for dying during the 2 years following the onset of NUP. Lesions consistent with a clinical diagnosis of NUP may also occur among individuals with severe malnutrition and other diseases leading to immunosuppression.

Given the strong association with HIV infection, HIV tests may be recommended for patients with either NUG or NUP. Referral for close medical follow-up may be indicated for HIV-infected patients with NUP as it may be an indicator of immune system deterioration.

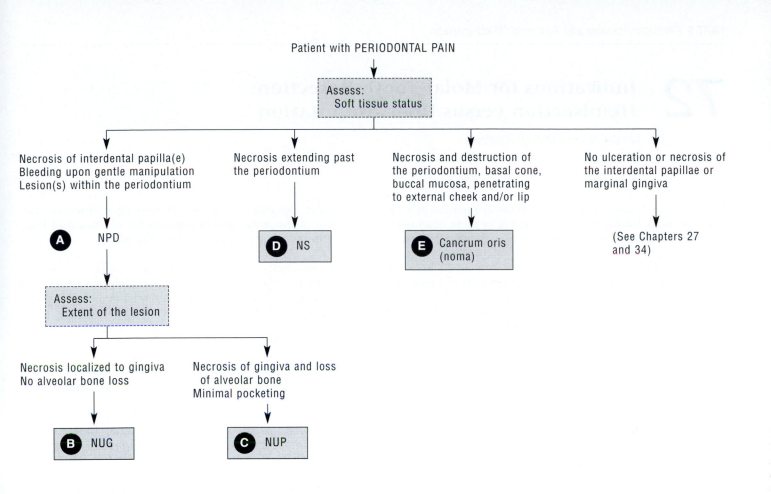

Patient with PERIODONTAL PAIN

Assess:
Soft tissue status

Necrosis of interdental papilla(e)
Bleeding upon gentle manipulation
Lesion(s) within the periodontium

A NPD

Assess:
Extent of the lesion

Necrosis localized to gingiva
No alveolar bone loss

B NUG

Necrosis of gingiva and loss
of alveolar bone
Minimal pocketing

C NUP

Necrosis extending past
the periodontium

D NS

Necrosis and destruction of
the periodontium, basal cone,
buccal mucosa, penetrating
to external cheek and/or lip

E Cancrum oris
(noma)

No ulceration or necrosis of
the interdental papillae or
marginal gingiva

(See Chapters 27
and 34)

D   Necrotizing stomatitis (NS) is characterized by necrosis extending past the periodontium into the surrounding oral tissues, soft and hard. Whether NS is a separate disease entity or a further progression of NUP is not known. It is possible that NS may be an intermediate step between NUP and cancrum oris.

E   Cancrum oris (noma) is an aggressive gangrenelike lesion characterized by necrosis and destruction of the periodontium that penetrates to the external cheek and lips. The disease begins as an NUG-like lesion and rapidly progresses to involve the alveolar process, basal bone, and face. The lesions, which result in permanent disfiguration and often in death, predominantly occur in malnourished children. Most reports of cancrum oris come from sub–Saharan Africa where the disease mainly affects children between the ages of 2 and 16 (mean age, 4 to 5 years). Lesions have also been reported to occur among neonates and other immunocompromised groups (eg, patients with leukemia

and diabetes). Cancrum oris is often preceded by systemic manifestations of herpes virus infection or measles. Whether these infections trigger the disease or are coincidental due to the depleted immune system of the host is unknown. The large areas of necrosis and tissue destruction are frequently colonized by *Fusobacterium necrophorum*, staphylococci, and anaerobic streptococci.

Additional Readings

Enwonwu CO, Falkler WA Jr, Idigbe EO, Savage KO. Noma (cancrum oris): questions and answers. Oral Dis 1999;5:144.

Listgarten MA. Electron microscopic observations on the bacterial flora of acute necrotizing ulcerative gingivitis. J Periodontol 1965;36:328.

Novak MJ. Necrotizing ulcerative periodontitis. Ann Periodontol 1999; 4:74.

Rowland RW. Necrotizing ulcerative gingivitis. Ann Periodontol 1999;4:65.

Consensus report: necrotizing periodontal diseases. Ann Periodontol 1999; 4:78.

72 Indications for Molar Tooth Resection: Hemisection versus Root Amputation

Jordi Cambra and Borja Zabelegui

Root resection is a technique for maintaining a portion of a diseased or injured molar by removal of one or more of its roots. Resection may be achieved by hemisection, in which the entire tooth is cut in half and one part is removed, or by root amputation, in which only a root or two are amputated from the remainder of the tooth (Figure 72-1). These surgical approaches may be useful in many situations. The selection of hemisection or root amputation depends on the status of the individual molar and its relationships to other teeth. Guided tissue regeneration (GTR) may be a viable option in many cases (see Chapter 79).

A If a molar has fused roots, neither hemisection nor root amputation is possible. If a Class II furcation is present (see Chapters 46 and 100), GTR may be attempted. If a Class III furcation is present (see Chapter 101), extraction or maintenance with a hopeless prognosis is an option.

B A maxillary molar with advanced involvement of a proximal furcation and separated roots in which root proximity is a problem should be treated by root amputation to facilitate access for débridement by the dentist. If root proximity is not a complicating factor, a Class II (definite) furcation involvement proximally may be treated by GTR or mucogingival-osseous surgery or maintained with frequent planing (see Chapter 100). The patient can establish plaque control with an interproximal brush. The same is true if the facial furcation has a Class II involvement; however, if the furcations join one another (Class III), root amputation is indicated, although GTR may be attempted in ideal cases.

C When the remaining bone support for a future implant would be jeopardized by retention of a badly involved molar, especially in the case of a younger patient, extraction of the molar would improve the likelihood of long-term success utilizing an implant alternative.

D A mandibular molar with advanced furcation involvement and separated roots that is an existing bridge abutment is a candidate for root amputation and retention of the existing bridge; however, a similarly involved mandibular molar that is not an existing bridge abutment should be treated by hemisection and crowning. In either case, if a Class II furcation is involved, GTR may be attempted. If a Class III furcation is present, hemisection or root amputation (if the tooth is part of an existing bridge) should be performed.

E If no endodontic involvement is evident, periodontal considerations assume paramount importance. Determine the roots to be amputated. If doubts exist, periodontal surgery with vital resection of the root selected during surgery should be performed before endodontic treatment. If the root to be removed is clearly indicated, endodontics should be done before amputation, but, if doubt exists, surgery and vital root amputation allow for clinical decisions to be made. If the molar is mandibular and is not an abutment for an existing fixed bridge, root amputation may permit retention of that bridge. If it is not an existing abutment, hemisection and then crowning are indicated.

F If necrotic pulp condition exists, initiate endodontic treatment before periodontal treatment. The differential diagnosis becomes difficult if the bone loss that is causing a deep pocket formation may be related to failure of the root canal therapy because of technical errors (leaking obturations). Perforations or vertical root fracture with no separation of fragments may cause bone loss defects that mask primary periodontal conditions.

G If the molar being considered has a cracked or perforated root, part of it may be salvaged by resection. If the tooth is nonsymptomatic, either maintenance with a guarded prognosis or a surgical approach may be considered. If the tooth is symptomatic and not of strategic (long-term) value, it may be extracted; however, if the tooth has strategic value, it should be treated. If the tooth is mandibular and is not an abutment for an existing bridge, tooth amputation should be considered if root canal therapy can be performed on the root that will be retained. If it is not an abutment for an existing bridge, hemisection is better. If the molar is a maxillary one and a single facial root is cracked or perforated, root amputation is better if root canal therapy can be performed on remaining roots. If both facial roots are cracked or perforated, hemisection with removal of both facial roots may be a reasonable choice.

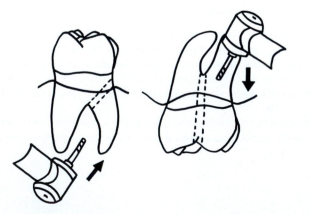

Figure 72-1 Illustrations of root amputation (removal of one root) and hemisection (removal of half a tooth).

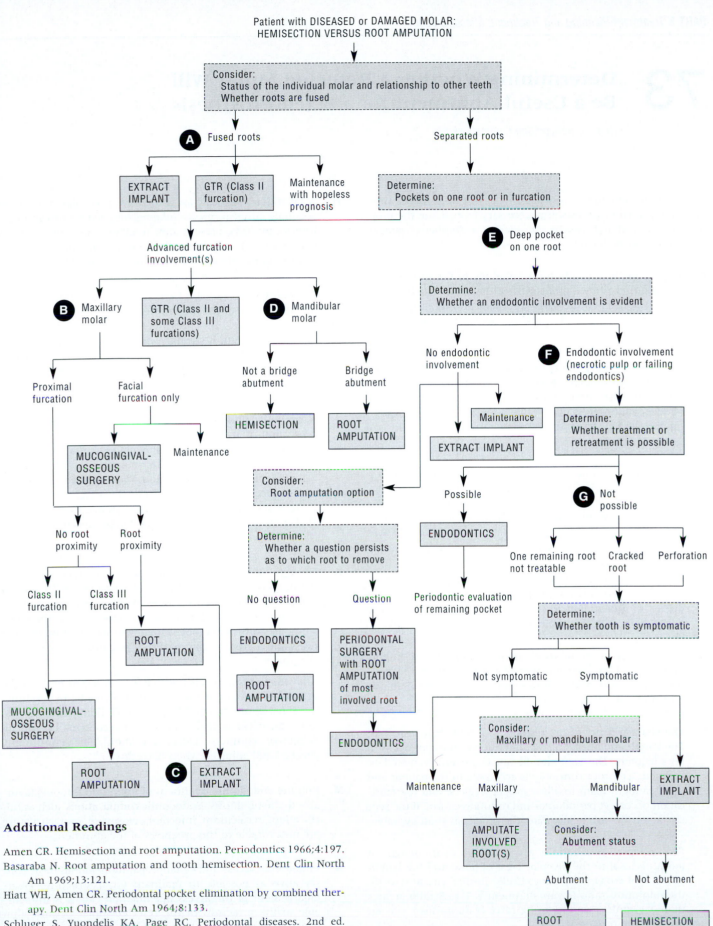

Patient with DISEASED or DAMAGED MOLAR:
HEMISECTION VERSUS ROOT AMPUTATION

Consider:
Status of the individual molar and relationship to other teeth
Whether roots are fused

A Fused roots

EXTRACT IMPLANT

GTR (Class II furcation)

Maintenance with hopeless prognosis

Separated roots

Determine:
Pockets on one root or in furcation

Advanced furcation involvement(s)

B Maxillary molar

GTR (Class II and some Class III furcations)

D Mandibular molar

Proximal furcation

Facial furcation only

MUCOGINGIVAL-OSSEOUS SURGERY

Maintenance

No root proximity

Root proximity

Class II furcation

Class III furcation

ROOT AMPUTATION

MUCOGINGIVAL-OSSEOUS SURGERY

ROOT AMPUTATION

C EXTRACT IMPLANT

Not a bridge abutment

Bridge abutment

HEMISECTION

ROOT AMPUTATION

Consider:
Root amputation option

Determine:
Whether a question persists as to which root to remove

No question

Question

ENDODONTICS

ROOT AMPUTATION

PERIODONTAL SURGERY with ROOT AMPUTATION of most involved root

ENDODONTICS

E Deep pocket on one root

Determine:
Whether an endodontic involvement is evident

No endodontic involvement

F Endodontic involvement (necrotic pulp or failing endodontics)

Maintenance

EXTRACT IMPLANT

Determine:
Whether treatment or retreatment is possible

Possible

ENDODONTICS

Periodontic evaluation of remaining pocket

G Not possible

One remaining root not treatable

Cracked root

Perforation

Determine:
Whether tooth is symptomatic

Not symptomatic

Symptomatic

Maintenance

Consider:
Maxillary or mandibular molar

Maxillary

Mandibular

EXTRACT IMPLANT

AMPUTATE INVOLVED ROOT(S)

Consider:
Abutment status

Abutment

Not abutment

ROOT AMPUTATION

HEMISECTION

Additional Readings

Amen CR. Hemisection and root amputation. Periodontics 1966;4:197.

Basaraba N. Root amputation and tooth hemisection. Dent Clin North Am 1969;13:121.

Hiatt WH, Amen CR. Periodontal pocket elimination by combined therapy. Dent Clin North Am 1964;8:133.

Schluger S, Yuondelis KA, Page RC. Periodontal diseases. 2nd ed. Philadelphia: Lea & Febiger; 1990. p. 548.

73 Determining Whether a Resected Molar Will Be a Useful Abutment for a Fixed Prosthesis

Brian J. Kenyon and Casimir Leknius

To determine whether a resected molar will be a useful abutment for a fixed prosthesis, it is necessary to evaluate the prognosis of the residual root by considering a number of general and tooth-specific factors.

A A good medical condition is favorable to the prognosis of the residual root. Significant health factors, such as diabetes, the use of anticonvulsant medications, a suppressed immune system, and smoking, are unfavorable to the prognosis.

B The genetic susceptibility of a patient to periodontal disease should be considered. A positive Periodontal Disease Susceptability Test (Medical Science Systems) indicates that the patient will progress more rapidly toward severe periodontal disease. This test result is unfavorable to the prognosis of a resected molar.

C The patient must be capable of proper oral hygiene and follow through with scheduled professional maintenance. After treatment, the site must have a periodontal and restorative form that facilitates adequate plaque control.

D The periodontal attachment needs to be assessed through oral examination, radiographs, and probing of the entire root circumference. Little loss of attachment (LOA) is favorable to the prognosis of the prosthetic abutment. A greater degree of attachment loss or a vertical component to the destruction, is unfavorable to the prognosis.

E The mobility of the tooth or the residual root is an important factor. Increased mobility is a sign of decreased periodontal support, and indicates that the root is unsuitable as an abutment.

F The characteristics of the residual root must be considered. The length and buccolingual dimension of the root needs to be adequate. The root should not be severely tapered or inclined. Any root concavity is accessible to the patient and the treatment team to allow proper hygiene and the fabrication of correct periodontal and restorative form. If the root characteristics are inadequate, the prognosis is unfavorable.

G The crown-to-root ratio is a comparison of the length of tooth occlusal to the alveolar crest of bone and the length of the root covered by bone. Under normal circumstances, the minimum ratio for an abutment is 1:1. A ratio greater than 1:1, unless the opposing force is diminished, has an unfavorable prognosis.

H A favorable prognosis for a resected molar depends on an adequate surgical result. Subgingival residual furcal lips or ledges cannot be present after resection. If osseous surgery is indicated, it must result in a positive periodontal architecture that facilitates adequate plaque control.

I The construction of the foundation restoration affects the prognosis. One of the major causes of resected molar failure is root fracture. The presence of a post, particularly in mandibular teeth, is strongly associated with root fracture. A post should not be used unless absolutely necessary. If required, post size should be minimized. The need for a post is unfavorable to the prognosis of the abutment.

J A favorable prognosis for a residual root depends on the fabrication of an adequate final prosthesis. The margins of the restoration should be well adapted, supragingival, and cleansable by the patient. If the margins extend subgingivally, the biologic space should not be violated. The proximal surfaces should emerge from the gingiva with a flat contour establishing interproximal contact. Buccal and lingual contours should sustain their flat profiles from the gingiva to the cusp tips.

K The type of prosthesis selected after root resection affects the prognosis of the abutment. Restorations with zero or one pontic supported by the residual root have a favorable prognosis. A residual root that supports more than one pontic has an unfavorable prognosis due to an increase in stress and a greater chance of root fracture.

L A favorable prognosis is possible for a resected molar if the occlusal forces can be satisfactorily managed and parafunctional habits are absent. The prosthesis should have vertical stops, an occlusal table narrowed buccolingually, and no deflective contacts. Occlusion should be continually checked and adjusted when necessary.

M Routine endodontic treatment of the residual root is favorable to the prognosis. Endodontic complications such as calcification, recalcitrant infection, or severe root curvature are unfavorable to the prognosis of the abutment.

N Endodontic access and canal preparation should be as conservative as possible to maintain tooth structure. Overenlargement of the access opening and canals is unfavorable to the prognosis of the resected molar because thin walls are susceptible to root fracture.

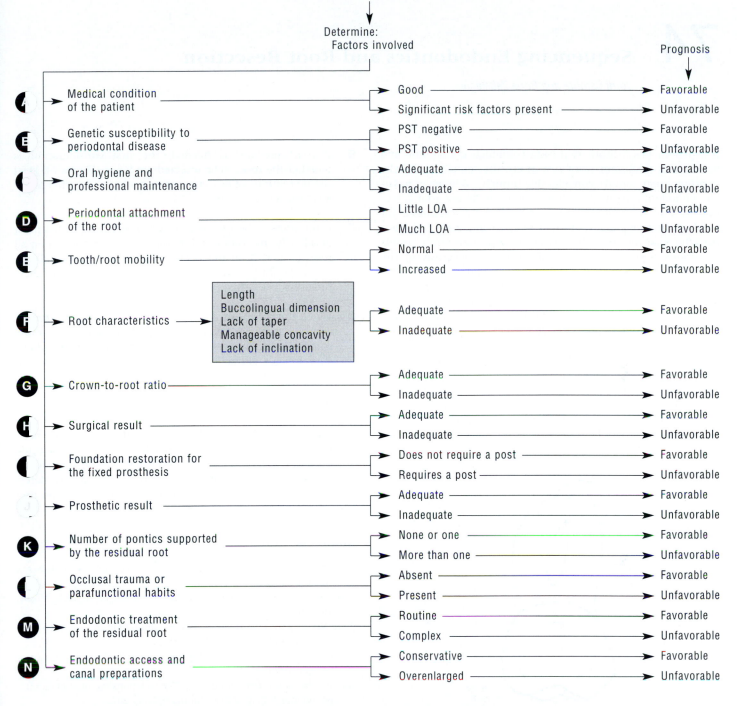

Patient with a DAMAGED OR DISEASED MOLAR

Determine:
Factors involved

Prognosis

A	Medical condition of the patient	Good → Favorable
		Significant risk factors present → Unfavorable
B	Genetic susceptibility to periodontal disease	PST negative → Favorable
		PST positive → Unfavorable
C	Oral hygiene and professional maintenance	Adequate → Favorable
		Inadequate → Unfavorable
D	Periodontal attachment of the root	Little LOA → Favorable
		Much LOA → Unfavorable
E	Tooth/root mobility	Normal → Favorable
		Increased → Unfavorable
F	Root characteristics → Length / Buccolingual dimension / Lack of taper / Manageable concavity / Lack of inclination	Adequate → Favorable
		Inadequate → Unfavorable
G	Crown-to-root ratio	Adequate → Favorable
		Inadequate → Unfavorable
H	Surgical result	Adequate → Favorable
		Inadequate → Unfavorable
I	Foundation restoration for the fixed prosthesis	Does not require a post → Favorable
		Requires a post → Unfavorable
J	Prosthetic result	Adequate → Favorable
		Inadequate → Unfavorable
K	Number of pontics supported by the residual root	None or one → Favorable
		More than one → Unfavorable
L	Occlusal trauma or parafunctional habits	Absent → Favorable
		Present → Unfavorable
M	Endodontic treatment of the residual root	Routine → Favorable
		Complex → Unfavorable
N	Endodontic access and canal preparations	Conservative → Favorable
		Overenlarged → Unfavorable

Additional Readings

Davarpanah M, Martinez H, Tecucianu J, et al. To conserve or implant: which choice of therapy? [review] Int J Periodontics Restorative Dent 2000;20:412.

Langer B. Root resections revisited. Int J Periodontics Restorative Dent 1996;16:200.

Schmitt SM, Brown FH. The hemisected mandibular molar: a strategic abutment. J Prosthet Dent 1987;58:140.

Shillingburg HT, Hobo S, Whitsett LD. Fundamentals of fixed prosthodontics. Chicago: Quintessence; 1997. p. 8990.

Svardstrom G, Weenstrom JL. Periodontal treatment decisions for molars: an analysis of influencing factors and long-term outcome. J Periodontol 2000;71:579.

74 Sequencing Endodontics and Root Resection

Jordi Cambra and Borja Zabelegui

If a patient has a tooth requiring combined endodontic and periodontal treatment (root resection), the sequencing of the treatment may require considerable thought. Whenever possible, endodontic treatment should be done before root resection so that difficulty in obtaining adequate anesthesia for comfortable root canal therapy does not complicate endodontics after vital root resection. Vital root resection rarely results in serious postoperative pain. However, as necrosis of the exposed pulp proceeds, the ability to obtain adequate anesthesia for comfortable root canal therapy is complicated by increasing acidity, which interferes with the efficacy of the local anesthetic; nevertheless, excellent reasons to accept and manage this problem do exist.

A   If the tooth is nonvital, the problem may be endodontic only (even if probing suggests that deep pockets are present), especially if the problem is severe and acute. If this appears to be the case, endodontics should be done first, because no need for root resection may arise later if pockets can no longer be probed.

B   If root resection is needed, the first consideration is whether the roots to be resected are fused (Figure 74-1). If so, the tooth must be extracted or maintained with a hopeless prognosis.

C   If the roots to be resected are not fused, the dentist must decide whether root canal therapy can be performed on all roots or not. If an untreatable root is to be retained, the tooth should be extracted or maintained with a hopeless prognosis if it is free of symptoms.

D   When the prognosis for success after root resection would continue to be poor because of significant bone loss, or one root is significantly cracked, or root canal therapy would be very difficult, extraction of the tooth and replacement with an implant would be the best long-term option.

E   If endodontics can be done on all roots or all roots to be retained, the next consideration relates to the certainty regarding the roots to be resected. If doubt exists, periodontal surgery with vital resection of the root selected during surgery should be performed before endodontic treatment. If the roots to be resected are clearly determinable before surgery, endodontic treatment should precede nonvital root resection.

Additional Readings

Basaraba N. Root amputation and tooth hemisection. Dent Clin North Am 1969;13:121.

Grant DA, Stern IB, Listgarten MA. Periodontics. 6th ed. St. Louis: Mosby; 1988. p. 916.

Hiatt WH, Amen CR. Periodontal pocket elimination by combined therapy. Dent Clin North Am 1964;8:133.

Schluger S et al. Periodontal diseases. 2nd ed. Philadelphia: Lea & Febiger; 1990. p. 549.

Simons HS, Glick DH, Frank AL. The relationship of endodontic–periodontal lesions. J Periodontol 1972;43:202.

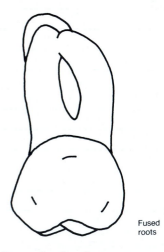

Fused roots

Figure 74-1 Roots that are fused at their apices are not candidates for root amputation.

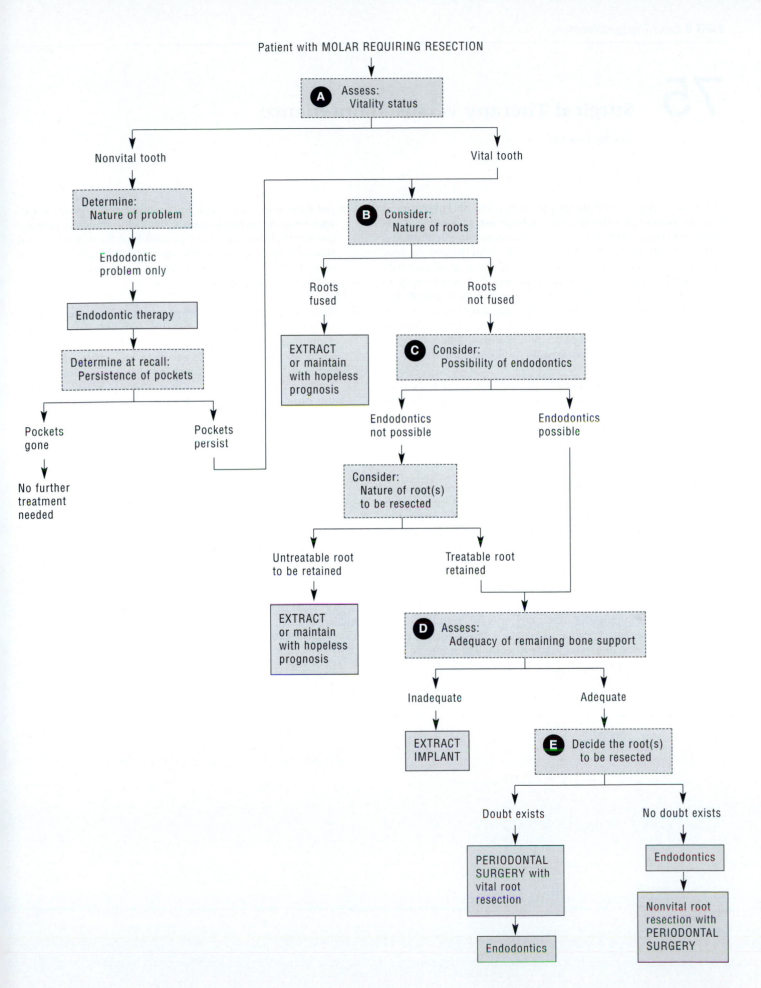

Patient with MOLAR REQUIRING RESECTION

A Assess: Vitality status

Nonvital tooth

Determine: Nature of problem

Endodontic problem only

Endodontic therapy

Determine at recall: Persistence of pockets

Pockets gone

No further treatment needed

Pockets persist

Vital tooth

B Consider: Nature of roots

Roots fused

EXTRACT or maintain with hopeless prognosis

Roots not fused

C Consider: Possibility of endodontics

Endodontics not possible

Consider: Nature of root(s) to be resected

Untreatable root to be retained

EXTRACT or maintain with hopeless prognosis

Treatable root retained

Endodontics possible

D Assess: Adequacy of remaining bone support

Inadequate

EXTRACT IMPLANT

Adequate

E Decide the root(s) to be resected

Doubt exists

PERIODONTAL SURGERY with vital root resection

Endodontics

No doubt exists

Endodontics

Nonvital root resection with PERIODONTAL SURGERY

149

75 Surgical Therapy versus Maintenance

Timothy F. Geraci

The goal of periodontal therapy is to develop an environment that the patient and the dentist can maintain in a stable status with ease. The possibilities of attaining this goal are determining factors in evaluating a case for surgery. If initial therapy (ie, root planing and plaque control) has attained the goal of an easily manageable case, maintenance planning and monitoring to determine continued stability may be all that is required. If a stable state cannot be attained or maintained with ease, surgical alteration may be useful in achieving this goal. The decision is made at the initial therapy evaluation, which should take place several weeks after completion of the initial treatment.

A If the patient's general health is good, surgery may be considered. If health is seriously compromised (eg, poorly controlled diabetes, high diastolic blood pressure), surgery may be contraindicated and the patient should be maintained as well as possible with frequent recall visits for instrumentation and oral hygiene.

B Plaque control by the patient is a key determining factor in deciding whether surgical therapy has merit. If the patient's plaque control on visible, accessible areas of the teeth is not good, mucogingival-osseous surgery is as likely to compromise the case as to help it. Initial therapy should be repeated. If the patient's plaque control is good (or overriding restorative demands are present), mucogingival-osseous surgery may be proposed.

C Bleeding or suppuration on probing is an indication that pocket areas inaccessible to plaque-control measures at home continue to exhibit active disease. If bleeding or suppuration does not occur on probing, recall maintenance may be an adequate means of stabilizing the case. Restorative needs, however, may be indications for surgery despite this stability. If plaque control on the visible, accessible parts of teeth is good, but bleeding or suppuration occurs on probing, consider surgery.

D Surgery is indicated if it may make areas more accessible for plaque control and root planing without compromising support of potentially maintainable teeth or creating unacceptable esthetic situations owing to root exposure. If additional support can be gained by regenerative means, the dentist should vigorously encourage the patient to consider the surgical alternative. If these objectives cannot be obtained surgically, recall maintenance is the approach of choice. If they can be obtained, propose the surgical alternative to the patient for acceptance or rejection.

Additional Readings

Carranza FA Jr, Newman MG. Clinical periodontology. 8th ed. Philadelphia: WB Saunders; 1996. p. 555.

Lindhe J. Textbook of clinical periodontology. 2nd ed. Copenhagen: Munksgaard; 1989. p. 386.

Lindhe J, Nyman S. The effect of plaque control and surgical pocket elimination on the establishment and maintenance of periodontal health: a longitudinal study of periodontal therapy in cases of advanced periodontal disease. J Clin Periodontol 1985;2:67.

Schluger S et al. Periodontal diseases. 2nd ed. Philadelphia: Lea & Febiger; 1990. p. 461.

Patient with RESIDUAL POCKET DEPTHS AT TIME OF INITIAL THERAPY EVALUATION

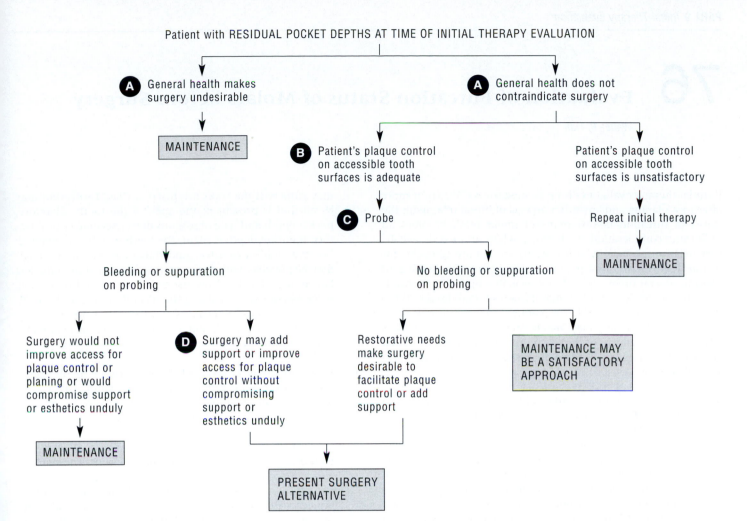

A General health makes surgery undesirable

MAINTENANCE

A General health does not contraindicate surgery

B Patient's plaque control on accessible tooth surfaces is adequate

Patient's plaque control on accessible tooth surfaces is unsatisfactory

Repeat initial therapy

MAINTENANCE

C Probe

Bleeding or suppuration on probing

No bleeding or suppuration on probing

Surgery would not improve access for plaque control or planing or would compromise support or esthetics unduly

MAINTENANCE

D Surgery may add support or improve access for plaque control without compromising support or esthetics unduly

Restorative needs make surgery desirable to facilitate plaque control or add support

MAINTENANCE MAY BE A SATISFACTORY APPROACH

PRESENT SURGERY ALTERNATIVE

76 Evaluation of Furcation Status of Molars before Surgery

Walter B. Hall

If initial therapy evaluation is performed several weeks or more after root planing and any other aspects of initial treatment, the status of furcation involvements of molar teeth becomes an important consideration in deciding whether surgery will be beneficial to the patient. If furcations are readily accessible for plaque removal and root planing, maintenance by regular root planing several times a year is a reasonable option for controlling the progression of inflammatory periodontal disease. If the furcations are not accessible for plaque removal and root planing, however, surgery may make them accessible, and thus improve the prognosis for the tooth. An individual molar should be treated on the basis of the worst furcation involvement present (Figure 76-1).

A   The type of furcation involvement must be assessed in deciding on treatment options. If the furcations are not involved, maintenance by root planing alone usually is a good option. The status of adjacent teeth and pocket depths on the individual molar may make surgery a desirable option in some cases even if furcations are not involved. Class I (incipient) and Class II (definite) involvements (see Chapters 99 and 100) require considerable decision making. Class III ("through and through") involvements are discussed in Chapter 101. Mandibular molars have two furcations that must be evaluated in deciding on further therapy at the time of initial therapy evaluation, whereas maxillary molars have three.

B   If the worst furcation involvement is incipient (Class I), maintenance with regular root planing several times a year

may suffice. If the roots are fused, a Class I furcation may be all that is present in the apex of the tooth; therefore, pocket depth and type of osseous defect become critical factors. If pocket depth is slight, the tooth may be maintained; however, if it is extensive, guided tissue regeneration (GTR) may be possible, with the exception of regenerating the lost attachment. Most defects associated with fused roots have three osseous walls, making them good candidates for GTR. Should the roots be tortuous and the defect not accessible to surgical instrumentation, extract the tooth or maintain it with a hopeless prognosis.

C   If the molar has a Class II (definite) furcation involvement, access—for plaque removal and root planing—is a most important consideration in deciding on the possible value of surgery. Because maxillary molars have proximal furcations, access is a greater problem than it is in the mandibular arch. If access is good, maintenance with regular root planing several times a year may be sufficient. The status of adjacent teeth, however, may make including molars with Class II furcations in surgery a desirable option even if they are accessible for maintenance. If access is not good, making adequate plaque removal and root planing difficult or impossible, loss of attachment (LOA) and type of osseous defect become the chief factors in deciding on treatment. If the defect is smaller than 3 mm, mucogingival-osseous surgery with an apically positioned flap approach should make the area accessible for instrumentation and plaque removal. If the defect is 3 mm or larger, a three-walled osseous defect usually is present on facial or lingual furcations, whereas proximal defects may be two walled or three walled. All are good candidates for GTR. If only one root is severely involved, root amputation or hemisection may be a better option (see Chapter 72).

D   Class III, "through-and-through" furcations are amenable to GTR now; however, the procedure is not likely to be successful because of the difficulty of removing all calculus and contaminated dentin due to the anatomy of the roots and furcations involved.

Additional Readings

Carranza FA Jr, Newman AG. Clinical periodontology. 8th ed. Philadelphia: WB Saunders; 1996. p. 610.

Genco RJ, Goldman HM, Cohen DW. Contemporary periodontics. St. Louis: Mosby; 1990. p. 3–44.

Hemp SE, Nyman S, Lindhe, J. Treatment of multi-rooted teeth: results after 5 years. J Clin Periodontol 1975;2:126.

Lindhe J. Textbook of clinical periodontology. 2nd ed. Copenhagen: Munksgaard; 1989. p. 515.

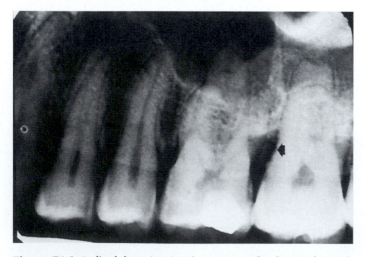

Figure 76-1 A distal furcation involvement on the first molar with apparent second-molar root proximity.

Patient with a MOLAR TOOTH WITH FURCATION INVOLVEMENT AT INITIAL THERAPY EVALUATION

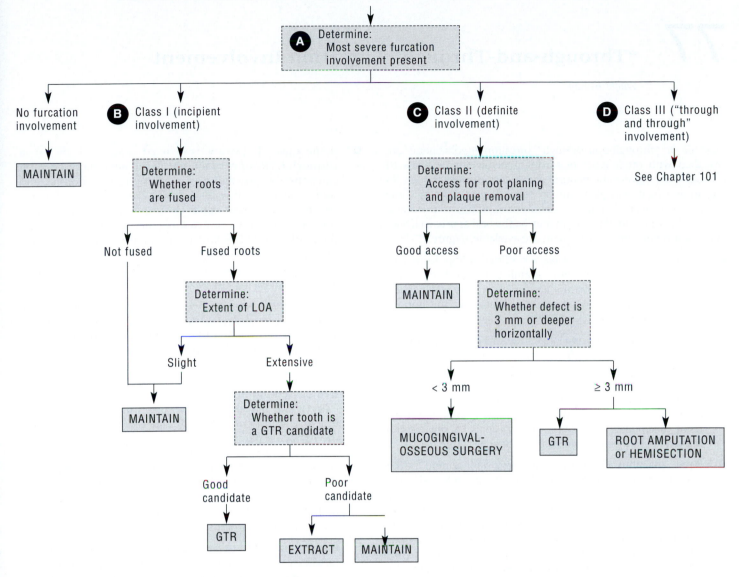

A Determine:
Most severe furcation involvement present

No furcation involvement

MAINTAIN

B Class I (incipient involvement)

Determine:
Whether roots are fused

Not fused

Fused roots

Determine:
Extent of LOA

Slight

MAINTAIN

Extensive

Determine:
Whether tooth is a GTR candidate

Good candidate

GTR

Poor candidate

EXTRACT

MAINTAIN

C Class II (definite involvement)

Determine:
Access for root planing and plaque removal

Good access

MAINTAIN

Poor access

Determine:
Whether defect is 3 mm or deeper horizontally

< 3 mm

MUCOGINGIVAL-OSSEOUS SURGERY

≥ 3 mm

GTR

ROOT AMPUTATION or HEMISECTION

D Class III ("through and through" involvement)

See Chapter 101

77   "Through-and-Through" Furcation Involvement

Walter B. Hall

Class III or "through-and-through" furcation involvements are described with other types of furcation involvements. Class III involvements require the dentist to give considerable thought in preparing a treatment plan. The prognosis for maintaining these teeth often is poor; therefore, a definitive approach to therapy is preferred. Extraction of the tooth may be the best approach if adequate abutments for a replacement are available (Figure 77-1).

A   If no abutments are available for a fixed bridge to replace the Class III involved tooth, retaining the tooth may be a valid approach. If potential abutments are available, their periodontal status and restoration determine the options open to the dentist.

B   If no abutments are available, the strategic value of the furcation-involved tooth to the overall treatment plan becomes the most important consideration. If the involved tooth is not important to the treatment plan, it may be either extracted or maintained with a hopeless prognosis. If the involved tooth is essential to the treatment plan, the treatment possibilities discussed in note D apply. A single tooth implant should be considered if an adequate bone exists.

C   If potential abutment teeth to support a replacement for the Class III involved tooth are available, the periodontal status of these teeth becomes the next important concern. If the potential abutment teeth are healthy, extract the badly involved tooth and place a fixed bridge replacement. If the potential abutment teeth have early or moderate periodontal involvement, notably loss of attachment (LOA), consider the value of the Class III involved tooth. If keeping the tooth would not add appreciably to the long-term prognosis of the case, extract the tooth, treat the abutment teeth periodontally, and place a replacement fixed bridge. If the Class III involved tooth may add to the long-term prognosis for the case, treatment options include guided tissue regeneration (GTR)—an approach that has become more successful in recent years—or endodontics with root amputation or hemisection (see Chapter 72).

D   If the Class III furcation-involved tooth is to be saved (through GTR) or partially saved, the next major decision concerns the possibility of performing endodontics and root resection. If endodontics cannot be performed (eg, because of root canal closure or root tortuosity) or the roots cannot be resected (eg, because of root fusion), the tooth should be extracted or maintained by root planing with a hopeless prognosis. The treatment options for mandibular and maxillary molars are different, and both are expensive.

E   If endodontics can be performed on both roots of the mandibular molars, and the roots can be resected, the two separated portions may be retained and crowned. If the roots are close together and orthodontic separation of the hemisected roots is not feasible, or if only one can be treated endodontically, then only one root should be fully treated endodontically; the other root should be extracted. If the root to be salvaged can be joined to a satisfactory abutment, a fixed bridge can be used to replace the extracted part of the molar. If the root to be salvaged is adjacent to an abutment and a bridge is not needed, it should be treated endodontically, the tooth hemisected, the other removed, and a crown placed on the salvaged half tooth. If possible, splinting the adjacent tooth to the half tooth and placing a cantilevered bridge may improve the overall case prognosis.

F   If endodontics can be performed on two of the roots of the maxillary molars that are to be retained and a badly involved third root can be resected, perform root amputation after endodontic therapy. The remaining portion of the tooth should be crowned in a manner to facilitate plaque removal. If endodontics cannot be performed on the roots to be retained, or if the roots are fused to the one to be amputated, extract the tooth or retain it with a hopeless prognosis. If all three furcations are of the Class III type, extraction or maintenance with a hopeless prognosis is also an option.

Additional Readings

Becker W et al. New attachment after treatment with root isolation procedures: report of treated Class III and Class II furcations and vertical osseous defects. Int J Periodontics Restorative Dent 1985;5:9.

Carranza FA Jr, Newman MG. Clinical periodontology. 8th ed. Philadelphia: WB Saunders; 1996. p. 643.

Genco RI, Goldman HM, Cohen DW. Contemporary periodontics. St. Louis: Mosby; 1990. p. 582.

Pontoviero R et al. Guided tissue regeneration in the treatment of furcation defects in mandibular molars: a clinical study of degree III involvements. J Clin Periodontol 1989;16:170.

Schluger S et al. Periodontal diseases. 2nd ed. Philadelphia: Lea & Febiger; 1989. p. 549.

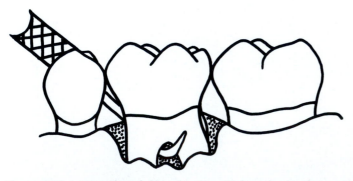

Figure 77-1 A "through-and-through" (Class III) furcation involvement with good adjacent abutments. The first molar should be considered for extraction.

Patient with a molar with a "THROUGH AND THROUGH" FURCATION INVOLVEMENT

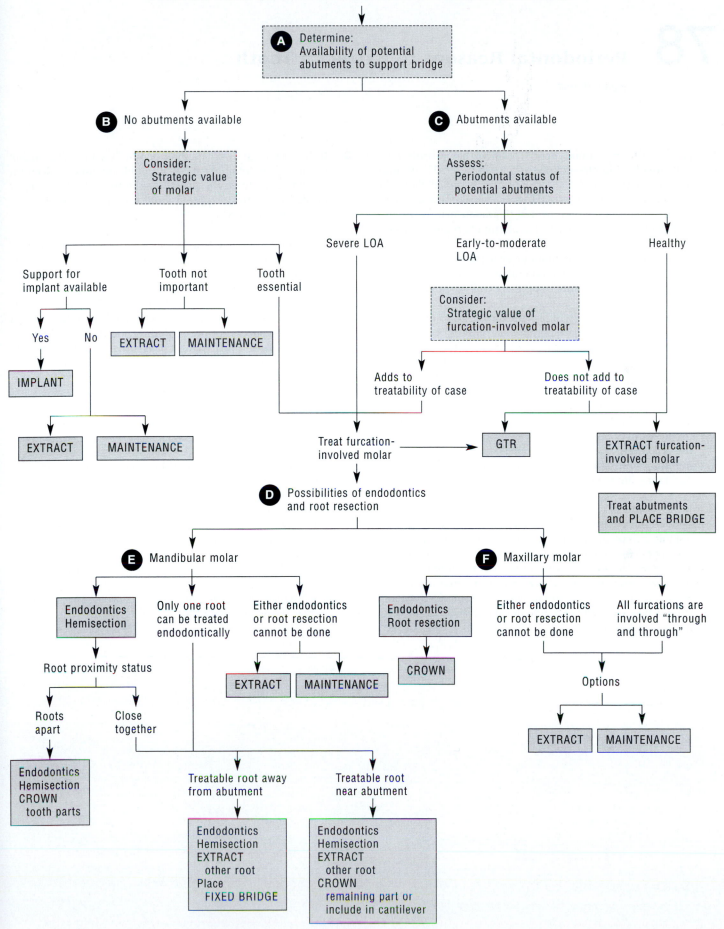

A Determine:
Availability of potential abutments to support bridge

B No abutments available

C Abutments available

Consider:
Strategic value of molar

Assess:
Periodontal status of potential abutments

Support for implant available

Tooth not important

Tooth essential

Severe LOA

Early-to-moderate LOA

Healthy

Yes   No

EXTRACT   MAINTENANCE

Consider:
Strategic value of furcation-involved molar

IMPLANT

Adds to treatability of case

Does not add to treatability of case

EXTRACT   MAINTENANCE

Treat furcation-involved molar → GTR

EXTRACT furcation-involved molar

Treat abutments and PLACE BRIDGE

D Possibilities of endodontics and root resection

E Mandibular molar

F Maxillary molar

Endodontics
Hemisection

Only one root can be treated endodontically

Either endodontics or root resection cannot be done

Endodontics
Root resection

Either endodontics or root resection cannot be done

All furcations are involved "through and through"

Root proximity status

EXTRACT   MAINTENANCE

CROWN

Options

Roots apart

Close together

EXTRACT   MAINTENANCE

Endodontics
Hemisection
CROWN
tooth parts

Treatable root away from abutment

Treatable root near abutment

Endodontics
Hemisection
EXTRACT
   other root
Place
   FIXED BRIDGE

Endodontics
Hemisection
EXTRACT
   other root
CROWN
   remaining part or include in cantilever

78 Periodontal Reasons to Extract a Tooth

Walter B. Hall

If a patient with a complex dental problem has a badly periodontally involved tooth—defined as a tooth with 50% or more loss of attachment (LOA)— a decision must be made about the consequences of extracting it. Making an assessment of the value of the individual tooth to the overall treatment plan is the first step in deciding whether to extract or attempt to retain the tooth.

A If the tooth has no crucial importance to the overall treatment plan, it should be extracted rather than maintained because it may compromise the success of the overall restorative plan.

B If the tooth is crucially important to the overall treatment plan, the role of the tooth in that plan must be clearly determined. Extraction may be the best option if the tooth is not a vital abutment. If the particular tooth may add to the likelihood of success of the treatment plan, its retention does not compromise other important teeth, and a "strategic retreat" (should it fail) is planned, surgical treatment may be a valid approach. Maintenance with a poor-to-hopeless prognosis may be considered if retention of the tooth does not jeopardize the overall plan or if the chances for retaining the tooth for a significant portion of the patient's remaining life seem good.

C If the tooth is a crucial abutment, the chances of treating it periodontally with reasonable likelihood of retaining it for a significant period should be assessed. If the prognosis does not appear good, the possibility of replacing the tooth with an implant should be considered. If this cannot be done because of the anatomy of the area or because the patient is unable or unwilling to consider an implant, the tooth should be extracted, and a removable prosthetic replacement plan devised.

D If the tooth can be treated periodontally with a reasonable chance of maintaining it for a significant time, a decision should be made on the need for splinting before surgery. If needed, temporary or provisional splinting should be performed before surgery.

E If splinting is not needed, the possibility of successful regeneration of LOA should be considered. If guided tissue regeneration (GTR) can be performed predictably (see Chapter 79), it should be done, and its success evaluated after 6 months. If the tooth is not amenable to GTR, the tooth has a guarded prognosis and may be treated by other surgical means; the success of the procedure should be evaluated 2 to 6 months later. If treatment is successful in improving the prognosis of the tooth, restoration may be instituted at this time. If the tooth's prognosis does not merit its inclusion in the plan at reevaluation, it should be extracted and an alternative plan instituted.

Additional Readings

Hall WB. Periodontal preparation of the mouth for restoration. Dent Clin North Am 1980;24:195.

Hall WB. Removal of third molars: a periodontal viewpoint. In: McDonald RE et al, editors. Current therapy in dentistry. St. Louis: Mosby; 1980. p. 225.

Laskin DM. Evaluation of the third molar problems. J Am Dent Assoc 1971;82:824.

Schluger S et al. Periodontal diseases. 2nd ed. Philadelphia: Lea & Febiger; 1989. p. 346.

Sorrin S, Burman LR. A study of cases not amenable to periodontal therapy. J Am Dent Assoc 1944;31:204.

Patient with a COMPLEX DENTAL PROBLEM AND A BADLY PERIODONTALLY INVOLVED TOOTH

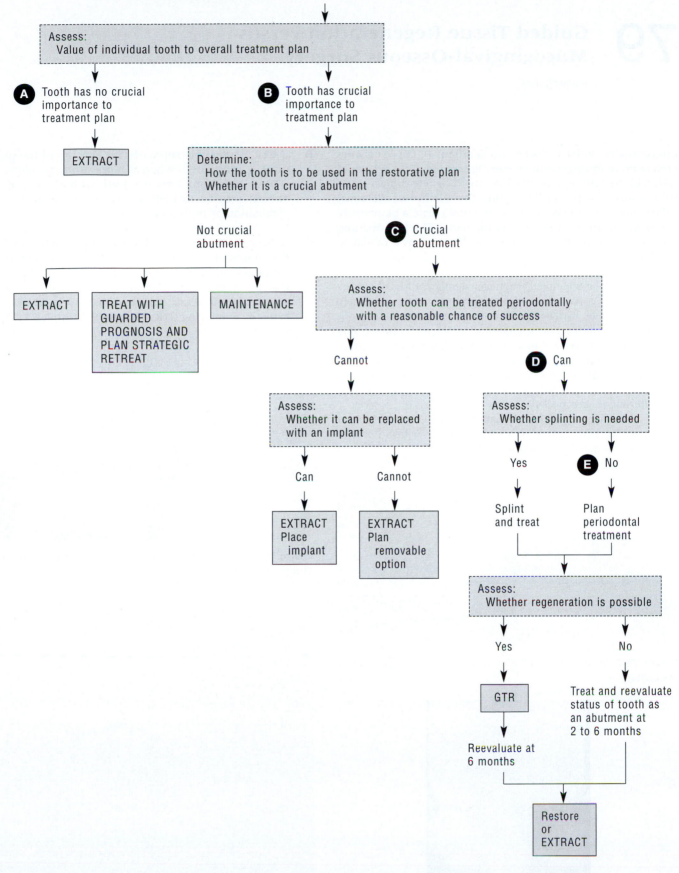

79 Guided Tissue Regeneration versus Mucogingival-Osseous Surgery

Walter B. Hall

Conceptually, guided tissue regeneration (GTR) is always preferable to mucogingival-osseous surgery, because successful GTR adds to existing support of the tooth, whereas mucogingival-osseous surgery usually requires the sacrifice of additional supporting tissue to eliminate pockets and create a more easily maintainable architecture around the tooth. The first decision, therefore, involves the assessment of the tooth as a candidate for GTR.

A   GTR may be attempted whenever significant loss of attachment (LOA) has occurred on a tooth; however, extremely periodontally involved teeth or those with additional problems(eg, untreatable endodontic problems, unrestorable crowns, deep vertical root cracks) may have to be extracted. Horizontal bone loss cannot be corrected by GTR on a predictable basis today. Nonstrategic teeth do not merit GTR in many cases, especially if less complicated or less expensive alternatives are available.

  If many or most of the patient's remaining teeth have extensive LOA, extraction or maintenance with a hopeless prognosis may be the necessary choice.

B   If GTR is a feasible approach, the severity of the problem must be considered. Whereas more severe problems merit GTR, minimal problems (eg, teeth with an LOA of 5 mm or less) may be treated quite satisfactorily with pocket-elimination or mucogingival-osseous surgery.

C   In the anterior segments of the mouth, even teeth with less than 5 mm of LOA may merit GTR rather than mucogingival-osseous surgery to improve the esthetic result; therefore esthetic requirements should be considered to determine whether the patient's esthetic demands would be satisfied better by employing GTR (Figures 79-1 through 79-7).

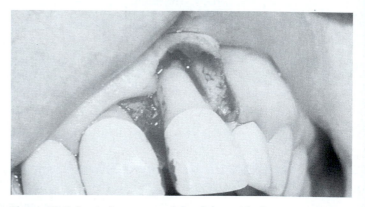

Figure 79-3 Surgical exposure of the defect with deepest readings of 11 mm from cementoenamel junction to bone.

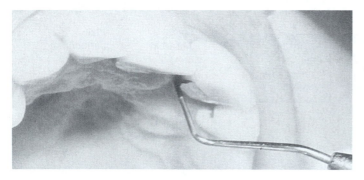

Figure 79-1 Preoperative view of an incisor with severe periodontal destruction.

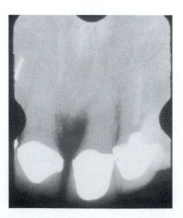

Figure 79-2 Radiographic view of the osseous defect.

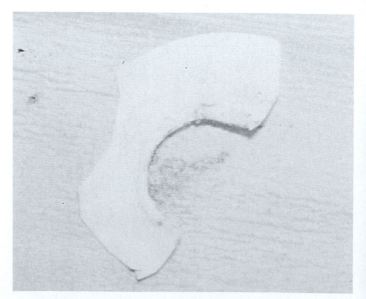

Figure 79-4 A Teflon membrane fashioned to surround the defect.

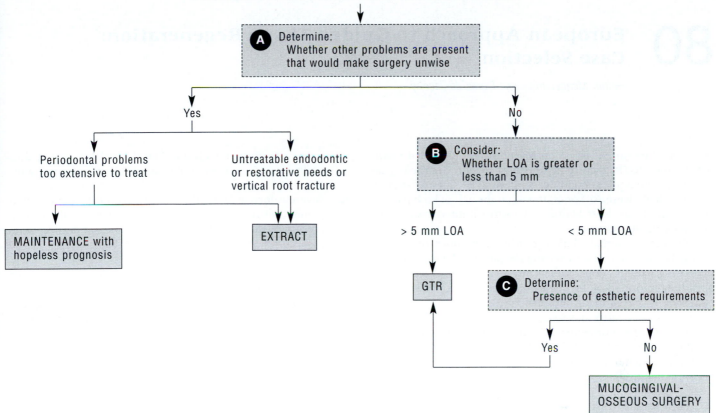

Patient with a PERIODONTAL PROBLEM THAT MERITS SURGERY

A Determine:
Whether other problems are present that would make surgery unwise

Yes

No

Periodontal problems too extensive to treat

Untreatable endodontic or restorative needs or vertical root fracture

B Consider:
Whether LOA is greater or less than 5 mm

MAINTENANCE with hopeless prognosis

EXTRACT

> 5 mm LOA

< 5 mm LOA

GTR

C Determine:
Presence of esthetic requirements

Yes

No

MUCOGINGIVAL-OSSEOUS SURGERY

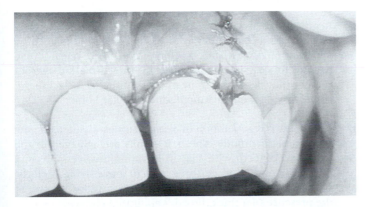

Figure 79-5 The membrane sutured in place and the flaps positioned to maximize esthetics.

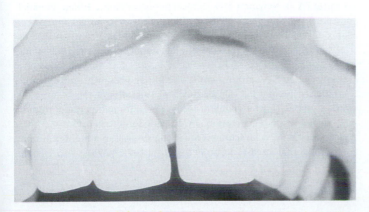

Figure 79-6 The healed area 9 months after surgery and before orthodontic movement.

Figure 79-7 Postorthodontic view with space closed, deepest crevice measurement of 3 mm, and only slight mobility 3½ years after surgery.

Additional Readings

Carranza FA Jr, Newman MG. Clinical periodontology. 8th ed. Philadelphia: WB Saunders; 1996. p. 615.

Genco RJ, Goldman HM, Cohen DW. Contemporary periodontics. St. Louis: Mosby; 1990. p. 585.

Schluger S et al. Periodontal diseases. 2nd ed. Philadelphia: Lea & Febiger; 1989. p. 332.

Smith DH, Ammons WF, Van Belle G. A longitudinal study of periodontal status comparing osseous recontouring with flap curettage: 1—results after 6 months. J Periodontol 1980;51:367.

Wilson TG, Kornman KS. Fundamentals of periodontics. Chicago: Quintessence Publishing; 1996. p. 372, 408.

80 European Approach to Guided Tissue Regeneration: Case Selection

Reiner Mengel and Lavin Flores-de-Jacoby

Periodontal treatment based on the principles of guided tissue regeneration (GTR) is currently the most advanced of the regenerative methods of periodontal surgery. GTR does, however, involve a high degree of commitment on the part of both patient and therapist, not least because two surgical interventions are necessary in all events.

To attain optimal clinical results, a number of criteria should be observed when selecting the patient, the most important being patient cooperation. Only those patients who have been fully informed of the possibilities and limits of GTR should be given this treatment. Competent work by the therapist ensures a good chance of success.

This chapter is designed to help the dentist decide whether a patient is suitable for GTR. Details such as selection of the appropriate membrane design are dealt with at another level of decision making.

A   Each patient with periodontitis is given preliminary treatment consisting of two detailed clinical examinations, a professional supragingival tooth-cleaning session, a subgingival scaling session, and oral hygiene instruction (OHI).

B   Clinical parameters such as probing attachment loss (PAL), bleeding on open probing, periodontal recession, tooth mobility, and furcation involvement are determined at the outset of treatment and on reevaluation after scaling and root planing. The findings are correlated with full-mouth radiographs. Patients with pocket depths as deep as 4 mm with no bleeding on probing may require no further treatment except regular recall maintenance. In cases of deeper pocket depths or furcation involvement, consider periodontal surgery. The decision in favor of surgery should be based on the efficacy of individual plaque control. For this purpose, a plaque index is recorded during each session. Plaque index values of less than 15% mean that plaque is found at less than 15% of the measuring points in the proximal area. Bleeding on probing is a sign of persistent periodontal inflammation. In conjunction with increased pocket depths, bleeding on probing is an indication for surgical intervention.

C   Vertical osseous defects and furcation involvements are detected by full-mouth radiography or probing. Use of a Nabers-type probe may be helpful in cases of furcation involvement. Only reflection of a flap provides proof that a defect amenable to GTR is present.

D   Nonvital teeth with necrotic pulps or irreversible pulpitis require endodontic treatment before surgery. Vitality testing must be performed with the utmost care because endodontically treated teeth are more susceptible to root resorption.

E   Severely increased tooth mobility (vertical or more than 1 mm horizontal) may cause problems in the healing process of the periodontal ligament and supporting bone. Perform splinting or occlusal grinding before GTR.

F   Microbiologic investigation is called for in clinically suspicious cases. Only those cases in which the extent or rate of destruction fails to correlate with the quantity of plaque or age of the patient are suspect. In these situations, testing for periodontopathogens such as *Haemophilus actinomycetemcomitans* or *Porphyromonas* and *Prevotella* may be helpful. Test kits such as the latex agglutination test are highly recommended for this purpose. Antibiotics are generally prescribed in accordance with accepted rules. Patients must take adequately high dosages of the appropriate drugs for a sufficiently long period (ie, at least 10 days).

G   Regenerative procedures are carried out to restore the original structure and function of tissue severely damaged by periodontal disease (eg, periodontitis). The regenerative healing process is characterized by the formation of root cementum, periodontal ligament, epithelial attachment, connective tissue attachment, and alveolar bone.

H   GTR permits regeneration of diseased or lost tissue using the membrane technique. The best results are achieved in the treatment of teeth with Class II furcation involvements and deep, narrow, two- to three-walled intraosseous defects. GTR also may be used to treat gingival recessions, subject to the presence of a thick, broad, keratinized gingiva.

Additional Readings

Carranza FA Jr, Newman MG. Clinical periodontology. 8th ed. Philadelphia: WB Saunders; 1996. p. 626.

Flores-de-Jacoby L. New perspectives in periodontal therapy: guided tissue regeneration [video cassette]. Berlin: Quintessence Publishing; 1989.

Gottlow J et al. New attachment formation as a result of controlled tissue regeneration. J Clin Periodontol 1984;11:494.

Gottlow J et al. New attachment formation in human periodontium by guided tissue regeneration. J Clin Periodontol 1986;13:604.

Nyman S et al. New attachment following surgical treatment of human periodontal disease. J Clin Periodontol 1982;9:290.

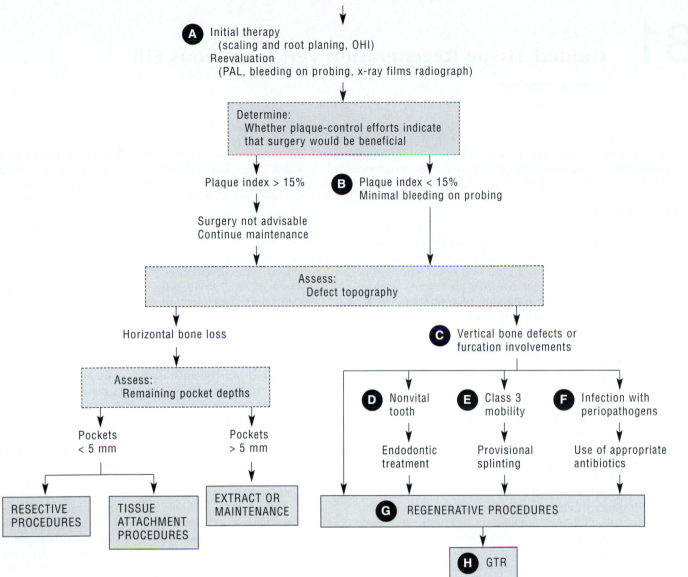

Patient with ADVANCED PERIODONTAL DISEASE

A Initial therapy
(scaling and root planing, OHI)
Reevaluation
(PAL, bleeding on probing, x-ray films radiograph)

Determine:
Whether plaque-control efforts indicate
that surgery would be beneficial

Plaque index > 15%

B Plaque index < 15%
Minimal bleeding on probing

Surgery not advisable
Continue maintenance

Assess:
Defect topography

Horizontal bone loss

C Vertical bone defects or
furcation involvements

Assess:
Remaining pocket depths

D Nonvital
tooth

E Class 3
mobility

F Infection with
periopathogens

Pockets
< 5 mm

Pockets
> 5 mm

Endodontic
treatment

Provisional
splinting

Use of appropriate
antibiotics

RESECTIVE
PROCEDURES

TISSUE
ATTACHMENT
PROCEDURES

EXTRACT OR
MAINTENANCE

G REGENERATIVE PROCEDURES

H GTR

81 Guided Tissue Regeneration versus Osseous Fill

Steven A. Tsurudome

The goal of guided tissue regeneration (GTR) is to regenerate lost periodontal structures. The lost periodontal structures include the alveolar bone, periodontal ligament, and cementum. The two most commonly used materials for GTR today are barrier membranes and graft materials.

A When a periodontal patient is evaluated for a GTR procedure, the radiographs must first be evaluated to assess the type of bone loss. Patients with a horizontal type of bone loss are usually not amenable to GTR procedures, whereas patients with vertical or intrabony type of bone loss are possible candidates for GTR procedures.

B If the patient has a vertical or intrabony radiographic defect, the clinician should consider a preliminary treatment plan that may consist of several different GTR technique options; however, the definitive treatment option should be made at the time of surgery when the surgical site is reflected, débrided, and the intrabony defect exposed for direct visual inspection. The overall defect depth, width, and the number of associated bony walls will ultimately dictate the type of regenerative technique used by the clinician.

C If the intrabony defect is narrow and deep with only one osseous wall, then the combination technique of a "bone graft and absorbable barrier membrane" is recommended for creation and maintenance of the critical space for regeneration. The use of barrier membranes alone may cause the membrane to collapse into the defect and obliterate this critical space. Currently, absorbable membranes are the preferred membranes over the nonabsorbable types because of the necessity of a secondary surgery for removal of nonresorbable membranes. This second procedure represents additional trauma to the patient and the newly regenerated tissues. Thus, most GTR procedures around natural teeth should benefit from using resorbable membranes.

D If the intrabony defect is narrow and deep with two or three walls, then the "membrane alone" technique may be considered. The two or three walls in narrow deep osseous defects should provide adequate space maintenance and wound stabilization for predictable regeneration without the additional use of a bone graft. Absorbable barrier membranes alone have shown consistent ability to promote periodontal regeneration because the unique epithelial exclusion afforded by the barrier membranes effectively inhibits the proliferation of the junctional epithelium into the periodontal defect. Upon visual inspection of the intrabony defect, if the membrane alone does not provide adequate space maintenance, then the clinician always has the option of the combination "bone graft and absorbable barrier membrane" technique, as described for the narrow, deep, one-walled intrabony defects.

E If the intrabony defect is narrow and shallow with only one wall, the benefits of GTR become minimal because the potential gain in regenerated periodontium in shallow defects is inconsequential. Considering the cost and inherent risks involved in GTR surgery, osseous resective surgery should be the treatment of choice because of its greater predictability in shallow, wide defect cases.

F If the intrabony defect is narrow and shallow with two or three walls, then a bone graft alone may be considered because the defect size is sufficient to accommodate the small quantity of autogenous bone usually harvested from the oral cavity. In addition, if bone grafts such as demineralized freeze-dried bone allografts are used, the predictability of the regenerative techniques caused by their possible release of bone-inducing proteins (known as bone morphogenic proteins), as well as maintaining the critical space for regeneration, can be helpful. The inorganic alloplastic graft materials, in contrast, may not be recommended because studies have shown encapsulation with little bone fill and periodontal regeneration; thus, they serve as space fillers only. In addition, barrier membranes are not recommended for shallow defects because the risks and benefits may not warrant their use. The cost of the membrane plus the inherent increased risk of complications may outweigh the potential benefit of only a slight gain in regenerated periodontium.

G If the intrabony defect is wide and deep with only one wall, the prognosis for the tooth decreases dramatically. The clinician must consider the possibility of extraction in these cases.

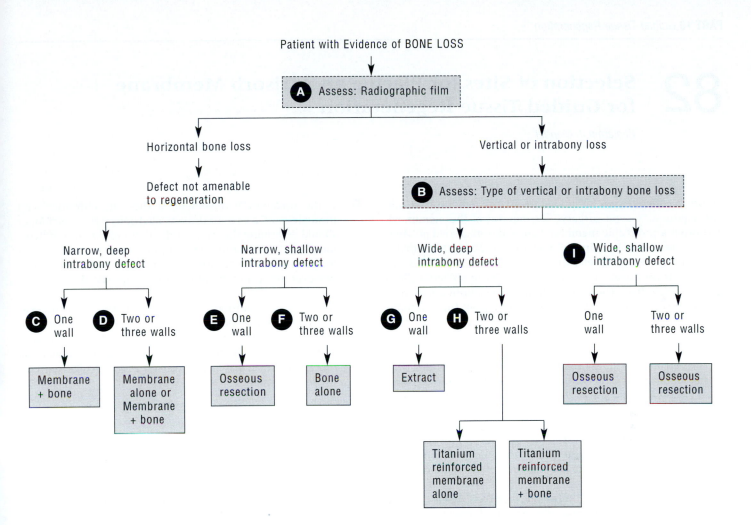

H   If the intrabony defect is wide and deep with two or three walls, the prognosis is only slightly better than that for a wide and deep defect with only one wall. Extraction again is a possible option, but if the tooth is strategically important, the clinician may consider the use of a titanium-reinforced membrane with or without the use of a bone graft to maintain the space and to stabilize the wound for possible regeneration to occur. However, the clinician must be aware that the predictability for regeneration of a wide and deep osseous defect is not great.

I   If the intrabony defect is wide and shallow with either one, two, or three walls, the recommended procedure is osseous resection. The rationale is similar to the recommendations given earlier for narrow, shallow intrabony defects.

In conclusion, the unique epithelial exclusion and wound stabilization afforded by the barrier membranes and the enhanced osteogenic, space-maintaining, and wound-stabilizing potential afforded by bone grafts (allogenic or autogenic) should increase the potential of regeneration; thus it is logical and prudent to combine the two techniques whenever possible to increase the predictability of regeneration of the periodontium destroyed by periodontal disease and to ultimately improve the clinical outcome.

Additional Readings

American Academy of Periodontology. Proceedings of the World Workshop in Clinical Periodontics; 1987 Aug; Princeton: The Academy; p. VI, 2.

Annals of Periodontology. 1996 World Workshop in Periodontics; 1996 Nov; Lansdowne. American Academy of Periodontology; p. 626.

Genco R, Goldman H, Cohen DW. Contemporary periodontics. St. Louis: Mosby; 1990. p. 585.

Wilson T, Kornman K. Fundamentals of periodontics. Chicago: Quintessence Publishing; 1996. p. 405.

82 Selection of Sites for Placing an Atrisorb Membrane for Guided Tissue Regeneration

Benjamin J. Mandel

Resorbable membranes for guided tissue regeneration (GTR) do not require a "second surgery" for removal of the membrane. Atrisorb is a resorbable membrane created from a solid polymer of lactic acid dissolved in a liquid carrier, NMP (N-methyl-2 pyrrolidone), which upon exposure to wetting becomes semisolid and is resorbable. It is used as a barrier to prevent cells of gingival origin from contacting prepared roots until a new connective tissue attachment to the root grows from the periodontal ligament coronally covering exposed root surfaces and eventually creating a new connective tissue attachment to them.

A For a patient with a localized periodontal problem that may be amenable to GTR, the number of osseous walls to the bony defects and the depth of those defects must be determined.

B For a one-walled osseous defect, determine the depth of the defect. If it is shallow (less than 5 mm deep), mucogingival-osseous surgery is indicated. For defects deeper than 5 mm, GTR with an Atrisorb resorbable membrane is indicated.

C For a two-walled or three-walled defect, determine the depth of the pocket and the class of furcation (if any) involved. If the pocket is less than 5 mm deep, mucogingival-osseous surgery is indicated. If the defect is 5 mm or more in depth, and no furcation or a shallow one is detected, GTR with an Atrisorb membrane may be employed. The same is true for Class II (definite) furcation involvements associated with two- or three-walled osseous defects.

D If the furcation involvement is Class III ("through and through") and a two- or three-walled defect, the practitioner should determine the value of the tooth in the overall treatment plan. If the tooth is critically important to the success of the plan, GTR with an Atrisorb membrane *may* be attempted; however, success of the procedure is unpredictable.

E Hemisection of a tooth with a Class III furcation involvement may be a viable option if the retained root is useful in the overall treatment plan; however, endodontic treatment and a crown will be necessary. In some cases, a remaining root's usefulness may be improved utilizing GTR with an Atrisorb membrane.

Additional Readings

Polson AM, Southard G, Dunn R, et al. Healing patterns associated with an Atrisorb barrier in guided tissue regeneration. Compend Educ Dent 1993;14:161–72.

Polson AM, Garret S, Stoller N. Guided tissue regeneration in human furcation defects after using a biodegradable barrier: a multicenter feasibility study. J Periodontol 1995;66:377–85.

Rosen P, Reynolds M, Bowers G. A technique report on the in situ application of Atrisorb as a barrier for combination therapy. Int J Periodontics Restorative Dent 1998;18:249–55.

Stower N, Johnson L. The use of the Atrisorb bio-absorbable barrier during guided tissue regeneration. Postgrad Dent 1997;4:13–22.

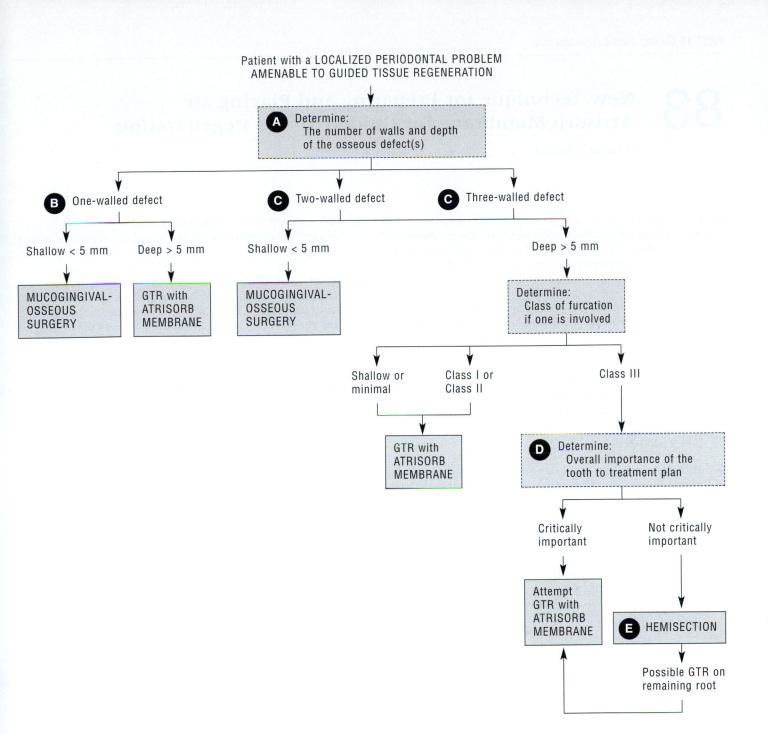

Patient with a LOCALIZED PERIODONTAL PROBLEM
AMENABLE TO GUIDED TISSUE REGENERATION

A Determine:
The number of walls and depth
of the osseous defect(s)

B One-walled defect

C Two-walled defect

C Three-walled defect

Shallow < 5 mm

Deep > 5 mm

Shallow < 5 mm

Deep > 5 mm

MUCOGINGIVAL-
OSSEOUS
SURGERY

GTR with
ATRISORB
MEMBRANE

MUCOGINGIVAL-
OSSEOUS
SURGERY

Determine:
Class of furcation
if one is involved

Shallow or
minimal

Class I or
Class II

Class III

GTR with
ATRISORB
MEMBRANE

D Determine:
Overall importance of the
tooth to treatment plan

Critically
important

Not critically
important

Attempt
GTR with
ATRISORB
MEMBRANE

E HEMISECTION

Possible GTR on
remaining root

83 New Technique for Preparing and Placing an Atrisorb Membrane for Guided Tissue Regeneration

Benjamin J. Mandel

Once the guided tissue regeneration (GTR) surgical site is exposed by flap reflection and débridement, the involved root surfaces are planed scrupulously and conditioned (eg, with citric acid) as the practitioner chooses. The Atrisorb membrane is prepared as follows:

A A sterile dappen dish (or small cup) is partially filled with sterile water or saline. The Atrisorb liquid's tube is opened, and the needle tip, which is provided, is placed over the opened tube.

B Determine whether a bone or bone substitute will be needed as the practitioner chooses, and have it available for use. Place the opened container and a sterile delivery device (eg, a periosteum elevator) and an amalgan plugger on the operating tray.

C Determine whether the bone or bone substitute will be placed in the defect alone first or totally incorporated into the Atrisorb plus.

D Place the sterile water or saline in the dappen dish and drip the Atrisorb liquid into it. Save about 20% of the liquid in the tube. Knead the solidifying mass continually until all of the liquid has become firm (the consistency of soft wax). This takes several minutes.

E Determine if the Atrisorb is to be used alone or mixed with bone or bone substitute, alone, mixed, or over bone placed initially.

F Place the Atrisorb, alone or mixed with bone or bone substitute, into the defect using the periosteum elevator and amalgan plugger. Fill or slightly overfill the defect and drip the Atrisorb fluid remaining in the tube over the defect and wet. Position the flap and suture in place.

By mixing the Atrisorb in the described manner, the defect can be filled with a firm membrane that will not collapse when suturing flaps in a more coronal position.

Additional Readings

Polson AM, Southard G, Dunn R, et al. Healing patterns associated with an Atrisorb barrier in guided tissue regeneration. Compend Educ Dent 1993;14:161–72.

Polson AM, Garret S, Stoller N. Guided tissue regeneration in human furcation defects after using a biodegradable barrier: a multicenter feasibility study. J Periodontol 1995;66:377–85.

Rosen P, Reynolds M, Bowers G. A technique report on the in situ application of Atrisorb as a barrier for combination therapy. Int J Periodontics Restorative Dent 1998;18:249–55.

Stower N, Johnson L. The use of the Atrisorb bio-absorbable barrier during guided tissue regeneration. Postgrad Dent 1997;4:13–22.

A patient for whom an ATRISORB GTR MEMBRANE IS TO BE PLACED

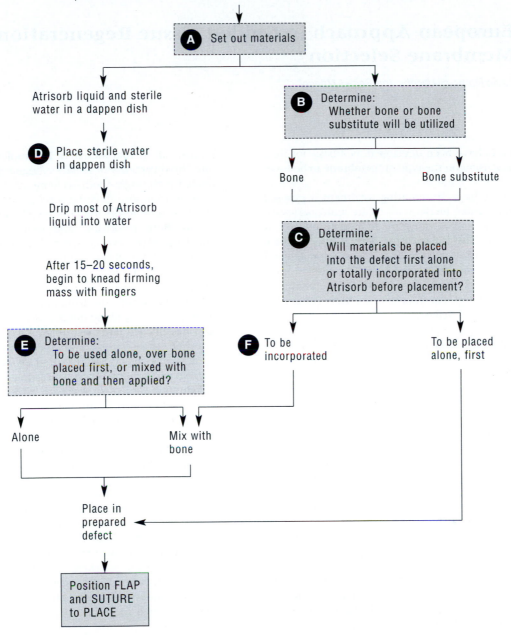

A Set out materials

Atrisorb liquid and sterile water in a dappen dish

D Place sterile water in dappen dish

Drip most of Atrisorb liquid into water

After 15–20 seconds, begin to knead firming mass with fingers

E Determine:
To be used alone, over bone placed first, or mixed with bone and then applied?

Alone

Mix with bone

B Determine:
Whether bone or bone substitute will be utilized

Bone

Bone substitute

C Determine:
Will materials be placed into the defect first alone or totally incorporated into Atrisorb before placement?

F To be incorporated

To be placed alone, first

Place in prepared defect

Position FLAP and SUTURE to PLACE

84 European Approach to Guided Tissue Regeneration: Membrane Selection

Lavin Flores-de-Jacoby and Reiner Mengel

The following criteria have been developed as a basis for final case selection and decision on the type of membrane to be used.

A The bone around the teeth requiring treatment is exposed using an intrasulcular incision to create mucoperiosteal flaps; vertical relief incisions are made at a distance of at least one premolar's width from the defects to be treated. The mucoperiosteal flap must extend at least 4 mm beyond the defect margin in an apical direction. The incision must be designed so that no suture runs across the membrane or an intra-alveolar defect. An unobstructed view is essential for optimal cleaning of defects.

B Use of a membrane and guided tissue regeneration (GTR) can be discontinued if an intraosseous defect is shallow and wide, bone resorption is found to be mainly horizontal, or Class I furcation involvement is detected. In these cases, the defect is cleaned thoroughly, any osseous resection is done, and the flaps are closed again. When teeth are involved in groups, the usual procedure is that some of the defects are treated in the standard way, and a few defects require the use of membranes. More complex cases, in which a number of adjacent defects require the use of membranes, should be treated only if the periodontal surgeon has sufficient experience in the field of GTR. The main problem is in the management of the flaps, which should cover the membrane as much as possible for the full 4-week period in which they remain in situ.

C Selection of the membrane design is based on the assumption that the following steps are to be taken in all events. As much as possible the membrane should be completely covered. Treat three-walled defects with a single-tooth-narrow or single-tooth-wide membrane depending on the size of the opening to be covered. If circular or semilunar defects on end-standing teeth (such as distal or second molars) are wide, use a wraparound barrier. All two-walled defects between teeth and some mixed one-walled and two-walled defects require the use of interproximal membranes. Class III ("through and through") furcation involvements on maxillary molars (although not predictably treatable today) may be treated with interproximal membranes. Mandibular Class III defects may be similarly treated if an adjacent tooth is available; if a single, isolated tooth is involved, use a wraparound membrane. In some cases with Class III furcation involvements on lower molars only, two single-

tooth-wide membranes may be employed. Class II (definite) involvements of facial or lingual furcations only are treated with single-tooth-wide membranes.

A decision also must be reached on whether the membrane is to be resorbable, nonresorbable, or titanium reinforced. Both resorbable and nonresorbable membranes may be used in cases of two-and three-walled intraosseous defects and furcation involvements. The precondition is that no risk of the membrane collapsing into the defect should be evident; the space-retaining function must be maintained during the healing phase. In case of doubt, a titanium-reinforced membrane should be used because this provides an adequate space-retaining function, especially in cases of single-walled and major two- to three-walled intraosseous defects and furcation involvements. The flap is secured with Gore-Tex suturing material. Nonresorbable membranes are left for 4 weeks, after which they must be removed in a second intervention. This is not necessary in the case of resorbable membranes. In the event of resorbable or nonresorbable membranes being exposed, an application of 0.12% solution of chlorhexidine gluconate twice a day for 4 weeks is prescribed.

D Hopeless teeth are those that are found during surgery to have functioning remaining periodontia of less than 3 mm. Multirooted molars in which more than half of the roots no longer are supported by bone also are considered hopeless. Grade III mobility does not make a tooth hopeless; corrective measures can be taken (eg, presurgical splinting, grinding). Therapeutic efforts may be considered worthwhile even for "hopeless" teeth, provided that the patient has given informed consent.

Additional Readings

Carranza FA Jr, Newman MG. Clinical periodontology. 8th ed. Philadelphia: WB Saunders; 1966. p. 627.

Flores-de-Jacoby L. New perspectives in periodontal therapy: guided tissue regeneration [video cassette]. Berlin: Quintessence Publishing; 1989.

Gottlow J et al. New attachment formation as a result of controlled tissue regeneration. J Clin Periodontol 1984;11:494.

Gottlow J et al. New attachment formation in human periodontium by guided tissue regeneration. J Clin Periodontol 1986;13:604.

Nyman S et al. New attachment following surgical treatment of human periodontal disease. J Clin Periodontol 1982;9:290.

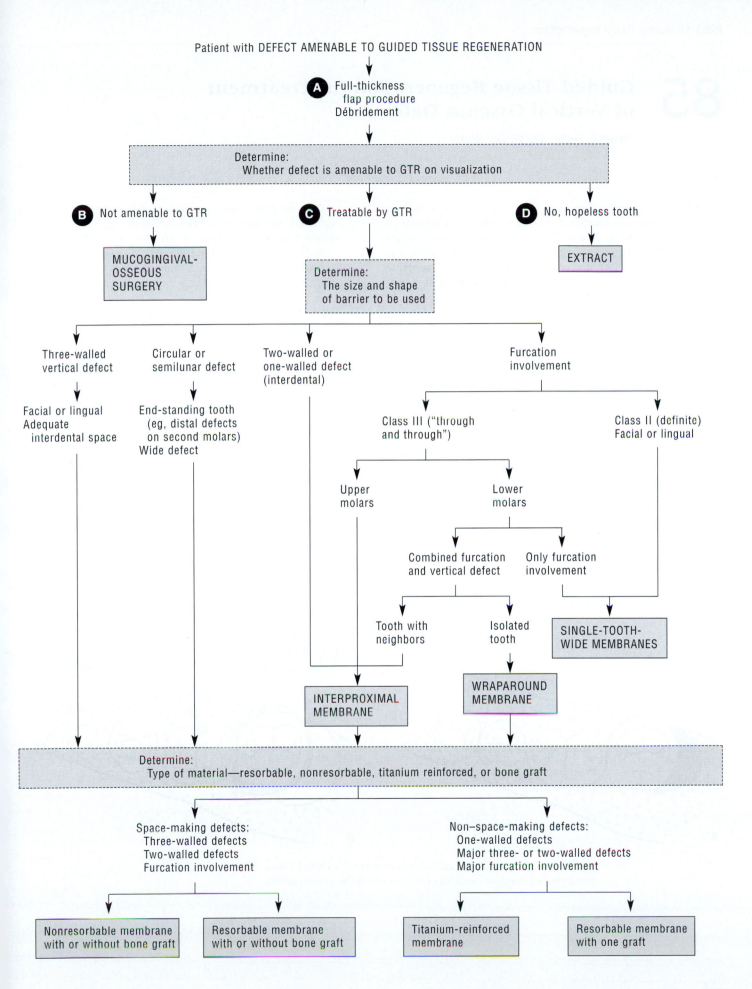

Patient with DEFECT AMENABLE TO GUIDED TISSUE REGENERATION

A Full-thickness
flap procedure
Débridement

Determine:
Whether defect is amenable to GTR on visualization

B Not amenable to GTR

C Treatable by GTR

D No, hopeless tooth

MUCOGINGIVAL-
OSSEOUS
SURGERY

Determine:
The size and shape
of barrier to be used

EXTRACT

Three-walled
vertical defect

Circular or
semilunar defect

Two-walled or
one-walled defect
(interdental)

Furcation
involvement

Facial or lingual
Adequate
interdental space

End-standing tooth
(eg, distal defects
on second molars)
Wide defect

Class III ("through
and through")

Class II (definite)
Facial or lingual

Upper
molars

Lower
molars

Combined furcation
and vertical defect

Only furcation
involvement

Tooth with
neighbors

Isolated
tooth

SINGLE-TOOTH-
WIDE MEMBRANES

INTERPROXIMAL
MEMBRANE

WRAPAROUND
MEMBRANE

Determine:
Type of material—resorbable, nonresorbable, titanium reinforced, or bone graft

Space-making defects:
Three-walled defects
Two-walled defects
Furcation involvement

Non–space-making defects:
One-walled defects
Major three- or two-walled defects
Major furcation involvement

Nonresorbable membrane
with or without bone graft

Resorbable membrane
with or without bone graft

Titanium-reinforced
membrane

Resorbable membrane
with one graft

85 Guided Tissue Regeneration for Treatment of Vertical Osseous Defects

Burton E. Becker and William Becker

The biologic principles of guided tissue regeneration (GTR) are based on epithelial exclusion and connective tissue exclusion. If the epithelium can be delayed from contacting the root surface long enough for the clot to organize, new cementum, periodontal ligament, and bone may have the potential to regenerate. The use of membranes to exclude the epithelium has been shown to achieve this clinically and histologically.

A GTR has been shown to be the most successful treatment for the deep vertical defect. The deep defect is detected best by probing depths greater than 5 mm, probing attachment loss (PAL) greater than 5 mm, and radiographic evidence of a vertical defect. The Teflon barrier excludes epithelial cells and flap connective tissues. GTR creates a space in which the clot may form and protects the clot during the early phases of wound healing. Teflon membranes made of expanded polytetrafluoroethylene (ePTFE, or Gore-Tex) and resorbable membranes have been used as barriers for GTR.

B A shallow defect is described as having pocket depths less than 5 mm, PAL less than 5 mm, and radiographic evidence of a small vertical defect. This type of defect may be treated with flap débridement or apically positioned flaps with or without osseous resection.

C If osseous defects that are greater than 5 mm in depth are exposed, the number of osseous walls that remain determine treatment options. A deep one-walled defect may require extraction or be amenable to maintenance (even with a poor prognosis) after mucogingival-osseous surgery. GTR may be attempted but is not totally predictable.

D Two- or three-walled defects that have pocket depths deeper than 5 mm and PAL greater than 5 mm can be treated with several modalities of therapy, including flap débridement, GTR, or GTR combined with either freeze-dried bone or synthetic grafting materials. GTR has been shown to achieve greater pocket reduction and gain of attachment than does flap débridement alone, but no evidence suggests that GTR with grafting creates any significant increase in attachment. Synthetic materials act as fillers. Although decreased probing depths have been demonstrated with their use, little or no attachment gain has been shown. Defects that have pocket depths greater than 5 mm, PAL greater than 5 mm, and, on entry, two- or three-walled vertical defects deeper than 5 mm with Class II furcations have several options for therapy. Flap débridement may be used; however, this type of defect responds well to GTR. Grafting materials may be used with GTR, but no evidence exists to suggest that allo-

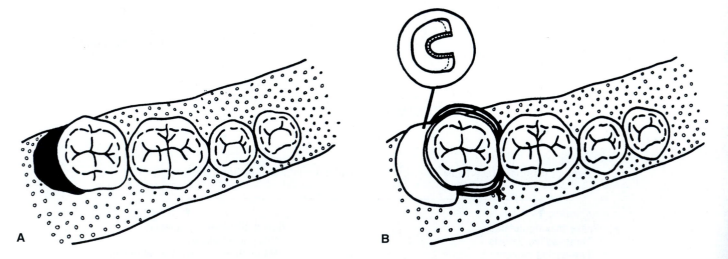

Figure 85-1 *A,* A deep, vertical, three-walled defect exposed before GTR. *B,* A wraparound membrane trimmed and sutured in place covering the vertical defect.

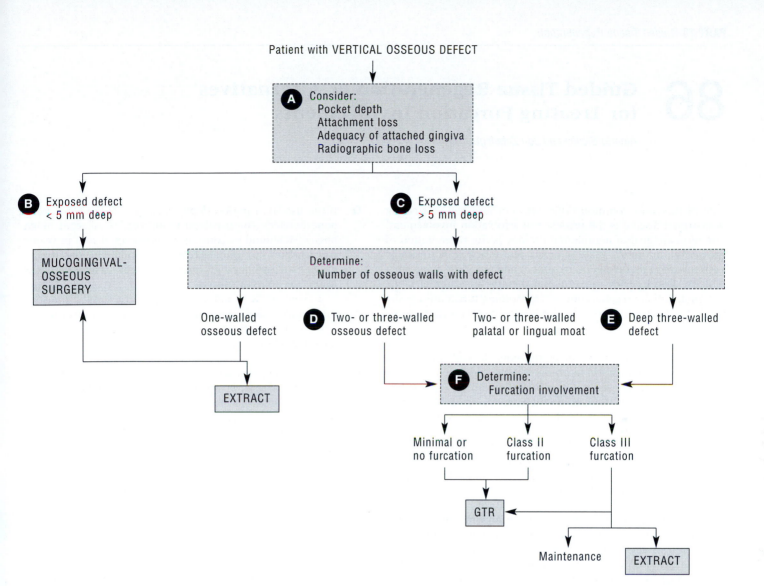

Patient with VERTICAL OSSEOUS DEFECT

A Consider:
Pocket depth
Attachment loss
Adequacy of attached gingiva
Radiographic bone loss

B Exposed defect
< 5 mm deep

C Exposed defect
> 5 mm deep

MUCOGINGIVAL-
OSSEOUS
SURGERY

Determine:
Number of osseous walls with defect

One-walled
osseous defect

D Two- or three-walled
osseous defect

Two- or three-walled
palatal or lingual moat

E Deep three-walled
defect

EXTRACT

F Determine:
Furcation involvement

Minimal or
no furcation

Class II
furcation

Class III
furcation

GTR

Maintenance

EXTRACT

---

genic or allographic grafting significantly improves the result. The presence of a deep Class II furcation makes this an ideal type of defect to treat with GTR.

E Most defects that have pocket depths greater than 5 mm and attachment loss greater than 5 mm may be treated with GTR. These defects, which usually are found to wrap around the lingual or palatal aspects of teeth, use the barrier to keep the space in the defect open for a clot to form. The deep three-walled intrabony defect is the ideal type of defect for treatment with GTR (Figure 85-1). This type of defect has been shown to heal with new bone after thorough débridement. GTR has been shown to provide a predictable reduction in pocket depth and pain and produce significant new attachment.

F The presence of a furcation may alter the likelihood of success with GTR. Class III furcations, however, do not have as good a prognosis as Class II furcations for successful GTR; therefore maintenance or extraction should be considered.

Additional Readings

Becker W et al. Clinical and volumetric analysis of three-walled intrabony defects following open flap debridement. J Periodontol 1986;57:277.

Becker W et al. New attachment after treatment with root isolation procedures: report for treated Class III and Class II furcations and vertical defects. Int J Periodontics Restorative Dent 1988;3:9.

Becker W et al. Root isolation for new attachment. J Periodontol 1987;58:819.

Cortellini P et al. Periodontal regeneration of human intrabony defects. V. Effect on oral hygiene and long-term stability. J Clin Periodontol 1994;21:606.

Gottlow J et al. New attachment formation in human periodontium by guided tissue regeneration. J Periodontol 1986;57:727.

Melcher HH. On the repair potential of periodontal tissues. J Periodontol 1976;47:256.

Schallhorn RG, McClain PR. Combined osseous composite grafting, root conditioning and guided tissue regeneration. Int J Periodontics Restorative Dent 1988;8:9.

86 Guided Tissue Regeneration or Alternatives for Treating Furcation Involvements

Alberto Sicillia and Jon Zabelegui

One of the most common difficulties encountered in treating periodontal disease is the presence of a furcation involvement. The ultimate goal of periodontal therapy is the regeneration of the periodontium to a state of health and function. Historically, with furcation involvement, treatment and prognosis have been difficult. Results with conventional therapy are unpredictable, but guided tissue regeneration (GTR) in some furcations consistently has been reported to be predictable if certain characteristics are found.

A A furcation involvement exists when loss of attachment exposes the furcation to probing. Depending on how much attachment has been lost, a furcation can be classified as Class I, II, or III. Furcation involvements are a periodontal hazard because they are difficult to clean even by professional means. Class I furcations are those where the tip of the probe does not catch within the furcation. This situation is easy to control; mild modification of the contour (odontoplasty) of the crown with a cylindrical finishing bur allows the tooth to be cleaned.

B When the probe catches in the furcation when moved coronally or in either lateral direction, a Class II or Class III furcation involvement is present. If an instrument goes into one furcation and comes out of another, a "through-and-through" or Class III furcation involvement is present; if it cannot do so, a definite or Class II furcation involvement is present.

C With Class II or III furcation involvement, a decision whether GTR or resective surgery should be performed is based on the apical depth of the furcation involvement in relation to the bone levels between the involved molar and adjacent teeth. This may be assessed radiographically and by probing.

D If the furcation pocket depth is deep to that of the crestal bone between the involved tooth and its adjacent neighbors, GTR should be considered; however, if root proximity (see Chapter 76) limits access for débridement (eg, there is only a narrow opening), resective surgery is a better option unless the roots are fused.

In some GTR situations, bone grafting to fill out a space into which regeneration tissue can grow (and prevent collapse of the membrane into the defect) may be helpful, or a coronal placement of the flap may be useful.

E If the furcation pocket depth is more shallow than the level of the crestal bone between the involved tooth and its adjacent neighbors, options include osseous surgery (see Chapter 79), hemisection or root amputation, (see Chapter 72), or extraction (see Chapter 78).

Additional Readings

Anderegg OR, Martin SJ, Gray JL, et al. Clinical evaluation of the use of decalcified freeze-dried bone allograft with guided tissue regeneration in the treatment of molar furcation invasions. J Periodontol 1991;62:264.

Becker W, Becker B, Berg L, et al. New attachment after treatment with root isolation procedures: report for treated Class III and Class II furcations and vertical osseous defects. Int J Periodontics Restorative Dent 1988;3:9.

Carranza FA, Newman MG. Clinical periodontology. 8th ed. Philadelphia: WB Saunders; 1996. p. 626.

Gottlow J, Nyman S, Karring T, Wennstrom J. New attachment formation in human periodontium by guided tissue regeneration. J Periodontol 1986;57:727.

Pontoriero R, Lindhe J, Nyman S, et al. Guided tissue regeneration in degree II furcation involved mandibular teeth. J Clin Periodontol 1988;15:247.

Patient with a COMPLEX DENTAL PROBLEM and a MOLAR with a FURCATION INVOLVEMENT

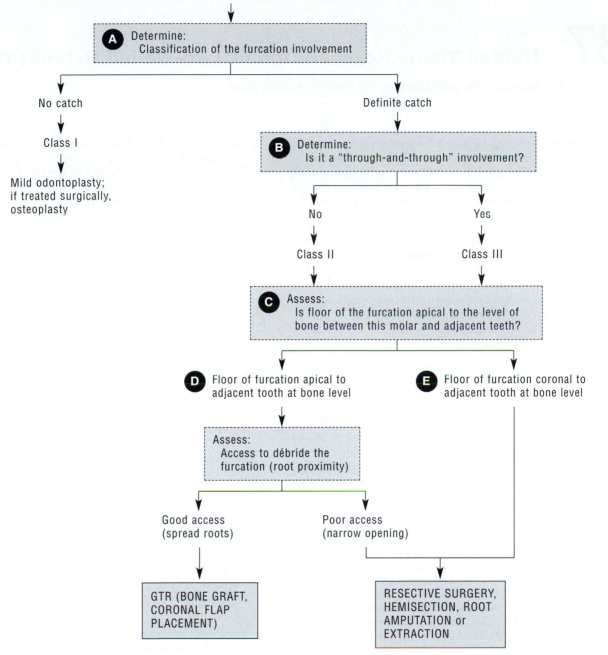

A Determine:
Classification of the furcation involvement

No catch

Definite catch

Class I

B Determine:
Is it a "through-and-through" involvement?

Mild odontoplasty;
if treated surgically,
osteoplasty

No

Yes

Class II

Class III

C Assess:
Is floor of the furcation apical to the level of
bone between this molar and adjacent teeth?

D Floor of furcation apical to
adjacent tooth at bone level

E Floor of furcation coronal to
adjacent tooth at bone level

Assess:
Access to débride the
furcation (root proximity)

Good access
(spread roots)

Poor access
(narrow opening)

GTR (BONE GRAFT,
CORONAL FLAP
PLACEMENT)

RESECTIVE SURGERY,
HEMISECTION, ROOT
AMPUTATION or
EXTRACTION

87 Guided Tissue Regeneration in Two-Walled Osseous Defects

Alberto Sicillia, John Zabelegui, and Francisco Enrile de Rojas

Before studying possible indications for a guided tissue regeneration (GTR) technique, the general condition of the patient should be evaluated. Factors such as systemic diseases or states that affect the patient's healing capacity, smoking, psychologic apects, and the manual dexterity (all of which may affect treatment and plaque control) must be considered.

A After this evaluation, the focus is on dental examination. The size of the intraosseous component of the defect (small, moderate, or large) must be determined. In shallow defects (< 2 mm), regeneration is difficult to achieve and often little regeneration may be obtained. The cost/benefit relationship compared with other kinds of treatment is unfavorable. GTR is not recommended.

B In moderate (2–4 mm) and deep defects (> 4 mm), the prognosis of the adjacent tooth or teeth must be evaluated, and if hopeless (see Chapter 37), the case is unfavorable for GTR on the middle tooth.

C If the tooth is treatable, analyze the local conditions. Positive findings include the following: (1) an adequate separation (> 2 mm) between the roots of the adjacent teeth, (2) an anatomy of the affected dental surface that allows a good adaptation of the membrane and closure of the defect, (3) a good quantity of healthy periodontium remaining close to the defect (such as occurs in narrow and deep defects), and (4) a thick periodontium and adequate vestibulum to facilitate viability and stability of the flap covering the membrane. If one or more negative conditions appear, the case should be considered unfavorable for GTR.

D If local conditions are positive, evaluate the anatomy of the defect. If anatomy permits the natural creation of space, a favorable situation exists. Evaluate the convenience of carrying out GTR in a conventional way with an expanded polytetrafluoroethylene membrane (ePTFE, or Gore-Tex) or decide whether a resorbable one* would be more efficacious (Figure 87-1).

E If the morphology of the defect does not follow the natural creation of space, the case is not as favorable; however, if the rest of the local conditions are favorable, GTR may be attempted using procedures to maintain the space below the barrier. In terms of predictability according to studies, these procedures use the following: (1) titanium-reinforced (TR) membranes, (2) TR membranes and bone grafts (BGs), (3) ePTFE membranes and BGs, or (4) resorbable membranes and BGs (Figure 87-2).

Additional Readings

Becker W, Becker BE. Treatment of mandibular 3-wall intrabony defects by flap debridement and expanded polytetrafluoroethylene barrier membranes. Long-term evaluation of 32 treated patients. J Periodontol 1993;64:1138.

Cortellini P, Pini-Prato G, Tonetti MS. Periodontal regeneration of human infrabony defects with titanium reinforced membranes. A controlled clinical trial. J Periodontol 1995;66:797.

Cortellini P, Pini-Prato G, Tonetti MS. Periodontal regeneration of human intrabony defects with bioresorbable membranes. A controlled clinical trial. J Periodontol 1996;67:217.

Laurell L et al. Clinical use of a bioresorbable matrix barrier in guided tissue regeneration therapy. Case series. J Periodontol 1994;65:967.

McClain PK, Shallhorn RG. Long-term assessment of combined osseous composite grafting, root conditioning, and guided tissue regeneration. Int J Periodontics Restorative Dent 1993;13:9.

Sanz M et al. Guided tissue regeneration in human Class II furcation and interproximal infrabony defects after using a bioabsorbable membrane barrier. Int J Periodontics Restorative Dent. [In press]

Tonetti MS, Pini-Prato G, Cortellini P. Factors affecting the healing response of intrabony defects following guided tissue regeneration and access flap surgery. J Clin Periodontol 1996;23:548.

* Short-term scientific data support the use of membranes made from pure lactide and glycolide polymers (Resolut) or a physical blend of poly-D, L-lactide, and poly-L-lactide softened with acetyl-μ-butyl citrate (Guidor).

Figure 87-1 Space-making defect treated with resorbable membrane (A) or Teflon membrane (B).

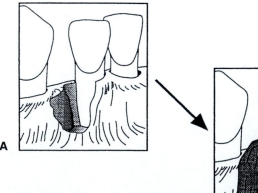

Patient with a TWO-WALLED OSSEOUS DEFECT FOR GTR SURGERY

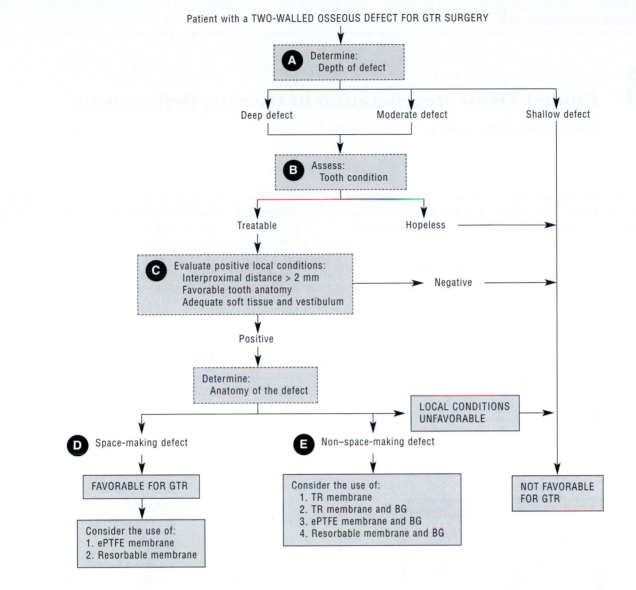

(A) Determine:
Depth of defect

Deep defect   Moderate defect   Shallow defect

(B) Assess:
Tooth condition

Treatable   Hopeless

(C) Evaluate positive local conditions:
Interproximal distance > 2 mm
Favorable tooth anatomy
Adequate soft tissue and vestibulum

Negative

Positive

Determine:
Anatomy of the defect

LOCAL CONDITIONS
UNFAVORABLE

(D) Space-making defect

(E) Non–space-making defect

FAVORABLE FOR GTR

NOT FAVORABLE
FOR GTR

Consider the use of:
1. ePTFE membrane
2. Resorbable membrane

Consider the use of:
1. TR membrane
2. TR membrane and BG
3. ePTFE membrane and BG
4. Resorbable membrane and BG

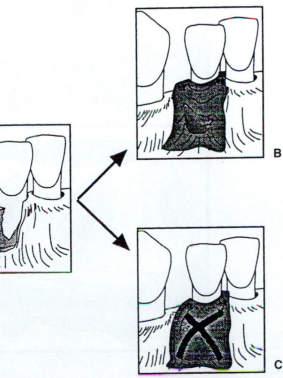

Figure 87-2 Non–space-making defect (A) treated with a collapsed ePTFE or resorbable membrane (B) or a titanium-reinforced ePTFE membrane (C).

88 Guided Tissue Regeneration in Osseous Dehiscences

Alberto Sicillia and Jon Zabelegui

After verifying the suitability of the patient for regenerative periodontal treatment and establishing the diagnosis of an osseous dehiscence using the usual methods (see Chapter 107), approach treatment in the following way:

A In shallow dehiscences (< 3 mm), regeneration is difficult to achieve or scant regeneration may be obtained. The cost/benefit relationship compared with other kinds of treatment is unfavorable. Guided tissue regeneration (GTR) is not recommended.

B In moderate (3–5 mm) and deep (> 6 mm) dehiscences, determine the prognosis of the affected tooth or teeth, and if hopeless (see Chapter 37), do not attempt GTR.

C If the tooth is treatable, evaluate the adequacy of the vestibulum and attached gingiva. If they are adequate, GTR is indicated because it is easier to keep the membrane covered during treatment, preventing gingival recession and contamination of the barrier, both of which may endanger regeneration. If desirable conditions do not exist, evaluate the need for mucogingival surgical procedures with or without membranes as alternatives.

D The anatomy of the osseous dehiscence and root prominence must permit adaptation of the membrane, ideally to the cementoenamel junction of the tooth, completely covering the defect and creating a space beneath the membrane (Figure 88-1).

E If the area is not spacious and the form of the osseous defect makes creating space easier, a favorable case exists. Use GTR with an expanded polytetrafluoroethylene (ePTFE, or GoreTex) or resorbable membrane.* Narrow dehiscences with thick bony walls make achieving these objectives easier because a greater quantity of adjacent donor cells exists near the surface in which regeneration takes place.

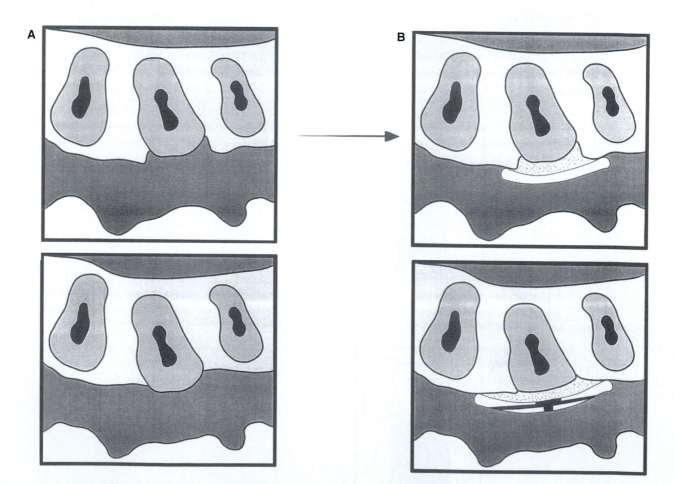

Figure 88-1 *A,* Space-making defect. *B,* Non–space-making defect using titanium-supported membrane.

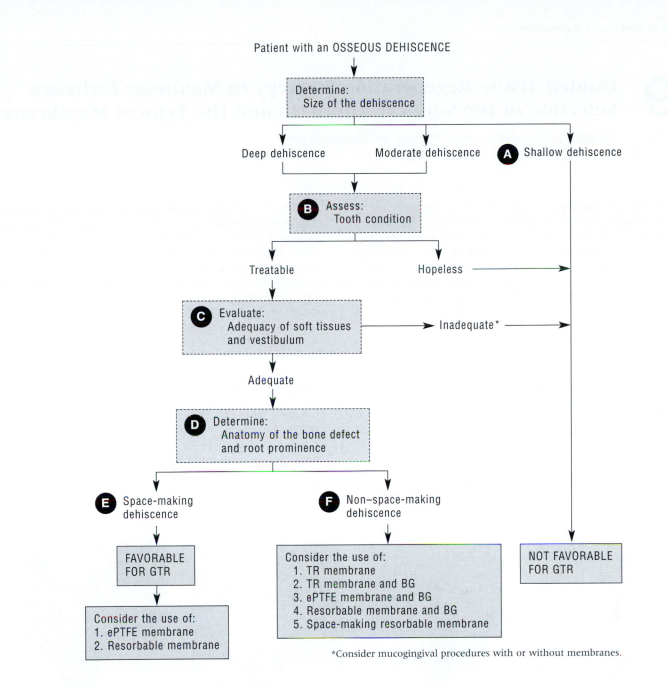

Patient with an OSSEOUS DEHISCENCE

Determine:
Size of the dehiscence

Deep dehiscence   Moderate dehiscence   **A** Shallow dehiscence

B Assess:
Tooth condition

Treatable   Hopeless

C Evaluate:
Adequacy of soft tissues
and vestibulum   → Inadequate*

Adequate

D Determine:
Anatomy of the bone defect
and root prominence

E Space-making
dehiscence   **F** Non–space-making
dehiscence

FAVORABLE
FOR GTR

Consider the use of:
1. TR membrane
2. TR membrane and BG
3. ePTFE membrane and BG
4. Resorbable membrane and BG
5. Space-making resorbable membrane

NOT FAVORABLE
FOR GTR

Consider the use of:
1. ePTFE membrane
2. Resorbable membrane

*Consider mucogingival procedures with or without membranes.

F If the osseous defect and morphology of the root do not allow creation of a space, a space may be created using titanium-reinforced (TR) membranes alone or with bone grafts (BGs); ePTFE membranes with osseous grafts (OGs), resorbable space-creating membranes (Guidor), or resorbable membranes with OGs also may be used.

---

* Short-term scientific data support the use of membranes made from pure lactide and glycolide polymers (Resolut), polyglactin 910 (Vicryl), or a physical blend of poly-D, L-lactide, and poly-L-lactide softened with acetyl-μ-butyl citrate (Guidor).

Additional Readings

Cortellini P, Clauser C, Pini-Prato GP. Histological assessment of new attachment following the treatment of a buccal recession by means of a guided tissue regeneration procedure. J Periodontol 1993;64:387.

Echeverrfa JJ, Manzanares C. Guided tissue regeneration in severe periodontal defects in anterior teeth. Case reports. J Periodontol 1995; 66:295.

Pini-Prato G et al. Resorbable membranes in the treatment of human buccal recession: a nine-case report. Int J Periodontics Restorative Dent 1995;15:259.

Rachlin G et al. The use of a resorbable membrane in mucogingival surgery. Case series. J Periodontol 1996;67:621.

Roccuzzo M et al. Comparative study of a bioresorbable and nonresorbable membrane in the treatment of human buccal gingival recessions. J Periodontol 1996;67:7.

Tinti C et al. Guided tissue regeneration in the treatment of human facial recession. A twelve case report. J Periodontol 1992;63:554.

Tinti C, Vincenzi G, Cocchetto R. Guided tissue regeneration in mucogingival surgery. J Periodontol 1993;64:1184.

89 Guided Tissue Regeneration Strategy to Maximize Esthetics: Selection of the Surgical Approach and the Type of Membrane

Pierpaolo Cortellini, Giovan Paolo Pini-Prato, and Maurizio Tonetti

Objectives of guided tissue regeneration (GTR) in esthetically sensitive sites include complete resolution of the periodontal defect and preservation of soft tissues. The selection of the proper regenerative strategy is aimed at overcoming common drawbacks of GTR such as the uncompleted filling of the bony defect and soft tissue dehiscence, both of which can result in impaired esthetics.

Deep intrabony defects benefit most from GTR therapy. Anatomic prerequisites for uneventful procedures include the presence of an adequate band of attached gingiva and the absence of frena in the area of treatment. GTR treatment should be initiated after completion of the initial therapy phase.

A The dentist selects the surgical procedure after considering the width of the interdental space and correlated thickness of the interdental tissues. The interdental space is considered wide if the interdental tissues exceed 2 mm mesiodistally. If the interdental tissues are less than 2 mm, the interdental space is classified as narrow.

B If the interdental space is wide, the surgical procedure of choice is the modified papilla preservation technique

(MPPT) (Cortellini and colleagues, 1995b). The interdental papilla is horizontally dissected at its base on the buccal side and elevated with a palatal full-thickness flap. After membrane positioning, the papilla is repositioned through the interdental space to cover the barrier and passively sutured to the buccal flap to obtain primary closure (Figure 89-1). If the interdental space is narrow, the simplified papilla preservation technique (SPPT) should be used. The interdental papilla is obliquely dissected to augment the connective tissue surface for the subsequent primary closure of the flap over the barrier membrane.

C The bony defect associated with the periodontal pocket may be a pure intrabony defect with the residual interproximal bone crest close to the cementoenamel junction (CEJ) or it may have a horizontal component on top of the intrabony component. In the latter case, the interproximal bone crest is located at a distance from the CEJ. The recognition of these two types of osseous defects is relevant for the selection of the barrier membrane.

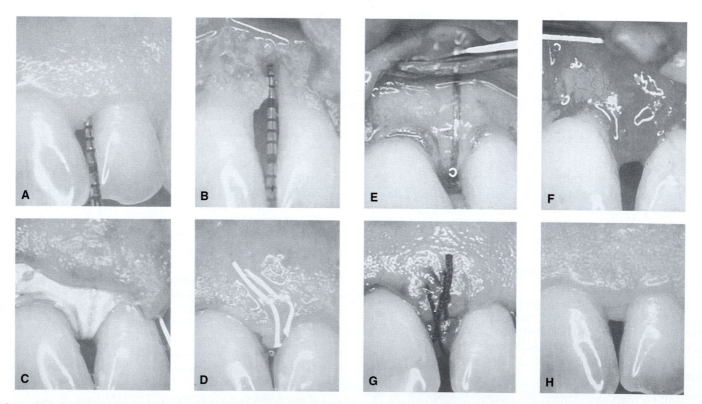

Figure 89-1 *A,* Preoperative view of a deep defect on the lateral incisor. *B,* The osseous defect has one-walled to three-walled components. *C,* A titanium-reinforced ePTFE interproximal membrane in place. *D,* The modified papilla preservation–designed flap sutured over the membrane. *E,* The membrane exposed 6 weeks after surgery. *F,* Regeneration tissue exposed after membrane removal. *G,* The sutured flaps covering the regeneration tissue. *H,* The healed result.

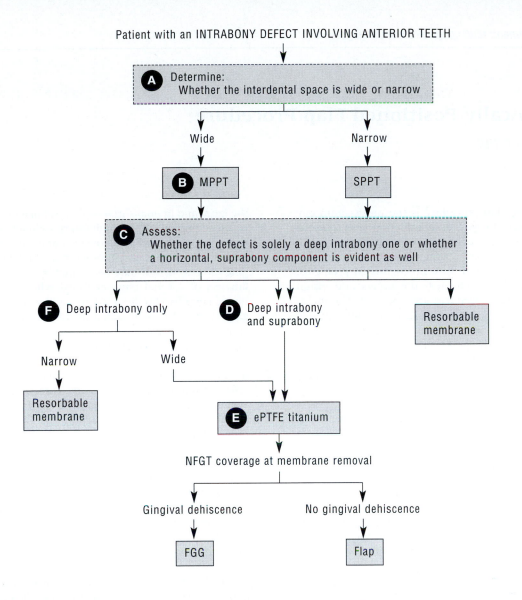

Patient with an INTRABONY DEFECT INVOLVING ANTERIOR TEETH

A Determine: Whether the interdental space is wide or narrow

Wide → **B** MPPT

Narrow → SPPT

C Assess: Whether the defect is solely a deep intrabony one or whether a horizontal, suprabony component is evident as well

F Deep intrabony only

D Deep intrabony and suprabony

Resorbable membrane

Narrow → Resorbable membrane

Wide

E ePTFE titanium

NFGT coverage at membrane removal

Gingival dehiscence → FGG

No gingival dehiscence → Flap

D   An expanded polytetrafluoroethylene (ePTFE, or Gore-Tex) titanium-reinforced membrane is selected if a horizontal component to the defect is present and the intrabony defect is wide (Cortellini and colleagues, 1995c). In such cases the self-supporting membrane may be positioned and maintained near the CEJ; it does not collapse into the wide defect after flap closure.

E   If a nonresorbable ePTFE titanium membrane is used, its removal is planned at about 6 weeks. At that time the tissue covering the membrane still may be preserved or may conversely be dehiscent. In the first instance, the newly formed gingival tissue (NFGT) may be properly covered by repositioning the flap. If a gingival dehiscence is present, NFGT coverage is difficult. Proper protection of the regenerated tissue may be achieved with a saddle-shaped free gingival graft (FGG) positioned in the interdental space (Cortellini and colleagues, 1995a).

F   A resorbable barrier membrane is preferred if a narrow, solely intrabony defect is to be treated (Cortellini and colleagues, 1996). The anatomy of this defect should allow positioning of the membrane near the CEJ and prevent its collapse into the defect.

If a resorbable membrane is used, a possible dehiscence of the flap cannot be treated in the early healing phase. An anatomic correction of the consequent soft-tissue deficiency should be postponed after completion of the healing until 9 to 12 months after the regenerative procedures.

Additional Readings

Cortellini P, Pini-Prato G, Tonetti M. Interproximal free gingival grafts after membrane removal in GTR treatment of infrabony defects. A controlled clinical trial indicating improved outcomes. J Periodontol 1995a;66:488.

Cortellini P, Pini-Prato G, Tonetti M. The modified papilla preservation technique. A new surgical approach for interproximal regenerative procedures. J Periodontol 1995b;66:261.

Cortellini P, Pini-Prato G, Tonetti M. Periodontal regeneration of human infrabony defects with titanium reinforced membranes. A controlled clinical trial. J Periodontol 1995c;66:797.

Cortellini P, Pini-Prato G, Tonetti M. The modified papilla preservation technique with bioresorbable barrier membranes in the treatment of intrabony defects. Case reports. Int J Periodontics Restorative Dent 1996;16:547.

Cortellini P, Pini-Prato G, Tonetti M. The simplified papilla preservation technique. A new surgical approach for the management of soft tissues in regenerative procedures. J Periodontol. [submitted]

Tonetti M, Pini-Prato G, Cortellini P. Periodontal regeneration of human intrabony defects. IV. Determinants of the healing response. J Periodontol 1993;64:934.

90 Apically Positioned Flap Procedure

Walter B. Hall

The apically positioned flap procedure is the most commonly used surgical approach to pocket elimination and osseous recontouring. Its advantages include its wide spectrum of usefulness, retention of most existing gingiva, and ability to solve both mucogingival-osseous and pure mucogingival problems. Because the flaps are fully reflected, the access and vision requirements for osseous procedures are achieved. The major disadvantages of the apically positioned flap procedure include possible unacceptable esthetic results in areas in which esthetics may be important and the greater likelihood of root sensitivity because of root exposure. Guided tissue regeneration (GTR) better resolves these problems with less esthetic compromise (see Chapter 79)

A   If the flap will extend to a canine tooth or another tooth with a similarly long crown, an envelope flap approach may be used. If access for visibility cannot be obtained adequately with that approach, vertical-releasing incisions may be used. Usually they are placed at the proximal line angle of the tooth at the end of a surgical segment.

B   If adequate attached gingiva will remain if the flap is positioned at the crest of the bone, the incision for the flap is made with an internal bevel to the crest of the alveolus on the facial and lingual surfaces. It is scalloped interdentally to retain additional gingiva to fit interproximally when the flap is sutured. It should be filleted so that its thickness is similar over the tooth root and interdentally. If additional attached gingiva is needed, it may be created by leaving several millimeters of coronal bone denuded when the flap is positioned apically. This denuded area will granulate and heal as gingiva, which, when added to the apically positioned old gingiva, will create a band of attached gingiva 2 to 5 mm high. Such a flap need not be scalloped to fulfill this need.

C   In the apically positioned flap approach, the flap is fully reflected into alveolar mucosa (in contrast to the modified Widman flap approach). Because the palate does not have alveolar mucosa, a gingival flap in that area cannot be apically positioned and is created differently (see Chapter 92). Next the remaining interdental and marginal tissue is removed with curets and chisels, exposing the bone and any osseous defects. These may be treated by osseous recontouring (see Chapter 93) or bone fill (see Chapter 95). If any defects are amenable to GTR, this technique should be employed preferentially to pocket elimination because it provides greater support, better esthetics, and easier cleansing of the area when healed.

D   When the flap is positioned and sutured, if no additional gingiva is to be created by denudation, it may be sutured tightly at the level of the crest of bone and the pack placed (Figure 90-1). If more attached gingiva is needed, the flap may be positioned so that some bone is exposed, and it may be sutured loosely with suspensory sutures to establish its position before pack placement. Healing is more rapid if the only bone left exposed is between teeth. Ideally performed, the apically positioned flap should result in pocket elimination with improved gingival form, facilitating plaque removal by the patient.

Additional Readings

Ariudo A, Tyrell H. Repositioning and increasing the zone of attached gingiva. J Periodontol 1957;28:106.

Carranza FA Jr, Newman MG. Clinical periodontology. 8th ed. Philadelphia: WB Saunders; 1996. p. 608.

Genco RJ, Goldman HM, Cohen DW. Contemporary periodontics. St. Louis: Mosby; 1990. p. 567.

Lindhe J. Textbook of clinical periodontology. 2nd ed. Copenhagen: Munksgaard; 1989. p. 405.

Nabers CL. Repositioning the attached gingiva. J Periodontol 1954;25:38.

Wilson JG, Kornman KS. Fundamentals of periodontics. Chicago: Quintessence Publishing; 1996. p. 383.

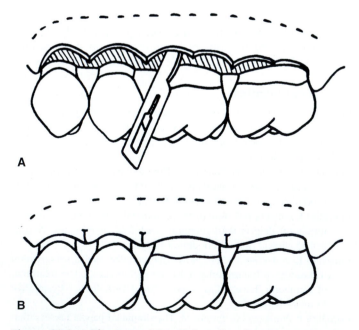

Figure 90-1 *A,* The internal bevelled, scalloped incision is used for pocket elimination through apical repositioning of the flap. *B,* The flap positioned apically for pocket elimination.

Patient scheduled for POCKET ELIMINATION SURGERY ON THE
MANDIBULAR ARCH OR THE FACIAL ASPECT OF THE MAXILLARY ARCH

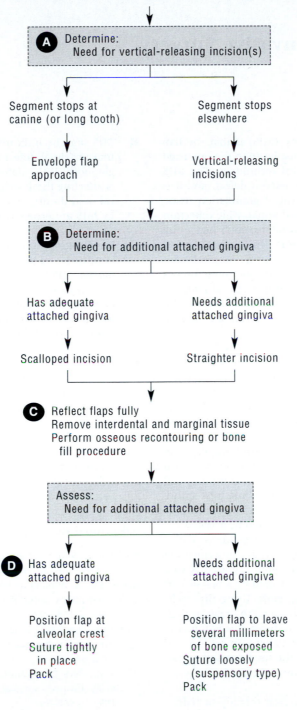

A Determine:
Need for vertical-releasing incision(s)

Segment stops at
canine (or long tooth)

Segment stops
elsewhere

Envelope flap
approach

Vertical-releasing
incisions

B Determine:
Need for additional attached gingiva

Has adequate
attached gingiva

Needs additional
attached gingiva

Scalloped incision

Straighter incision

C Reflect flaps fully
Remove interdental and marginal tissue
Perform osseous recontouring or bone
fill procedure

Assess:
Need for additional attached gingiva

D Has adequate
attached gingiva

Needs additional
attached gingiva

Position flap at
alveolar crest
Suture tightly
in place
Pack

Position flap to leave
several millimeters
of bone exposed
Suture loosely
(suspensory type)
Pack

91 Minimally Invasive Surgery

Stephen K. Harrel

The basis of minimally invasive surgery (MIS) is that the flap used for access to the defect is much smaller than the one used in other, traditional periodontal surgical techniques. The MIS flap is confined to an area of a single osseous defect, and it is reflected just enough to permit removal of granulation tissue and root débridement of that defect. Traditional, wide reflection for "visualization" is avoided. MIS can be accomplished using standard operating lights, small mirrors (judiciously), small curets, and small scalpels. Magnification using surgical telescopes with high-intensity headlights and/or fiber-optic probes will improve visualization, and the use of mechanical granulation tissue-removing instruments will speed débridement of the defect. Endoscopic cameras that can be placed into the surgical site can also be used to facilitate MIS.

The MIS flap is reflected only to the mucogingival junction. No vertical incisions are used. Care is taken that the flaps are not folded during retraction, and strict caution is used to minimize soft-tissue trauma. All of these steps are based on the goal of causing the least amount of damage to the blood supply of the soft tissue. By working carefully, it is possible to retain all or most of the soft-tissue height (papilla) for improved postsurgical esthetics. Maintenance of the blood supply during surgery may improve regenerative procedures and also help in the retention of soft tissue. To maintain the blood supply to the soft tissue and to minimize soft-tissue trauma, a single vertical mattress suture is used to close interproximal flaps. The use of multiple sutures—even if those sutures are extremely fine—should be avoided.

MIS can be used for flap débridement or flap curettage procedures, but it is most often used for regenerative procedures in isolated sites. The MIS technique most often reported is that using freeze-dried demineralized bone covered by a polyglactin 910 membrane (Vicryl) to stabilize the graft. Using this technique yields regenerative results that are equal to or better than those from using traditional surgical procedures. In addition, the small incision seems to produce far less patient discomfort and little or no recession is reported. Due to the small surgical access, MIS is not applicable for use with osseous surgery.

A The patient has undergone nonsurgical therapy to reduce or eliminate pockets and, after a suitable length of time, periodontal status is reevaluated. If isolated defects of 5 mm or greater are still present, MIS may be considered.

B MIS may be indicated if the defect is isolated, such as an interproximal defect or the mesial or distal aspect of a single tooth. If the defect continues around multiple teeth or is affecting three surfaces on a single tooth (ie, mesial, buccal, and distal), access incisions larger than those afforded by MIS are probably indicated.

C In MIS procedures the incisions are isolated to the area of bone loss, and they do not extend beyond the interproximal papilla. MIS flaps are freed with sharp dissection only. Granulation tissue is carefully removed to visualize the osseous defect. Care is taken to preserve as much blood supply to the soft tissue as possible (eg, with minimal retraction and preservation of the periosteal–soft-tissue attachment).

D If the osseous defect does not have a vertical component, an open débridement can be performed with the soft tissue returned to its original position. The MIS flap is closed using a vertical mattress suture.

E If the osseous defect contains a vertical component, a regenerative procedure is performed. This can be an osseous graft stabilized with Vicryl or the use of a growth enhancer (Emdogain), or a combination of both. The MIS flap is closed using a vertical mattress suture.

Additional Readings

Harrel SK. A minimally invasive surgical approach for bone grafting. Int J Periodontics Restorative Dent 1998;18:161–9.

Harrel SK. A minimally invasive surgical approach for periodontal regeneration: surgical technique and observations. J Periodontol 1999;70:1547–57.

Harrel SK, Nunn M, Belling CM. Long-term results of minimally invasive surgical approach for bone grafting. J Periodontol 1999;70: 1558–63.

Harrel SK, Rees TD. Granulation tissue removal in routine and minimally invasive surgical procedures. Compend Cont Educ Dent 1995;16:960–967.

Harrel SK, Wright JM. Treatment of periodontal destruction associated with a cemental tear using minimally invasive surgery. J Periodontol 2000;71.

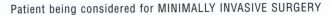

Patient being considered for MINIMALLY INVASIVE SURGERY

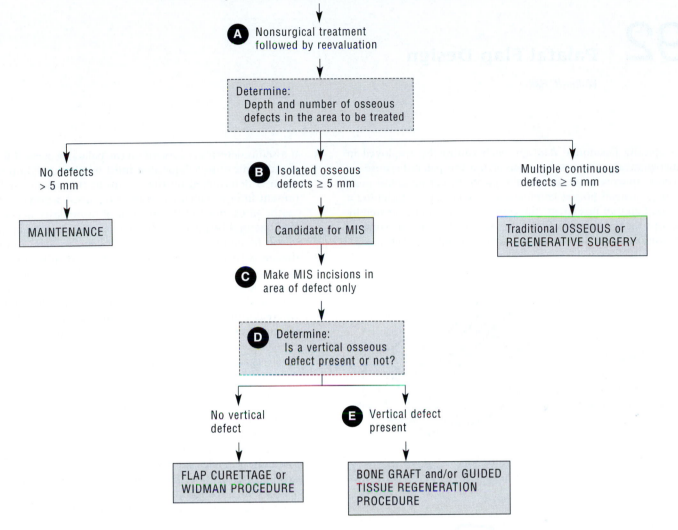

A Nonsurgical treatment followed by reevaluation

Determine:
Depth and number of osseous defects in the area to be treated

No defects > 5 mm

B Isolated osseous defects ≥ 5 mm

Multiple continuous defects ≥ 5 mm

MAINTENANCE

Candidate for MIS

Traditional OSSEOUS or REGENERATIVE SURGERY

C Make MIS incisions in area of defect only

D Determine:
Is a vertical osseous defect present or not?

No vertical defect

E Vertical defect present

FLAP CURETTAGE or WIDMAN PROCEDURE

BONE GRAFT and/or GUIDED TISSUE REGENERATION PROCEDURE

92 Palatal Flap Design

Walter B. Hall

An apically positioned flap approach cannot be employed in mucogingival-osseous surgery involving the palate because no alveolar mucosa is present on the palate to permit apical positioning. Instead pocket elimination is achieved by designing a palatal flap that just covers the contours of the bone created by osseous recontouring to eliminate osseous defects. The conceptualization of the flap design requires skill and experience.

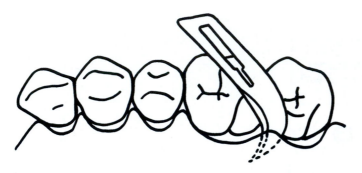

Figure 92-1 Initial incision thinning of the flap.

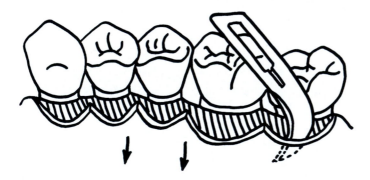

Figure 92-2 Exposure of the underlying connective tissue with the flap.

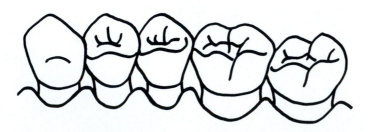

Figure 92-3 Flap repositioned after removal of connective tissue of pocket walls.

A If osseous defects are present on the palatal aspects of teeth, the amount of soft tissue that must be eliminated on each tooth is determined by the nature of the osseous defects present interproximally and on the palatal aspects of each tooth, an estimate of the amount of osteoplasty needed to facilitate oral hygiene and flap adaptation, and the amount of soft tissue to be eliminated in creating a flap of uniform thickness to cover the reshaped bone and just cover the new osseous crests (Figures 92-1 and 92-2). Narrow three-walled defects (1 mm or less horizontally from the crest of bone to the tooth) usually will "fill" when fully débrided, whereas other defects—if not treatable by guided tissue regeneration—require elimination by ostectomy.

B If defects are sufficiently narrow that bone fill should occur, the margin of the flap should be cut apically to the existing crest of the bone at a distance that depends on the amount of osteoplasty anticipated to create osseous form (to enhance plaque control and flap adaptation) and the bulk of connective tissue to be removed in creating a uniformly thick flap. If little osteoplasty or soft-tissue–bulk reduction is anticipated, the flap edge should be cut only a little apically to the existing crest of bone. The greater the amount of osteoplasty or soft-tissue reduction anticipated, the further apically to the existing osseous crest the flap edge should be cut.

C If the defects are not amenable to osseous fill, ostectomy is required to eliminate the osseous defects. In deciding the degree to which to scallop the flap so that it just covers the new bone margin on suturing, the dentist must estimate the approximate amount of ostectomy required and correlate those expectations with an estimate of the amount of osteoplasty or soft-tissue–bulk reduction needed to facilitate plaque control and flap adaptation (Figure 92-3). If little osteoplasty or bulk reduction is anticipated, the scalloping is less dramatic; the greater the amount of bone or soft-tissue bulk to be removed, the more severely apically the scalloping should be placed.

Additional Readings

Carranza FA Jr, Newman MG. Clinical periodontology. 8th ed. Philadelphia: WB Saunders; 1996. p. 602.

Nevins M, Mellonig JT. Periodontal therapy: clinical approaches and evidence of success. Chicago: Quintessence Publishing; 1998. p. 170.

Oschsenbein C, Bohannon HM. Palatal approach to osseous surgery. I. Rationale. J Periodontol 1963;34:60.

Oschsenbein C, Bohannon HM. Palatal approach to osseous surgery. II. Clinical applications. J Periodontol 1964;35:54.

Rateitshak KH et al. Color atlas of periodontology. Stuttgart: Thieme-Verlag; 1985. p. 199.

Schluger S et al. Periodontal diseases. 2nd ed. Philadelphia: Lea & Febiger; 1990. p. 469.

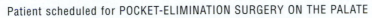

Patient scheduled for POCKET-ELIMINATION SURGERY ON THE PALATE

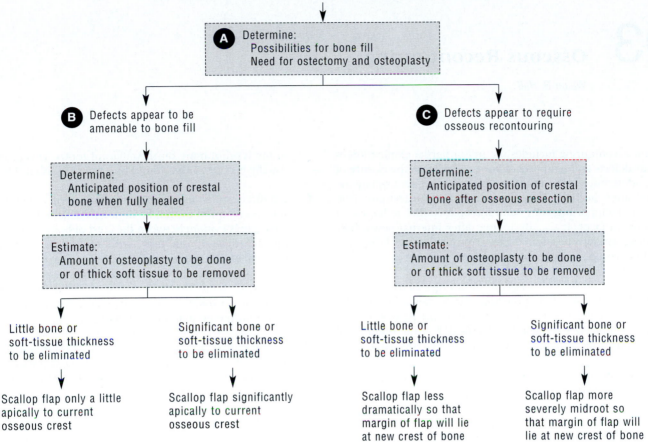

A Determine:
Possibilities for bone fill
Need for ostectomy and osteoplasty

B Defects appear to be amenable to bone fill

Determine:
Anticipated position of crestal bone when fully healed

Estimate:
Amount of osteoplasty to be done or of thick soft tissue to be removed

Little bone or soft-tissue thickness to be eliminated

Significant bone or soft-tissue thickness to be eliminated

Scallop flap only a little apically to current osseous crest

Scallop flap significantly apically to current osseous crest

C Defects appear to require osseous recontouring

Determine:
Anticipated position of crestal bone after osseous resection

Estimate:
Amount of osteoplasty to be done or of thick soft tissue to be removed

Little bone or soft-tissue thickness to be eliminated

Significant bone or soft-tissue thickness to be eliminated

Scallop flap less dramatically so that margin of flap will lie at new crest of bone

Scallop flap more severely midroot so that margin of flap will lie at new crest of bone

93 Osseous Recontouring

Walter B. Hall

Osseous recontouring includes the full or partial elimination of osseous defects and sculpting of bone to facilitate the closure of flaps and permit the most ideal access for plaque removal by the patient after healing. It may include both ostectomy (the removal of supporting bone) and osteoplasty (the reshaping of the bony surface). It usually is used after internal bevel, full-thickness, apically positioned flap exposure of the bone surrounding periodontally involved teeth.

A If pocket-elimination surgery employing osseous contouring has been selected as the appropriate method of treating a case, the need for ostectomy relates to the type of osseous defect involved, which is described by the number of osseous walls remaining (see Chapters 99, 100, 101).

B If no osseous defects are present, the only ostectomy necessary is to correct "reversed architecture."

C If one- and two-walled intrabony defects are present, they are ramped out by eliminating the remaining osseous walls

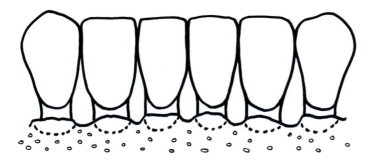

Figure 93-1 Reversed osseous architecture created by periodontitis (preoperative).

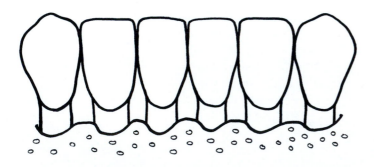

Figure 93-2 Corrected reversed architecture.

to the level of bone on the adjacent tooth. This procedure usually is done with a round bur and various chisels.

D If a three-walled intrabony defect is present and guided tissue regeneration cannot be done (see Chapter 101), and a wide gap is evident between the crest of bone and the tooth (greater than 1 mm from crest of tooth), it should be ramped in the same manner until a narrow (less than 1 mm) gap remains. Narrow three-walled defects routinely "fill" with bone from the walls of the defect, and new attachment usually occurs as the connective tissue regenerates from the periodontal ligament.

E Interproximal grooving (osteoplasty) is performed to create a festooned form to the fully healed area, facilitate closure of the flaps interproximally, and permit greater interproximal penetration of toothbrush bristles during brushing.

F If exostoses or ledges are present, they are ramped to create an even, flowing surface to facial and lingual bone to facilitate flap closure and improve plaque removal possibilities for the patient.

G If reversed architecture (the more coronal positioning of bone facially or lingually rather than interproximally) is present or occurs after ostectomy (Figure 93-1), it should be corrected with a chisel to create positive architecture (the more apical positioning of bone facially or lingually rather than interproximally). Creating positive architecture from reversed architecture is discussed later (Figure 93-2).

H On completion of osseous recontouring, the roots are planed to remove any nicks created by the instrumentation, the flaps are sutured in place, a dressing is placed, and postoperative instructions are given to the patient.

Additional Readings

Grant DA, Stern IB, Listgarten MA. Periodontics. 6th ed. St. Louis: Mosby; 1988. p. 838.

Heins PG. Osseous surgery: an evaluation after twenty years. Dent Clin North Am 1969;13:75.

Newman MG, Takei HH, Carranza FA. Carranza's clinical periodontology. 9th ed. Philadelphia: WB Saunders; 2002. p. 790–802.

Prichard JF. A technique for treating intrabony pockets based on alveolar process morphology. Dent Clin North Am 1968;85.

Schluger S. Osseous resection—a basic principle in periodontal surgery. Oral Surg 1949;2:316.

Schluger S et al. Periodontal diseases. 2nd ed. Philadelphia: Lea & Febiger; 1990. p. 501.

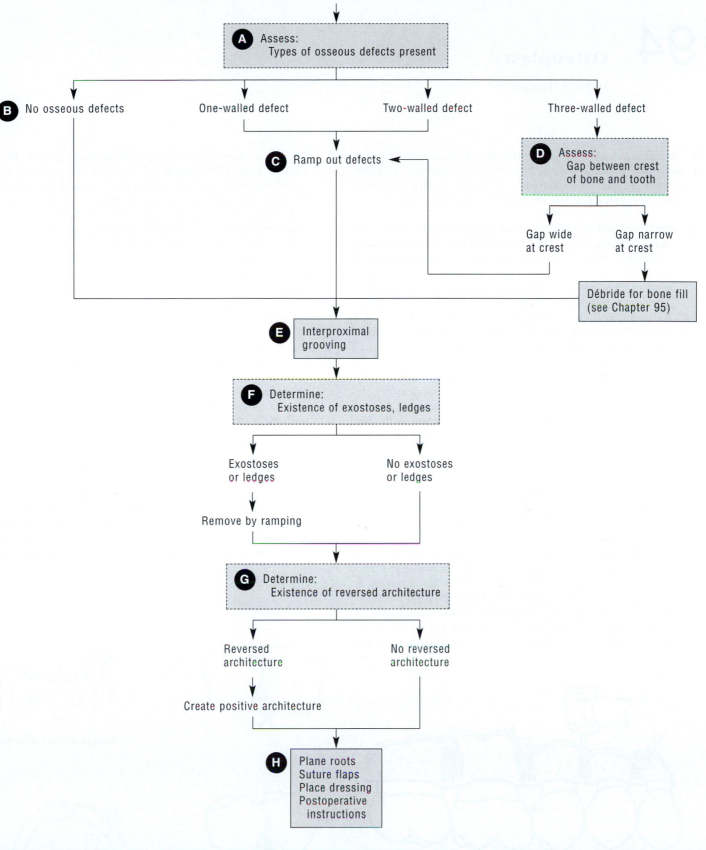

Patient for POCKET-ELIMINATION SURGERY WITH FLAPS REFLECTED

A Assess:
Types of osseous defects present

B No osseous defects   One-walled defect   Two-walled defect   Three-walled defect

C Ramp out defects

D Assess:
Gap between crest of bone and tooth

Gap wide at crest   Gap narrow at crest

Débride for bone fill (see Chapter 95)

E Interproximal grooving

F Determine:
Existence of exostoses, ledges

Exostoses or ledges   No exostoses or ledges

Remove by ramping

G Determine:
Existence of reversed architecture

Reversed architecture   No reversed architecture

Create positive architecture

H Plane roots
Suture flaps
Place dressing
Postoperative instructions

94 Osteoplasty

Luther H. Hutchens Jr

By definition, *osteoplasty* is the reshaping of the alveolar process to achieve a more physiologic form without removal of alveolar (supporting) bone. Osteoplasty is used frequently in periodontal therapy to reshape osseous structures around the teeth.

A Maxillary and mandibular facial or lingual exostoses or tori often are present as a result of hereditary anatomic bony variations, heavy occlusal loading, and parafunctional habits. The presence of exostoses or tori may necessitate bone reshaping to improve periodontal health and patient comfort. Normal crestal alveolar bone also may require reshaping in some clinical situations in which heavy marginal ledges and increased cortical plate thickness are evident in interproximal and interradicular areas.

B Patient discomfort often is a chief complaint because of the presence of exostoses or tori. These bony prominences are subject to trauma, aphthae, and herpetic ulcerations. Reduction of these bony contours may be achieved with flap access and osteoplasty using rotary surgical burs and hand instruments.

C Osteoplasty may be required to facilitate pocket reduction or elimination, flap placement, oral hygiene, and restorative procedures. If the therapist determines that intrabony pockets should be eliminated and supportive osseous structures removed to create a normal parabolized osseous architecture (ostectomy), osteoplasty of the crestal bone height and thickness often is required before ostectomy. Also, interproximal and interradicular vertical grooving is sometimes necessary to create a physiologic form to which the gingival tissues may adapt (Figure 94-1). Reshaping of cortical projections and facial and lingual ledges also facilitates flap placement when efforts are being made to obtain primary closure in the interproximal space (Figure 94-2). Ideal closure of the interdental area facilitates pocket reduction and allows good flap adaption. The use of the modified Widman flap often requires some osteoplasty to allow for tight closure in the repositioning of the flap. Marginal bone osteoplasty also is used to facilitate procedures and improve the patient's oral hygiene. Patients who are unable to achieve optimal plaque control in marginal areas because of excessive contours of bone or deep subgingival restorative margins may benefit from osteoplasty of the crestal bone. This situation is particularly true in Class II furcation areas in which access for oral hygiene is difficult.

D Edentulous ridge modifications often are required to facilitate the placement of fixed prosthetic pontics and increase access for patient oral hygiene after the prosthesis is placed. Decreased ridge height and excessive ridge thickness may require reshaping of the alveolar ridge before prosthetic placement. Ridge modification in the anterior part of the mouth often improves restorative esthetics. Osteoplasty to flatten the edentulous ridge often is required to facilitate the surgical placement of root-form implants.

E Extensive subgingival caries, faulty restorations, pin perforations, and root proximity are some clinical situations that require surgical exposure of the tooth to facilitate adequate restoration. Although both ostectomy and osteoplasty are usually required in this procedure, many times osteoplasty

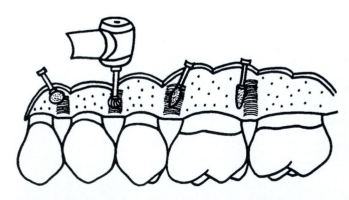

Figure 94-1 Osseous grooving, performed with various rotating burs or stones, permits better adaptation of flaps to facilitate plaque removal after healing. Illustration shows diamond stones and round bur being used for grooving.

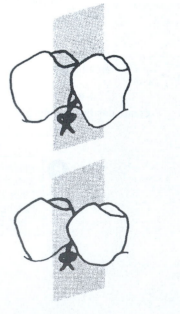
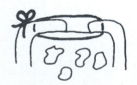
Closure without grooving

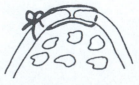
Closure with grooving

Figure 94-2 Illustration of closure with and without grooving.

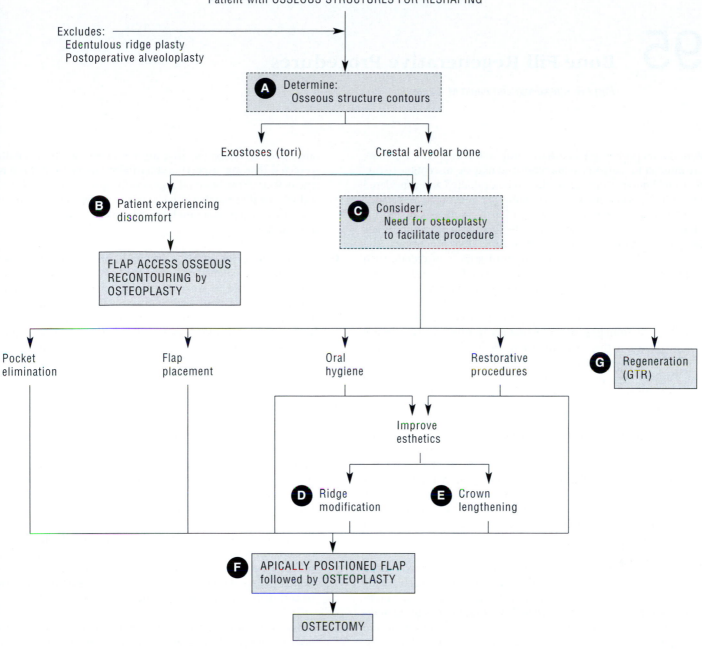

Patient with OSSEOUS STRUCTURES FOR RESHAPING

Excludes:
Edentulous ridge plasty
Postoperative alveoloplasty

A Determine:
Osseous structure contours

Exostoses (tori)   Crestal alveolar bone

B Patient experiencing discomfort

C Consider:
Need for osteoplasty
to facilitate procedure

FLAP ACCESS OSSEOUS
RECONTOURING by
OSTEOPLASTY

Pocket elimination   Flap placement   Oral hygiene   Restorative procedures   **G** Regeneration (GTR)

Improve esthetics

D Ridge modification   **E** Crown lengthening

F APICALLY POSITIONED FLAP followed by OSTEOPLASTY

OSTECTOMY

of the crestal areas facilitates apical flap placement and allows for better access for the restoration. Exposure of short clinical crowns by osseous reshaping and apical flap positioning often may improve anterior esthetics.

F   Exostosis and torus removal, ridge modifications, and most osteoplasty procedures are preceded by apical positioning of the flap at the osseous margin. Osteoplasty done in conjunction with pocket elimination of crown extension procedures usually requires removal of supportive bone (ostectomy) and apically positioned flaps.

G   Regeneration procedures using implant materials (osseous autografts, allografts, and alloplastic grafts) may require osteoplasty to improve the coronal positioning of the flap for

implant coverage. Guided tissue regeneration (GTR) also may require osteoplasty to improve flap coverage of synthetic membranes.

Additional Readings

Friedman N. Periodontal osseous survey: osteoplasty and ostectomy. J Periodontol 1955;26:257.

Genco RJ, Goldman HM, Cohen DW. Contemporary periodontics. St. Louis: Mosby; 1990. p. 569, 629.

Schulger S et al. Periodontal diseases. 2nd ed. Philadelphia: Lea & Febiger; 1990. Ch. 3.

Yuodelis RA, Smith DH. Corrections of periodontal abnormalities as a preliminary phase of oral rehabilitation. Dent Clin North Am 1976;20:181.

95 Bone Fill Regenerative Procedures

Perry R. Klokkevold and Paulo M. Camargo

Periodontal pockets greater than 5 mm following phase I therapy are difficult for patients to maintain and may be susceptible to further breakdown. These areas should be evaluated and considered for either pocket reduction or bone fill regenerative surgery. Increased success can be achieved with a decision-making process aimed at controlling those clinical factors that contribute to less favorable outcomes with bone fill regenerative procedures. The decision pathway includes evaluation of important criteria such as plaque control, amount and type of bone loss, tooth mobility, degree of furcation involvement, and root proximity.

A Initial therapy should precede these surgical approaches so that inflammation and infection are minimized. The control of plaque is the most important determinant of success in all surgical procedures used to treat periodontal defects. Patients with poor plaque control should be managed with nonsurgical therapy and oral hygiene instruction (OHI) until an acceptable level of plaque control is achieved.

B Patients with periodontal pockets that are not associated with vertical bone loss (ie, intraosseous defects) should be managed with surgery directed at reducing the suprabony pockets, such as flap curettage, open flap débridement, or gingivectomy. In the anterior portion of the mouth, it may be better to maintain these areas with a nonsurgical approach if postsurgical gingival recession would create an esthetic compromise.

C Teeth with advanced bone loss will become more mobile after periodontal surgery that may be more problematic and lead to loss of teeth sooner. In cases with a poor prognosis, the teeth are best treated with maintenance. In addition to scaling and root planing, occlusal adjustment and splint therapy aimed at reducing occlusal trauma and stabilizing mobile teeth can be helpful.

D If a tooth has lost 80% or more of its supporting bone volume and has significant mobility (class 2+ or greater) following initial therapy, then bone fill regenerative procedures have little, if any, chance of success. In these hopeless situations, extraction should be considered, and the area should be evaluated for prosthetic replacement with implants or conventional dentistry.

E Horizontal defects have not responded well to bone fill regenerative procedures. Until evidence of successful bone regeneration in horizontal bone loss becomes available, these areas are best treated with pocket-elimination flap procedures with or without osseous resective surgery.

F Crater defects are best managed with nonregenerative surgical procedures such as osseous resection and apically positioned flaps. Extremely deep craters that are not amenable to complete osseous resection can be partially resected (coronal aspect) and partially regenerated (base of the defect) using bone fill regenerative procedures. The apical end of these crater defects, which is typically narrower with three walls, respond favorably to bone fill regenerative procedures.

G Vertical bone loss with a resultant intrabony defect can result in moat-shaped defects. A wide variety of approaches have been used to treat intrabony defects. These lesions, especially those with two or three walls, respond well to bone fill regenerative procedures. Most notably, guided tissue regeneration (GTR) with or without bone graft materials (eg, autogenous bone, decalcified freeze-dried bone, hydroxyapatite, bovine bone) has yielded favorable results when used to treat intrabony defects.

H In areas with furcations where there has been bone loss extending apically less than 4 mm from the crotch of the furca, the defect can be well managed with osseous surgery and apically positioned flaps. This will result in a papilla-like projection of gingival tissue in the furcation with pocket depths of 2 to 3 mm. Bone fill regenerative procedures do not provide significant advantages for the Class I furcation defect with minimal bone loss.

I There have been a number of reports of successful treatment of Class II furcation defects using such bone fill regenerative procedures as GTR, osseous grafts, and coronally repositioned flaps. Combinations of bone graft materials and GTR or coronally repositioned flaps have been beneficial.

J Class III furcation defects in lower molars generally have a poor prognosis. If the appropriate anatomic conditions are present, such as adequate root separation, a short root trunk, treatable root canals, and an adequate residual bone-encased root volume, then hemisection with the use of one or both roots is indicated.

K Class III furcation defects do not respond well to bone fill regenerative procedures. Exposed root surfaces, especially in the furcation, are at increased risk of caries. Any surgical approach to these areas will carry a guarded prognosis for the future periodontal health of the affected teeth. Surgical therapy for Class III furcation defects tends to be limited to open flap débridement with or without exposure of the furcation for postsurgical maintenance (tunnel procedure).

L The ultimate success and management of periodontal osseous defects following any surgical (bone fill regenerative or nonregenerative) procedure must emphasize control of bacterial plaque in order to maintain the beneficial results of the surgery. Generally, postsurgical patients

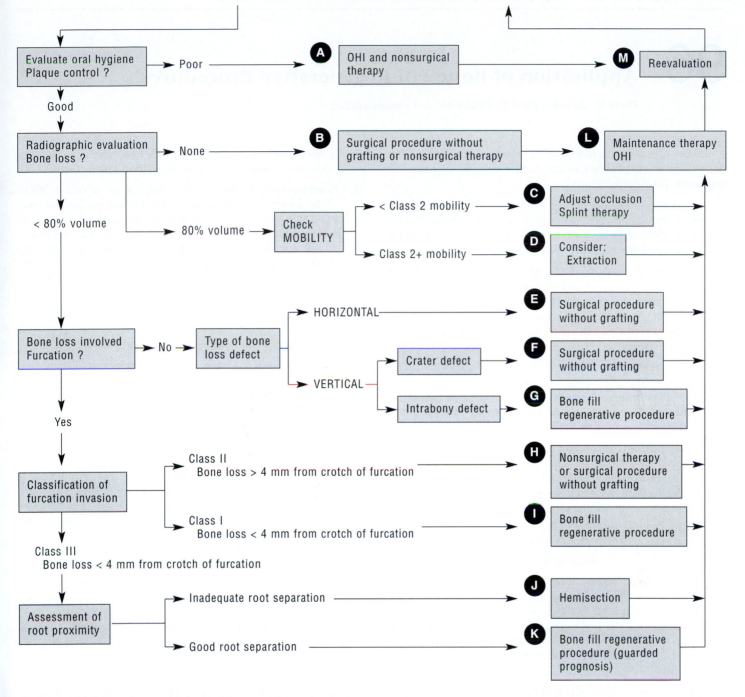

Patient with a 5 mm POCKET FOLLOWING PHASE I THERAPY

should be seen frequently (every 2 or 3 months) for maintenance scaling, polishing, and OHI during the first year after therapy. Thereafter, maintenance intervals can be adjusted according to the patient's varying ability to maintain good oral hygiene.

M   All patients, regardless of therapeutic modality, should be reevaluated annually. Using the same decision-making pathway, areas with 5 mm or greater pockets should be evaluated and treated appropriately.

Additional Readings

Gantes B, Martin M, Garrett S, et al. Treatment of periodontal furcation defects. II. Bone regeneration in mandibular class II defects. J Clin Periodontol 1988;15:232.

Garrett S, Bogle G. Periodontal regeneration with bone grafts. Curr Opin Periodontol 1994;168.

Hamp S, Nyman S, Lindhe J. Periodontal treatment of multirooted teeth: results after 5 years. J Clin Periodontol 1976;2:126.

Lekovic V, Kenney EB, Carranza FA, et al. Treatment of grade II furcation defects using porous hydroxylapatite in conjunction with a polytetrafluoroethylene membrane. J Periodontol 1990;61:575.

Levokvic V, Klokkevold P, Camargo P, et al. Evaluation of periosteal membranes and coronally positioned flaps in the treatment of class II furcation defects: a comparative clinical study in humans. J Periodontol 1998;69:1050.

Mellonig JT. Autogenous and allogenic bone grafts in periodontal therapy. Crit Rev Oral Biol Med 1992;3:333.

Pontoriero R, Lindhe J, Nyman S, et al. Guided tissue regeneration in the treatment of furcation defects in man. J Clin Periodontol 1987; 14:619.

96 Application of Bone Fill Regenerative Procedures

Paulo M. Camargo, Perry R. Klokkevold, and Vojislav Lekovic

A number of procedures have proven to be clinically successful in the treatment of intrabony defects with a bone fill-regeneration approach. They are as follows:

1. Extraoral autogenous bone graft: Sites such as the iliac crest, even though of high osteogenic potential, have limited application because of complexities involved in performing an additional surgical procedure outside the mouth.

2. Intraoral autogenous bone graft: This is the primary source of bone fill material. The main limitation of this technique is the amount of bone available to be used for donation. Areas that can be used as sources are retromolar regions, healed extraction sockets, and mandibular tori and exostoses.

3. Freeze-dried bone (FDB) and decalcified freeze-dried bone (DFDB) allografts: These are substitutes for autogenous bone that ensure sufficient volume of the graft material. Donor screening and graft processing make the risk of disease transmission essentially zero.

4. Xenografts: Bovine porous bone mineral (BPBM) is a graft material prepared by protein extraction of bovine bone that results in a trabecular structure of hydroxyapatite (HA) similar to human cancellous bone and that has the ability to enhance bone formation.

5. Synthetic bone substitutes: HA is the most popular example of this category. Although it facilitates bone formation, it is not predictable in stimulating new cementum formation.

6. Guided tissue regeneration (GTR): This technique uses either nonabsorbable membranes made of expanded polytetrafluoroethylene (ePTFE) or absorbable membranes made of polylactic acid, collagen, glycolide and lactide polymers, or calcium sulfate. GTR has been shown to result in true restoration of the periodontal unit including the formation of new cementum.

7. Growth factors: Recently, there has been interest in examining the role played by growth factors in periodontal regeneration. Most of these agents are still in their developmental and testing stages. Enamel matrix derivative (EMD) is a product that contains proteins derived from porcine enamel that have been shown to be important in the development of the dental organ including the formation of cementum, periodontal ligament (PDL), and aveolar bone. Of all growth factors being studied, EMD is the only one that is commercially available and has been shown to be effective in periodontal regenerative procedures. Autologous platelet-rich plasma (PRP) is a blood preparation that contains high concentrations of transforming growth factor-β (TGF-β) and platelet-derived growth factor (PDGF). TGF-β and PDGF have been shown to increase proliferation and differentiation of PDL cells in vitro. Since this opseparation is derived from the patient's own blood, it is available for current use. Although PRP has shown promise in promoting periodontal

regeneration, more clinical trials are necessary to confirm its effectiveness and substantiate its indications for use.

8. Combination techniques: The combination of two or more of the materials and techniques listed above has been shown to be at least as effective, and, in most instances, superior to any materials or techniques used alone. A general summary of the research done in regenerative procedures utilizing two or more materials and/or techniques indicates that the combination of a graft material with GTR and/or EMD will result in the most favorable postsurgical outcomes.

A The presence of a furcation invasion is based on exploring the furcation area on clinical examination with a curved (Nabers) periodontal probe and radiographic evaluation.

B An early Class II furcation can be treated by osseous resective surgery combined with apical displacement of the soft tissues. A moderate or advanced Class II furcation invasion can be treated with an intraoral autograft if enough material is available, with FDB or DFDB, with BPBM, or with HA. The combination of GTR with one of the osseous grafts described above has been shown to result in the most favorable postsurgical outcome, particularly with regard to bone fill.

C A Class III furcation invasion is difficult to resolve with bone fill regenerative procedures. Procedures employing bone grafts and GTR do not provide the clinician with predictable bone fill regeneration results in Class III furcation invasions. Consideration should be given to the creation of a tunnel, hemisection, root amputation, and tooth extraction.

D Shallow (< 2 mm) intrabony defects can be treated with osseous resection combined with apical positioning of the soft tissue. Resective therapy is indicated as long as it does not result in bone removal in furcation areas and it does not require excessive ostectomy resulting in tooth mobility.

E Bone fill regenerative therapy for deeper (> 3 mm) intrabony defects is dictated by the geometry of the lesion. As a general rule, success in bone fill regeneration procedures is directly related to the bone surface surrounding the defect and inversely proportional to the root surface present in the defect area. Also, narrow defects are more suitable to bone fill regenerative procedures than wide defects because graft retention is facilitated. The graft materials of choice are autografts, FDB/DFDB allografts, BPBM, or HA. Combining GTR with osseous grafts may not be as advantageous as it is in furcations, but may aid in graft retention in wider defects. EMD will also have its most efficacious results if combined with an osseous graft or with GTR plus an osseous graft.

F If an autograft site is available, compatibility and cost of the graft materials will be best. If not, allographic bone, xenograft bone, or an alloplast must suffice.

G Many resorbable materials are available for use in GTR. They include the following: polylactic acid, collagen, glycolide and lactide polymers, and calcium sulfate. The only

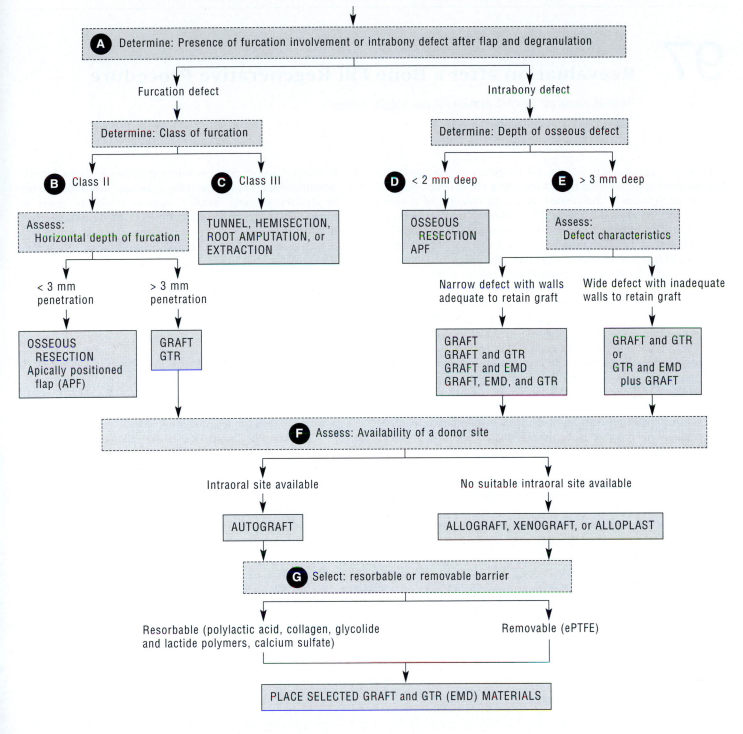

Patient with an OSSEOUS DEFECT and > 5 mm POCKET DEPTH AFTER INITIAL THERAPY

A Determine: Presence of furcation involvement or intrabony defect after flap and degranulation

Furcation defect

Intrabony defect

Determine: Class of furcation

Determine: Depth of osseous defect

B Class II

C Class III

D < 2 mm deep

E > 3 mm deep

Assess: Horizontal depth of furcation

TUNNEL, HEMISECTION, ROOT AMPUTATION, or EXTRACTION

OSSEOUS RESECTION APF

Assess: Defect characteristics

< 3 mm penetration

> 3 mm penetration

Narrow defect with walls adequate to retain graft

Wide defect with inadequate walls to retain graft

OSSEOUS RESECTION Apically positioned flap (APF)

GRAFT GTR

GRAFT
GRAFT and GTR
GRAFT and EMD
GRAFT, EMD, and GTR

GRAFT and GTR or GTR and EMD plus GRAFT

F Assess: Availability of a donor site

Intraoral site available

No suitable intraoral site available

AUTOGRAFT

ALLOGRAFT, XENOGRAFT, or ALLOPLAST

G Select: resorbable or removable barrier

Resorbable (polylactic acid, collagen, glycolide and lactide polymers, calcium sulfate)

Removable (ePTFE)

PLACE SELECTED GRAFT and GTR (EMD) MATERIALS

available removable membranes at this time are made of ePTFE. The practitioner must select the combination that experience indicates has the best success.

Additional Readings

Camargo PM, Lekovic V, Weinlaender M, et al. A controlled reentry study on the effectiveness of bovine porous bone mineral used in combination with a collagen membrane of porcine origin in the treatment of intrabony defects in humans. J Clin Periodontol 2000;27:889.

Lekovic V, Camargo PM, Weinlaender M, et al. The effectiveness of bovine porous bone mineral in combination with enamel matrix proteins or with an autologous fibrinogen/fibronectin system in the treatment of intrabony defects in humans: a reentry study of twenty-four cases. J Clin Periodontol 2001;72:1157–63.

Garrett S. Periodontal regeneration around natural teeth. In: Newman MG, editor. Annals of periodontology. Vol 1. Chicago: American Academy of Periodontology; 1996. p. 621.

Lekovic V, Camargo PM, Weinlaender M, et al. A comparison between enamel matrix proteins used alone or in combination with bovine porous bone mineral in the treatment of intrabony defects in humans. J Periodontol 2000;71:110.

Lekovic V, Camargo PM, Weinlaender M, et al. Combination use of bovine porous bone mineral, enamel matrix proteins, and a bioabsorbable membrane in intrabony periodontal defects in humans. J Periodontol 2001;72:583–9.

97 Reevaluation after a Bone Fill Regenerative Procedure

Paulo M. Camargo, Perry R. Klokkevold, and Vojislav Lekovic

Periodontal regeneration includes the following: regeneration of lost supporting periodontal tissues including bone, development of new cementum in the treated area, and creation of a new attachment periodontal ligament (PDL). *Bone fill* means the clinical restoration of bone tissue in the treated periodontal defect. Bone fill does not evaluate the presence or absence of histologic evidence of true periodontal regeneration; therefore, bone fill *can* be evaluated clinically and radiographically, whereas periodontal regeneration can be evaluated histologically only. At 12 months postsurgery, clinical pocket depths and attachment levels can be compared with original values to determine success. New radiographs, taken in as similar a manner as possible, can be compared with the presurgical ones as an additional measurement of "success." Depending upon these comparisons, a choice among maintenance, a resective surgical procedure, or a repeat bone fill guided tissue regeneration (GTR) procedure can be made.

A Clinical measurements and subjective evaluations and new radiographs must be made and compared with the presurgical data.

B If minimal pocket depths and other clinical findings and new radiographs indicate new bone filling the defect, the patient can be placed on regular maintenance (usually at 3- to 4-month intervals) for a year and then placed on a schedule based upon varying oral hygiene achievement levels over the long term.

C If residual pocket depth is detected and/or a residual defect remains visible on radiographs, a decision for maintenance or further surgery, usually osseous resection, must be made. If pockets are less than 4 mm in depth, maintenance is a justifiable choice. If pockets are greater than 5 mm in depth, osseous resection should be considered to improve the outcome.

D If residual pocket depths are little changed from the initial ones and/or radiographic evaluation shows little improvement, the practitioner should consider repeating the bone fill GTR procedure.

Additional Readings

Garrett S. Periodontal regeneration around natural teeth. In: Newman M, editor. Annals of periodontology. Vol 1. Chicago: American Academy of Periodontology; 1966. p. 621.

Lekovic V, Klokkevold P, Camargo P, et al. Evaluation of periosteal membranes and coronally positioned flaps in the treatment of Class II furcation defects: a comparative clinical study in humans. J Periodontol 1998;69:1050.

Poptoriero R, Lindhe J, Nyman S. Guided tissue regeneration in the treatment of furcation defects in man. J Clin Periodontol 1987;14:619.

Patient for REEVALUATION 1 YEAR AFTER A BONE FILL REGENERATION PROCEDURE

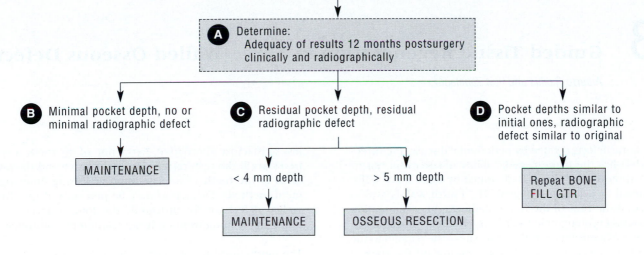

98 Guided Tissue Regeneration in Three-Walled Osseous Defects

Alberto Sicillia and Jon Zabelegui

Of all the bone defects created by periodontal disease, the three-walled defect has the highest predictability of successful regeneration. A three-walled defect is delimited by three bony walls: buccal, mesial or distal, and lingual. The fourth wall is always the surface of the root of the tooth. Radiographic examination and periodontal probing help to diagnose a three-walled defect; two different osseous levels at the same site—one parallel to the pattern to bone level and the other aiming toward the apex of the root—suggest a three-walled defect. Probings on a possible three-walled defect are shallow at the line angles and deep in the interproximal area under the contact.

A If the defect is shallow (1 or 2 mm deep) and wide, possible approaches include an apically positioned flap (APF) with osseous recontouring of the architecture or an open flap débridement.

B If the defect is deep and wide with deep surrounding vestibular depth, perform guided tissue regeneration (GTR). Choose the wraparound configuration that best covers the defect, overlapping 2 to 3 mm over the osseous walls. An autograft or allograft of autogenous bone is sometimes used. Denudation with secondary intention healing may be useful with narrow defects.

C If the defect is deep with shallow surrounding vestibular depth, perform GTR. Choose the wraparound configuration that best covers the defect, overlapping 2 to 3 mm over the osseous walls. An autograft or allograft of autogenous bone may be used so that the gingival tissue does not push the GTR membrane into the defect because this would not allow enough space for the regenerative tissue to form. Denudation with secondary intention healing is a less satisfactory alternative. Extraction of the tooth may be necessary if the restorative plan is extensive and the prognosis of the tooth cannot be improved using other treatment methods. Extraction may be necessary if the three-walled defect totally surrounds the four surfaces of the tooth and trauma from occlusion cannot be controlled.

The most critical factor in obtaining maximum results with GTR is the availability of good access for root débridement. The periodontal membrane used should not be allowed to collapse into the defect, and with this in mind the sutures and surrounding (hard and soft) tissues-to-membrane relationships must be managed. The flap should be elevated so that no tension occurs at the time of closure; either vertically releasing incisions or extending two teeth to each side of the treated area is recommended for this purpose.

Additional Readings

Becker W, Becker B, Berg L, Sansom O. Clinical and volumetric analysis of three-walled intrabony defects following open flap débridement. J Periodontol 1986;57:277.

Becker W, Becker B, Berg L, et al. New attachment after treatment with root isolation procedures: report for treated Class III and Class II furcations and vertical defects. Int J Periodontics Restorative Dent 1988;8:9.

Carranza FA, Newman MG. Clinical periodontology. 8th ed. Philadelphia: WB Saunders; 1996. p. 626.

Gottlow J, Nyman S, Karring T, Wennstrom J. New attachment formation in human periodontium by guided tissue regeneration. J Periodontol 1986;57:727.

Shallhorn RC, McClain PR. Combined osseous composite grafting, root conditioning and guided tissue regeneration. Int J Periodontics Restorative Dent 1988;8:9.

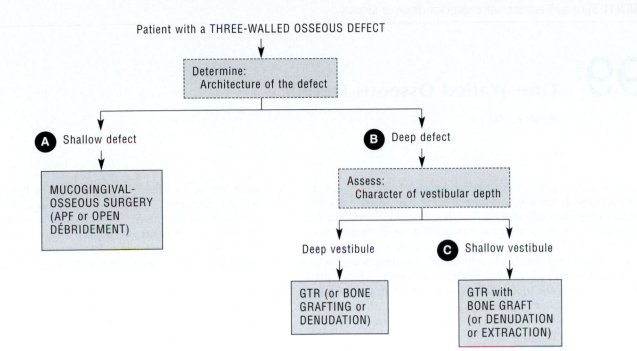

Patient with a THREE-WALLED OSSEOUS DEFECT

Determine:
Architecture of the defect

A Shallow defect

MUCOGINGIVAL-
OSSEOUS SURGERY
(APF or OPEN
DÉBRIDEMENT)

B Deep defect

Assess:
Character of vestibular depth

Deep vestibule

C Shallow vestibule

GTR (or BONE
GRAFTING or
DENUDATION)

GTR with
BONE GRAFT
(or DENUDATION
or EXTRACTION)

99 One-Walled Osseous Defect

Walter B. Hall

A one-walled osseous defect may be detected by careful probing and evaluation of radiographs. Radiographs alone are not sufficient to diagnose such defects, but in conjunction with careful probing they are helpful in conceptualizing them (Figures 99-1 and 99-2). The one osseous wall of such a defect always supports the adjacent tooth; therefore, the interproximal pocket depth on the affected tooth is several millimeters deeper than that on the adjacent tooth. Probing does not indicate less bone loss at the line angles of the affected tooth than it does interproximally (as is the case with a three-walled defect).

A   A tooth with a one-walled defect may be an essential tooth or it may not be important to a treatment plan for the patient. For example, canine teeth usually are essential to restorative treatment plans; therefore, guided tissue regeneration (GTR) should be employed to improve a canine tooth's support. A less important tooth such as a maxillary lateral incisor may be sacrificed if it is not important to the restorative plan; however, the use of extensive guided tissue procedures, if successful, may make extensive restorative plans unnecessary. The treatment plan that the dentist and patient agree on determines whether a tooth is essential and GTR should be employed.

B   After deciding that a tooth is not essential, the dentist should assess the risk to adjacent teeth in keeping the badly involved tooth. If good abutments on adjacent teeth are available, or the affected tooth may easily be replaced with a removable device, extraction of that tooth often is the best approach. A patient who has decided to retain the tooth should be made aware of the need for frequent planing and of the signs and symptoms of a periodontal abscess so that immediate dental treatment may be sought if they appear.

C   If the affected tooth jeopardizes adjacent teeth that are potentially good abutments, it should be extracted. If the adjacent teeth are themselves potentially poor abutments, GTR should be employed.

D   If the tooth with the one-walled osseous defect is an essential tooth (eg, a canine), the depth of the defect is important in deciding among treatment alternatives.

E   For essential teeth with shallow-to-moderate one-walled defects (ie, 1 mm from osseous crest to maximal depth), osseous resection on the adjacent tooth or teeth is a reasonable approach to eliminating the defect. The importance of the adjacent tooth may be such that removing any bone from its support creates a greater overall problem (eg, if the tooth is an abutment for an existing bridge). GTR should be employed.

F   If the one-walled defect on an essential tooth is a deep one (4 mm or more), GTR should be employed.

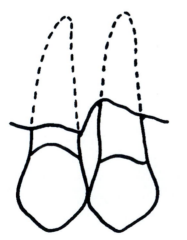

Figure 99-1 A hemiseptum in half of an interdental septum. The bone remaining against the adjacent, less-involved tooth constitutes the one remaining osseous wall.

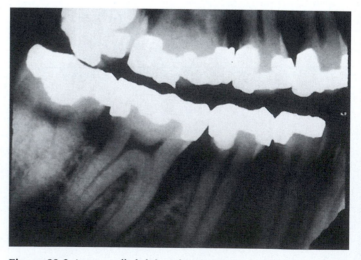

Figure 99-2 A one-walled defect (hemiseptum) on the mesial side of the first molar.

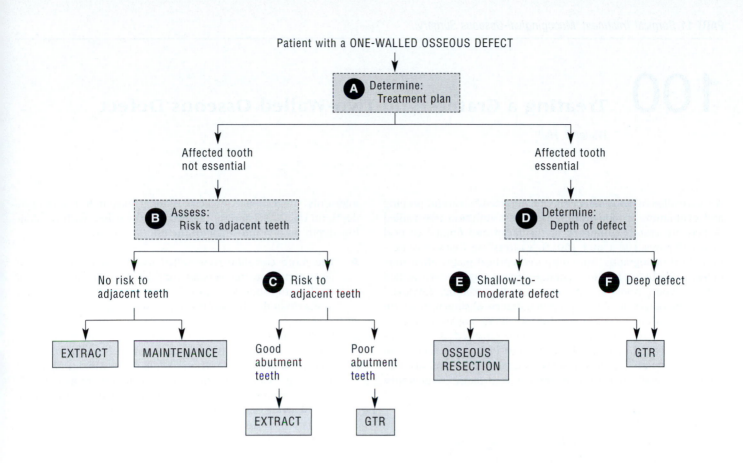

Patient with a ONE-WALLED OSSEOUS DEFECT

A Determine: Treatment plan

Affected tooth not essential

Affected tooth essential

B Assess: Risk to adjacent teeth

D Determine: Depth of defect

No risk to adjacent teeth

C Risk to adjacent teeth

E Shallow-to-moderate defect

F Deep defect

EXTRACT

MAINTENANCE

Good abutment teeth

Poor abutment teeth

OSSEOUS RESECTION

GTR

EXTRACT

GTR

Additional Readings

Genco RJ, Goldman HM, Cohen DW. Contemporary periodontics. St. Louis: Mosby; 1990. p. 569.

Heins PS. Osseous surgery: an evaluation after twenty-five years. Dent Clin North Am 1960;4:75.

Nevins M, Mellonig JT. Periodontal therapy: clinical approaches and evidence of success. Chicago: Quintessence Publishing; 1998. p. 255.

Ochsenbein C. Rationale for periodontal osseous surgery. Dent Clin North Am 1960;4:27.

Schluger S et al. Periodontal diseases. 2nd ed. Philadelphia: Lea & Febiger; 1990. p. 522.

100 Treating a Crater-Type Two-Walled Osseous Defect

Walter B. Hall

A two-walled osseous defect may be detected by careful probing and evaluation of radiographs. The most common two-walled defects are craters composed of the facial and lingual cortical plates (Figures 100-1 and 100-2). Craters are easily misinterpreted on radiographs. Superimposed cortical plates often hide defects. Slight angulation changes may suggest two-walled defects when none are present. Careful probing, however, allows the detection of interproximal defects of similar depth on adjacent teeth and shallow readings at all line angles in areas in which the cortical plates have not been resorbed. A less common two-walled defect is the noncrater type, occurring when one cortical plate has been resorbed but the other remains with an osseous wall against one of the adjacent teeth. Radiographs

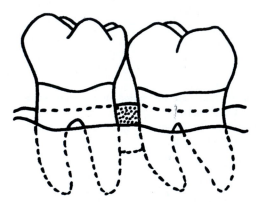

Figure 100-1 A crater is a two-walled infrabony defect in which facial and lingual cortical plates remain as the two osseous walls.

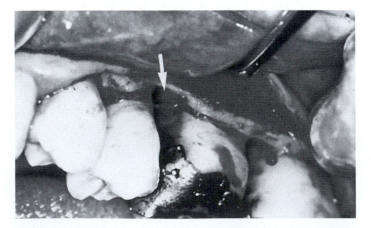

Figure 100-2 Two-walled infrabony defect (crater).

may only suggest such defects. Probing may detect a shallow depth on one tooth and more depth on the other, with no shallow depth on one line angle of the affected tooth.

A   The more common two-walled osseous defects in which both cortical plates remain may be divided into those of shallow-to-moderate depth (ie, 1–3 mm from osseous crest to maximal depth) and those that are deeper.

B   Shallow-to-moderate defects are readily eliminated by osseous resection with minimal removal of facial and lingual bone on adjacent teeth. This provides the advantage of ease of access for cleaning by the patient or dentist compared with alternative procedures, in which cleaning to the bottom of the pockets with oral hygiene devices is impossible, and instrumentation at the angles at which the cortical plates meet the floor of the defects is difficult or impossible to achieve.

C   Deep defects are not good candidates for osseous resection because too much facial and lingual bone must be sacrificed to achieve "positive" architecture. Uninvolved furcations in molar teeth may be treated using this process. Deep craters are amenable to guided tissue regeneration (GTR). If GTR is possible, and the patient is willing to undergo such surgery, it is a predictable means of building back lost attachment and minimizing or eliminating Class II furcation involvements. Successful GTR is the least expensive and most readily maintainable approach to managing the problems of deep craters.

D   GTR is not feasible in all deep crater situations. If the roots of the adjacent involved teeth are only 1 to 2 mm apart, a root proximity problem may make barrier design impossible because the "isthmus" portion will be too narrow to act as an effective epithelial barrier. A resorbable membrane can greatly improve prospects for regeneration in these cases. In such a case, extraction of the most badly involved tooth is a sound approach if good abutments remain or an implant is feasible. If either of the adjacent teeth has a Class III ("through and through") furcation involvement, extraction of the involved tooth is a good approach if satisfactory abutments remain or an implant is feasible. Alternatively, root resection may be employed, possibly with GTR, if poor abutments would remain if extraction were to be used. Maintenance of a "hopeless" situation may be a necessary last resort.

If the patient is unable or unwilling to proceed with these approaches, either one tooth may be extracted or the area may be maintained with a hopeless prognosis.

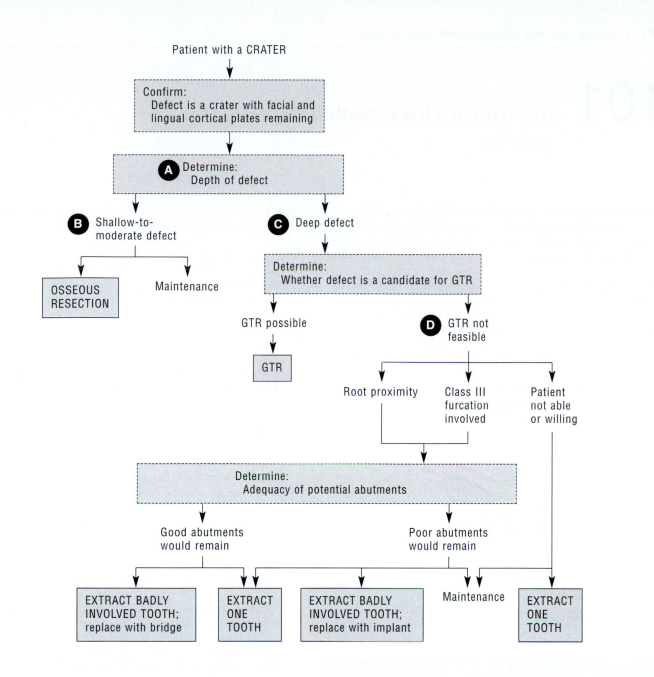

Additional Readings

Nevins M, Mellonig JT. Periodontal therapy: clinical approaches and evidence of success. Chicago: Quintessence Publishing; 1998. p. 178, 249.

Ochsenbein C, Bohannon HM. Palatal approach to osseous surgery. I. Rationale. J Periodontol 1960;34:60.

Ochsenbein C, Bohannon HM. Palatal approach to osseous surgery. II. Clinical application. J Periodontol 1961;35:54.

Schluger S et al. Periodontal diseases. 2nd ed. Philadelphia: Lea & Febiger; 1990. p. 513.

101 Treating a Three-Walled Osseous Defect

Walter B. Hall

A three-walled osseous defect is detected best by careful prob-ing; however, radiographs often are useful in suggesting the presence of such defects (Figures 101-1 and 101-2). An inter-proximal three-walled defect has a deep interproximal reading with shallow facial and lingual readings at line angles in which cortical plates remain intact. The interproximal depth on any adjacent teeth also is shallow. Palatal three-walled defects elicit a deep reading with shallower readings on both sides. If the palate is flat, the presence of a third wall palatally may be assumed. In other areas, "sounding" (probing to bone with anesthetic) may be necessary to detect a third wall situated away from the tooth. Despite their depth, many three-walled defects are amenable to regenerative procedures.

A Because such defects often occur on an endodontically involved tooth or a "cracked tooth," testing to ensure that these problems do not coexist is necessary before proceed-ing with periodontal treatment (see Chapter 35). If the tooth is endodontically involved, but does not have a long vertical crack, endodontics should be used and the peri-odontal status reassessed after an appropriate interval. If endodontics cannot be performed, extract the tooth. If a vertical crack is present and is extensive, the tooth should be extracted or maintained with a hopeless prognosis.

B Narrow defects—ones in which the crest of the bone is 1 mm or less from the tooth horizontally at the widest point of the coronal aspect of the defect—are treated with predictable success by complete débridement and readaptation of the flap to cover the defect. Such regenerative osseous proce-dures are among the most successful means of adding lost support to a tooth. Such surgery therefore is far preferable to attempts to maintain such areas in which curets cannot be placed or manipulated easily. Regenerative procedures in the case of narrow, three-walled defects (< 1 mm from tooth to crest of bone horizontally) have a very high predictability of successful regeneration with new attachment.

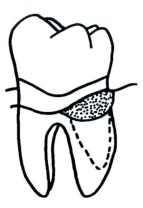

Figure 101-1 A wide, three-walled infrabony defect amenable to guided tissue regeneration.

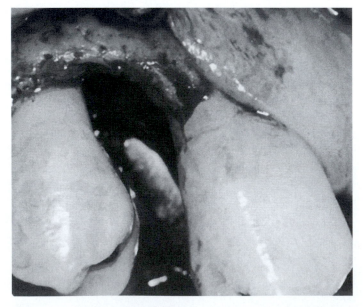

Figure 101-2 A three-walled infrabony defect mesial to the premolar.

C Shallow three-walled defects (ie, 1–2 mm deep) are amenable to osseous resection for pocket elimination. Some moderately deep, wide, three-walled defects (2–3 mm deep) may be treated by eliminating the wider three-walled portion by osseous resection and treating the deeper, narrow portion as a narrow defect in which new attachment is predictable.

D Wide, deep, three-walled osseous defects are excellent can-didates for guided tissue regeneration (GTR) (see Chapter 98). So strong is the likelihood of regeneration with new attachment that GTR always should be emphasized as the treatment of choice. Numerous three-walled defects on the distal of second molars have been treated through extrac-tion of an impacted or partially erupted third molar that lay close to the root of the second molar. These are among the most predictably successful situations in which to employ GTR. Similar defects on isolated abutment teeth may rou-tinely be treated with GTR. Palatal three-walled defects also have high predictability for successful restoration of support by GTR. Because this approach is highly predictable and inexpensive compared with alternatives such as mainte-nance and extraction and replacement with a bridge or implant, GTR should be employed routinely for treating deep, wide, three-walled defects.

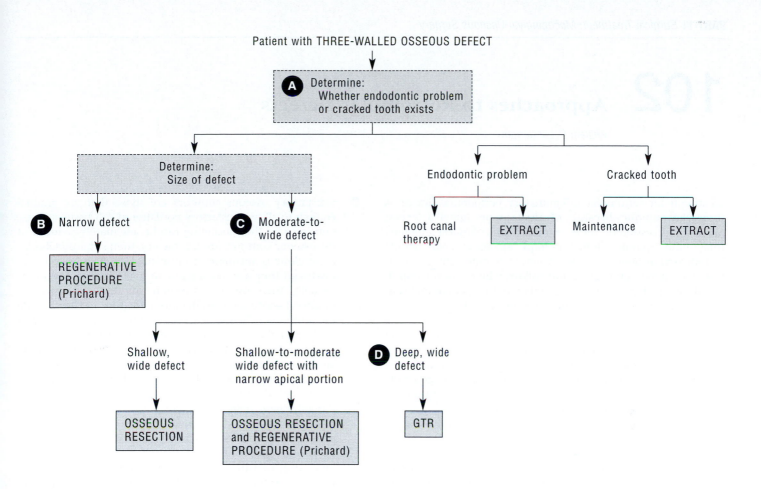

Patient with THREE-WALLED OSSEOUS DEFECT

A Determine: Whether endodontic problem or cracked tooth exists

Determine: Size of defect

B Narrow defect

C Moderate-to-wide defect

Endodontic problem

Cracked tooth

Root canal therapy

EXTRACT

Maintenance

EXTRACT

REGENERATIVE PROCEDURE (Prichard)

Shallow, wide defect

Shallow-to-moderate wide defect with narrow apical portion

D Deep, wide defect

OSSEOUS RESECTION

OSSEOUS RESECTION and REGENERATIVE PROCEDURE (Prichard)

GTR

Additional Readings

Becker W et al. New attachment after treatment with root isolation procedures: report for treated Class III and Class II furcations and vertical defects. Int J Periodontics Restorative Dent 1988;3:9.

Gottlow J et al. New attachment formation in human periodontics by guided tissue regeneration. J Periodontol 1986;57:727.

Lindhe J. Textbook of clinical periodontology. 2nd ed. Copenhagen: Munksgaard; 1989. p. 450.

Nevins M, Mellonig JT. Periodontal therapy: clinical approaches and evidence of success. Chicago: Quintessence Publishing; 1998. p. 174, 249.

Prichard JF. The infrabony technique as a predictable procedure. J Periodontol 1957;28:202.

Schallhorn RG, McClain PK. Combined osseous composite grafting, root conditioning and guided tissue regeneration. Int J Periodontics Restorative Dent 1988;8:9.

102 Approaches to Retromolar Defects

William P. Lundergan

Treatment for retromolar inflammatory periodontal disease is somewhat unique because of tissue type (gingiva versus mucosa), accessibility (often limited), and surgical anatomy (may limit options). Initial therapy for these areas should include oral hygiene instructions, closed débridement, and control of secondary etiologic factors followed by a reevaluation. If initial therapy fails to control the inflammatory periodontal condition, then surgical therapy must be considered.

A   Treatment planning for retromolar defects should consider the nature of the defect. Gingival defects (no bone loss or apical migration of the junctional epithelium) and suprabony defects (horizontal bone loss) are generally addressed differently from infrabony defects (vertical bone loss). Deeper infrabony defects (3–4 mm) may be treatable with regeneration techniques, whereas suprabony, shallow infrabony, and gingival defects generally are not.

B   The type of soft tissue can influence the treatment of retromolar defects. If the tissue is gingiva (often seen in maxilla), and the osseous contours are satisfactory, then a gingivectomy or a flap approach can be considered to allow improved access for débridement. If the tissue is mucosa (often seen in the mandible), then a flap approach is appropriate using a wedge procedure. The type of incision (linear incision versus "trolley" incision) for the flap will vary with the tissue type, difficulty of access, and goal of the procedure. Triangular incisions are preferable for the mandible and "trolley" incisions for the maxilla. Once surgical access is achieved, the bone contours should be evaluated.

C   Satisfactory osseous contours are those that are gradual enough to allow satisfactory postsurgical soft tissue adaptation in order that pocketing can be adequately reduced. If the osseous contours are satisfactory, then surgical débridement alone is adequate. If unsatisfactory osseous contours exist, and they are too shallow to make regeneration predictable, then osseous resection should be considered. Common anatomic considerations for the maxilla include the position of the maxillary sinus, the shape of the palatal vault, and the length of the tuberosity. These could limit access or the extent of osseous resection. Common limiting anatomic considerations for the mandible include the external oblique ridge and the anterior border of the ramus.

D   For infrabony defects that are deeper than 3 to 4 mm, regeneration should be considered as an alternative to débridement and osseous resection. Favorable conditions for regeneration can include patient factors (healthy, well motivated, nonsmoker), defect type (three-walled defect is most predictable), and lack of tooth mobility. Regeneration procedures can include the use of bone grafts, membranes, and growth factors (eg, Emdogain, bone morphogenetic proteins, platelet rich plasma)—singly or in combination. Generally, a linear distal incision is preferred when regeneration is attempted.

Additional Readings

Sato N. Periodontal surgery: a clinical atlas. Tokyo: Quintessence Publishing; 2000. p. 54–5.

Patient with a RETROMOLAR DEFECT IN NEED OF TREATMENT

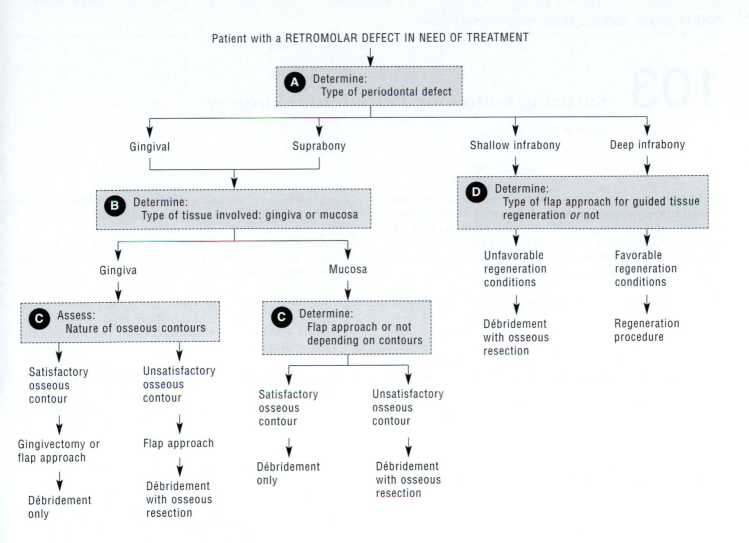

103 Suturing Following Periodontal Surgery

Walter B. Hall

Many innovative types of sutures may be used to close periodontal surgical wounds; however, here only a small number of suture techniques adequate for closing surgical sites are discussed. Mastery of these techniques permits the dentist to manage just about all contingencies. The type of suturing to be used depends on the surgery performed.

A   For pure mucogingival procedures such as connective tissue grafts and free gingival grafts, simple interrupted sutures usually are all that is required. Suturing in these cases usually is done using 4.0 or 5.0 gut or 5.0 Ethibond (braided Dacron-coated Teflon) suture material and a small, round, malleable needle such as the V5 needle by Ethicon.

B   For mucogingival-osseous surgery, a wider armamentarium of sutures is needed. Usually 4.0 black silk with a back-cutting needle is used here.

C   For guided tissue regeneration (GTR) procedures in which flaps are replaced in a more coronal position, simple inter-rupted sutures approximating facial and lingual flaps at each interdental papilla commonly are used.

D   For distal wedge or trapdoor procedures, surgical sites normally may be completely closed with one to several simple interrupted sutures.

E   Ridgeplasty procedures always involve the use of simple interrupted sutures. Occasionally, single-sling sutures around abutment teeth are used as well. Such sutures also may be used in extensive and posterior tooth procedures.

F   For apically positioned flap procedures in which only one to three teeth are included, single-sling sutures (Figure 103-1) are an excellent choice for use in approximating palatal or lingual flaps close to the teeth at the level of the crest of bone. On the facial flap, a single sling may be used as a suspensory suture; however, skillful architects of the osseous form often use no sutures on the facial flap. If a full sextant of teeth is treated by means of apically repositioned flaps, a continuous-sling suture (see Figure 103-1) is the best choice to adapt palatal and lingual flaps close to the teeth. If the tissue is thin or needs to be stretched to gain full closure, a mattress type of continuous-sling suture may be necessary. In routine cases a simple continuous sling suffices. The facial flap may be suspended with a single-sling suture or, if well adapted, no sutures are needed.

G   When vertically releasing incisions are used to permit adequate reflection or positioning of a flap, simple interrupted sutures are used to approximate the flap in its new position in relation to adjacent tissue.

Additional Readings

Dahlberg. WH. Incisions and suturing: some basic considerations about each in periodontal flap surgery. Dent Clin North Am 1969;13:149.

Lindhe. Textbook of clinical periodontology. 2nd ed. Copenhagen: Munksgaard; 1989. p. 416.

Newman MG, Takei HH, Carranza FA Jr. Carranza's clinical periodontology. 9th ed. Philadelphia: WB Saunders; 2002. p. 767–93.

Schluger S et al. Periodontal diseases. 2nd ed. Philadelphia: Lea & Febiger; 1990. p. 479.

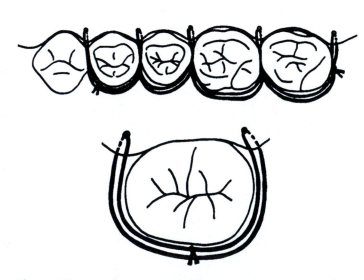

Figure 103-1 Continuous or single-sling sutures may be used to close posterior areas of mucogingival-osseous surgery.

Patient for SUTURING FOLLOWING PERIODONTAL SURGERY

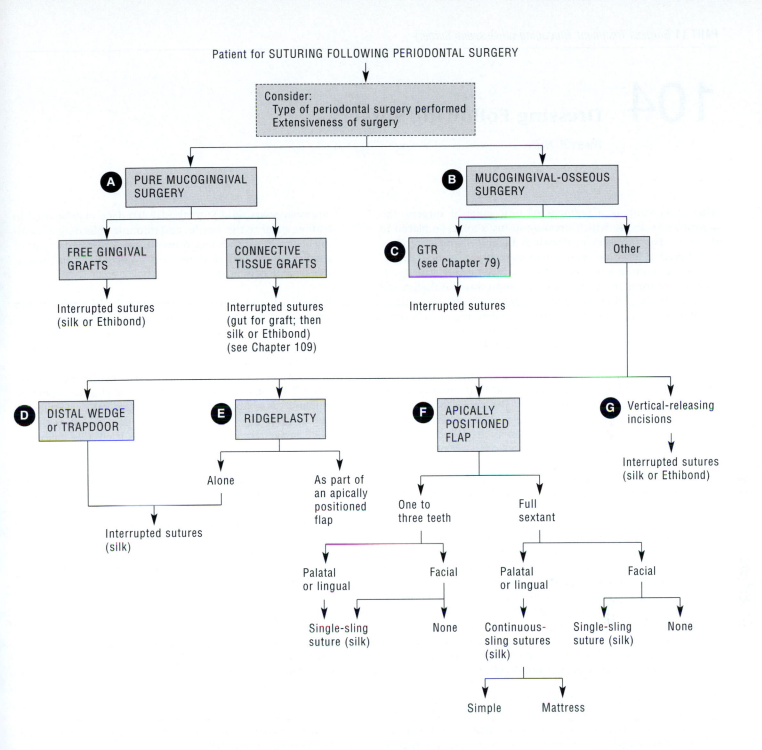

Consider:
  Type of periodontal surgery performed
  Extensiveness of surgery

A PURE MUCOGINGIVAL SURGERY

B MUCOGINGIVAL-OSSEOUS SURGERY

FREE GINGIVAL GRAFTS

CONNECTIVE TISSUE GRAFTS

C GTR (see Chapter 79)

Other

Interrupted sutures (silk or Ethibond)

Interrupted sutures (gut for graft; then silk or Ethibond) (see Chapter 109)

Interrupted sutures

D DISTAL WEDGE or TRAPDOOR

E RIDGEPLASTY

F APICALLY POSITIONED FLAP

G Vertical-releasing incisions

Interrupted sutures (silk or Ethibond)

Alone

As part of an apically positioned flap

One to three teeth

Full sextant

Interrupted sutures (silk)

Palatal or lingual

Facial

Palatal or lingual

Facial

Single-sling suture (silk)

None

Continuous-sling sutures (silk)

Single-sling suture (silk)

None

Simple

Mattress

104 Dressing Following Surgery

Walter B. Hall

After completion of a segment of mucogingival surgery, the dentist must decide which dressing if any should be placed in the area. The purposes of dressings include better control of postoperative bleeding, better patient comfort during eating, and stabilization of loose teeth during early healing. The disadvantages of using dressings include compromised esthetics and delay in healing after the first few postoperative days. Great variability in determining the need for a dressing and choosing the appropriate one exists. The following are conservative guidelines that should work well for most dentists.

A Anterior segments of mucogingival-osseous surgery may present esthetic problems that should be considered in the decision to dress the wound and the choice of dressings. This is especially true in the maxillary anterior region. Because these areas lend themselves to full closure and suturing, not placing a dressing is a reasonable option. Placing a Stomahesive bandage that dissolves in 8 to 24 hours (depending on the activity of the tongue against it) minimizes early postoperative bleeding and further stabilizes the flaps. It is simple to place, requiring only a minute or two.

B Mandibular anterior segments usually do not present esthetic problems, but the mandibular incisors often are quite mobile and have considerable bone loss; therefore, Coe Pak or another nondissolvable "pack" often is a good choice. If a mandibular anterior segment of mucogingival-osseous surgery may be completely closed with sutures and the teeth have little mobility, Stomahesive bandage or even no dressing may be sufficient; however, if closure is incomplete (leaving exposed areas) or mobility is significant, Coe Pak or an alternative pack is preferable.

C In posterior segments of mucogingival-osseous surgery, the objectives of surgery and the scope of the area to be treated vary more. Tuberosity or retromolar pad surgery may be the only surgery to be performed in a posterior region. Good closure of the flaps is attainable in these distal ridge procedures if the procedure is done alone. A dressing may

be unnecessary, or a Stomahesive bandage may be used to further stabilize the wound and minimize bleeding as healing begins. If a distal ridge procedure is performed as part of surgery on adjacent posterior teeth, Coe Pak or an alternative pack usually is used.

D Ridgeplasty and crown lengthening may be performed in any part of the mouth, but they are performed more frequently as isolated procedures in posterior segments. In anterior segments, they usually are dressed with Stomahesive bandage. In posterior segments, if good closure of the flaps may be attained with sutures a Stomahesive bandage or no dressing at all works well. If good closure cannot be obtained (as under existing bridges), Coe Pak or an alternative is preferable. If adjacent areas are treated with the ridgeplasty areas or if gingivectomy is used, Coe Pak or an alternative is preferred.

E In posterior segments, if the closure is incomplete, especially between molar teeth, Coe Pak or an alternative is preferred to control bleeding and stabilize the flaps. If pocket-elimination surgery (apically positioned flap, gingivectomy) is used in posterior segments, Coe Pak or an alternative is preferred to minimize bleeding, help stabilize teeth, minimize initial sensitivity to temperature change, and improve comfort in eating.

Additional Readings

Carranza FA Jr, Newman MG. Clinical periodontology. 8th ed. Philadelphia: WB Saunders; 1996. p. 571.

Grant DA, Stern IB, Listgarten MA. Periodontics. 6th ed. St. Louis: Mosby; 1988. p. 731.

Hall WB. Pure mucogingival problems. Berlin: Quintessence Publishing; 1984. p. 107.

Lindhe J. Textbook of clinical periodontology. 2nd ed. Copenhagen: Munksgaard; 1989. p. 418.

O'Neil TCA. Antibacterial properties of periodontal dressings. J Periodontol 1975;46:469.

Patient with COMPLETED SEGMENT OF MUCOGINGIVAL-OSSEOUS SURGERY

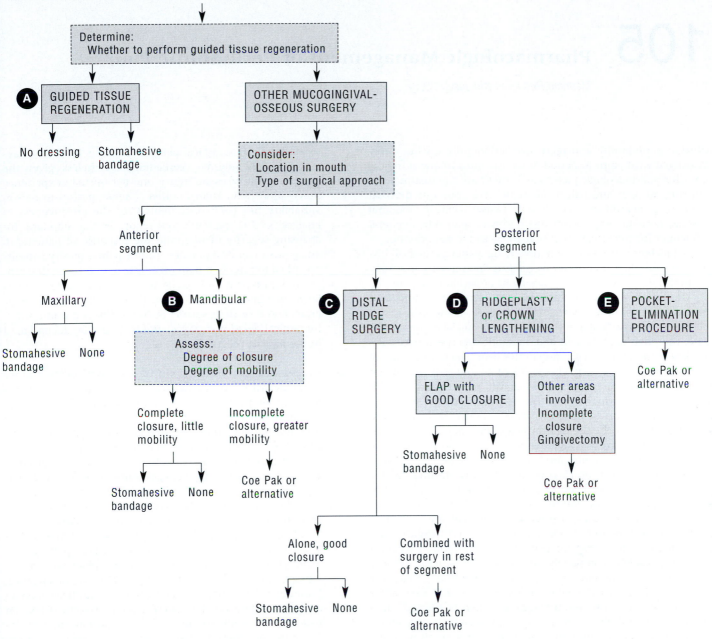

105 Pharmacologic Management of Periodontic Pain

Mauricio Ronderos and Joseph Levy

Chronic periodontitis and aggressive periodontitis are but rarely associated with pain. In periodontics, the most frequent indications for pharmacologic pain management are the treatment of postsurgical pain and pain from acute periodontal or mucosal lesions (eg, necrotizing periodontal diseases, acute periodontal abscess, herpetic gingivostomatitis). This chapter offers general guidelines for the selection of oral analgesics in periodontics.

Clinicians should carefully review the patient's medical history to assess contraindications or drug interactions that may influence the protocol for management of periodontic pain.

In managing pain associated with acute periodontal or mucosal lesions, begin by treating the cause. If the pain is secondary to a periodontal abscess or necrotizing periodontal disease, thorough débridement and antibiotic therapy, if necessary, are key to the prompt resolution of this pain. The frequent use of topical anesthetics (eg, 2% viscous lidocaine solution), in addition to oral analgesics, may give additional pain relief to patients with aphthae, herpetic gingivostomatitis, or other ulcerative lesions.

It is important to prevent inflammation and to minimize postsurgical pain. The use of atraumatic surgical techniques that are minimally invasive, together with local cold packs or ice during the first 24 hours after surgery, is helpful to prevent inflammation. Short-term use of steroid drugs, starting the day prior to surgery, may keep to a minimum inflammation after large autogenous bone grafting or other extensive surgical procedures. Local measures to protect the surgical site, including surgical dressings and stents, minimize the postsurgical pain from gingivectomies, soft-tissue grafting, or procedures where it was not possible to completely close a flap. It is easier to prevent pain than to eliminate it after onset. Therefore, analgesics should be prescribed at fixed intervals (eg, every 6 hours) rather than at patient-controlled intervals (ie, taken as needed). It is useful to administer a long-acting local anesthetic (eg, etidocaine), immediately after the completion of a surgical procedure, for the control of pain while adequate blood levels of a systemic analgesic are obtained.

A This decision-making protocol is founded on the concept that clinicians should be conservative in their initial selection of analgesics. Based on an assessment of pain severity or invasiveness of the procedure performed, together with the patient's medical history, clinicians will select a pain management protocol and escalate to higher dosages or more powerful drugs if required (see Algorithm). As healing advances and pain subsides the clinician should consider safer medications.

Most patients report negligible or mild pain for 24 hours after nonsurgical procedures that include scaling and root planing. The pain associated with acute periodontal lesions and periodontal surgical procedures, including osseous surgery, mucogingival surgery, guided tissue regeneration, small bone grafts, and implant placement, is generally mild

to moderate. Postsurgical pain usually lasts for 3 to 4 days and gradually subsides thereafter. Nevertheless, given the same amount of tissue injury one person may experience much more pain than another. Similar person-to-person variability has been documented for the effectiveness of analgesics. The patient's self-report is the standard for assessing severity of pain and the response of patients to analgesics in clinical practice. To rate pain intensity patients are asked to rate their pain on a scale of 0 to 10 (with 0 representing no pain and 10 the worst possible pain). Ratings between 1 and 3 are considered as mild pain, 4 to 7 as moderate, and 8 to 10 as severe. Such information is important for clinical decision-making, and it should be documented in the patient record.

B Unless contraindicated, nonsteroidal anti-inflammatory drugs (NSAIDs) are the medications of choice for the management of pain that is mild to moderate. By blocking prostaglandin synthesis, these medications reduce pain and minimize inflammation. NSAIDs also inhibit platelet aggregation and, in high dosages, may increase the risk for postoperative bleeding. These medications should be avoided in patients with recent history of gastrointestinal disease (bleeding or ulcers) or those receiving anticoagulants, and they should be used with caution after surgical procedures where there is a significant risk of postoperative bleeding (eg, freestanding soft-tissue grafts). The potency of NSAIDs is frequently underestimated. These drugs have been proven to be as effective as a combination of weak opioids and acetaminophen in the management of pain after minor surgeries. Furthermore, NSAIDs have fewer undesirable effects than do analgesics acting on the central nervous system (CNS). In patients with a mild to moderate risk of postoperative bleeding or treated gastrointestinal ulcers, cyclooxygenase-2 (Cox-2) inhibitors, a new class of NSAIDs, should be preferred over other NSAIDs. By selectively inhibiting the action of Cox-2, these medications reduce pain and inflammation with minimum effect on platelet function and minimum risk for postoperative or gastrointestinal bleeding.

C The management of mild-to-moderate pain in patients where all NSAIDs are contraindicated starts by subdividing them into those who report or are expected to have mild pain and those with moderate pain. For the management of pain after nonsurgical therapy and after minor surgical procedures, acetaminophen is the drug of choice. Acetaminophen does not affect platelet aggregation. However, the analgesic effect of acetaminophen is not as potent as that of NSAIDs, and it does not have anti-inflammatory properties. For the management of moderate pain, the combination of acetaminophen and centrally acting analgesics (eg, codeine, tramadol) is recommended.

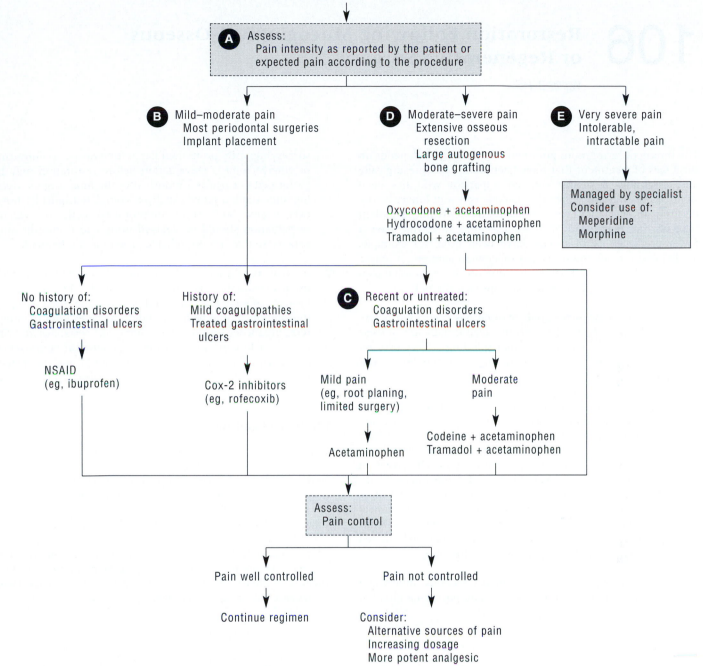

Patient requiring PHARMACOLOGIC MANAGEMENT OF PERIODONTAL PAIN

A Assess:
Pain intensity as reported by the patient or expected pain according to the procedure

B Mild–moderate pain
Most periodontal surgeries
Implant placement

D Moderate–severe pain
Extensive osseous resection
Large autogenous bone grafting

Oxycodone + acetaminophen
Hydrocodone + acetaminophen
Tramadol + acetaminophen

E Very severe pain
Intolerable, intractable pain

Managed by specialist
Consider use of:
Meperidine
Morphine

No history of:
Coagulation disorders
Gastrointestinal ulcers

NSAID
(eg, ibuprofen)

History of:
Mild coagulopathies
Treated gastrointestinal ulcers

Cox-2 inhibitors
(eg, rofecoxib)

C Recent or untreated:
Coagulation disorders
Gastrointestinal ulcers

Mild pain
(eg, root planing, limited surgery)

Moderate pain

Acetaminophen

Codeine + acetaminophen
Tramadol + acetaminophen

Assess:
Pain control

Pain well controlled

Continue regimen

Pain not controlled

Consider:
Alternative sources of pain
Increasing dosage
More potent analgesic

D Centrally acting drugs should only be used after surgical procedures in which very extensive osseous resection is performed or when peripherally acting analgesics have failed. The addition of NSAIDs or acetaminophen to an opioid reduces the needed dosage of the opioid, thus reducing its possible side effects (eg, respiratory depression, constipation). Tolerance and dependence are rare when mild opioids are used for short periods. Tramadol is a centrally acting non-narcotic synthetic opioid analgesic that is as potent as many other oral opioids; tramadol has minimum cardiovascular side effects, does not result in respiratory depression, and minimizes the risk of dependency. This analgesic is generally well tolerated and has relatively mild side effects, that include nausea and dizziness.

E Periodontal pathologies and surgical procedures rarely result in pain that is intolerable. If despite adequate dosages of analgesics the pain cannot be controlled, the presence of some additional pathology should be considered (eg, pain of endodontic origin, neuropathic pain). General dentists should refer such cases to a specialist who will evaluate the source of pain and may prescribe higher dosages of medications or short courses of strong opioids (eg, meperidine). Such patients should be closely monitored.

106 Restoration Following Mucogingival-Osseous or Regenerative Surgery

Walter B. Hall

The timing of restorations after periodontal surgery depends on the types of treatment that have been done both presurgically and surgically. A dentist treating a patient who has been splinted presurgically generally speaking can wait longer before deciding on permanent restorations than one treating a patient who has not been splinted. If surgical procedures that have a lower predictability of success have been used, for example, guided tissue regeneration (GTR) or new attachment, a longer time should be allowed before deciding on the restorative plan than is allowed if a more definitive approach is employed.

A　If temporary or provisional splinting has been used before periodontal surgery, the teeth involved usually are so loose that the dentist has decided that splinting is necessary for comfort and function during the surgical period. Provisional splinting is done for as long as 2 years in cases that ultimately require extensive reconstruction and in which some of the teeth have guarded prognoses. Temporary splinting often is extracoronal (requiring a night guard or wire and composite splint); in these cases, restorative decisions may be made 3 months or more after the final surgery unless a new attachment or bone regeneration approach is used, in which case a 6-month wait is indicated. If intracoronal temporary or provisional splinting is used, a minimal waiting period of 6 months after surgery before reevaluation is necessary. If the provisionally splinted case is extensive, a waiting period as long as 2 years after surgery may be indicated before reevaluation and permanent restoration.

B　If a patient who has had mucogingival-osseous surgery and has not required splinting also has had pocket-elimination surgery (apically positioned flap with osseous recontouring or gingivectomy), reevaluation before restoration may be performed as early as 1 month after the final surgery. Healing after such surgery usually is completed quickly; however, if any significantly compromised teeth are evident, reevaluation should be delayed until 3 to 6 months after surgery so that a more reliable prognosis can be made.

C　If a new attachment procedure or GTR procedure has been used, reevaluation before restoration should not be performed sooner than 6 months after the final surgery. Restoration should be delayed in these cases until the long-term prognoses for these teeth are clearly established. With new attachment and osseous regeneration approaches, extensive, expensive restorations should not be placed unless the teeth have a reasonable prognosis 6 months after surgery.

Additional Readings

Carranza FA Jr, Newman MG. Clinical periodontology. 8th ed. Philadelphia: WB Saunders; 1996. p. 710.

Nyman S, Lindhe J. A longitudinal study of combined periodontal and prosthetic treatment of patients with advanced periodontal disease. J Periodontol 1979;50:163.

Schluger S et al. Periodontal diseases. 2nd ed. Philadelphia: Lea & Febiger; 1990. p. 612.

Seibert JS, Cohen DW. Periodontal considerations in preparation for fixed and removable prosthodontics. Dent Clin North Am 1987;31:529.

Wilson TG, Kornman KS. Fundamentals of periodontics. Chicago: Quintessence Publishing; 1996. p. 469.

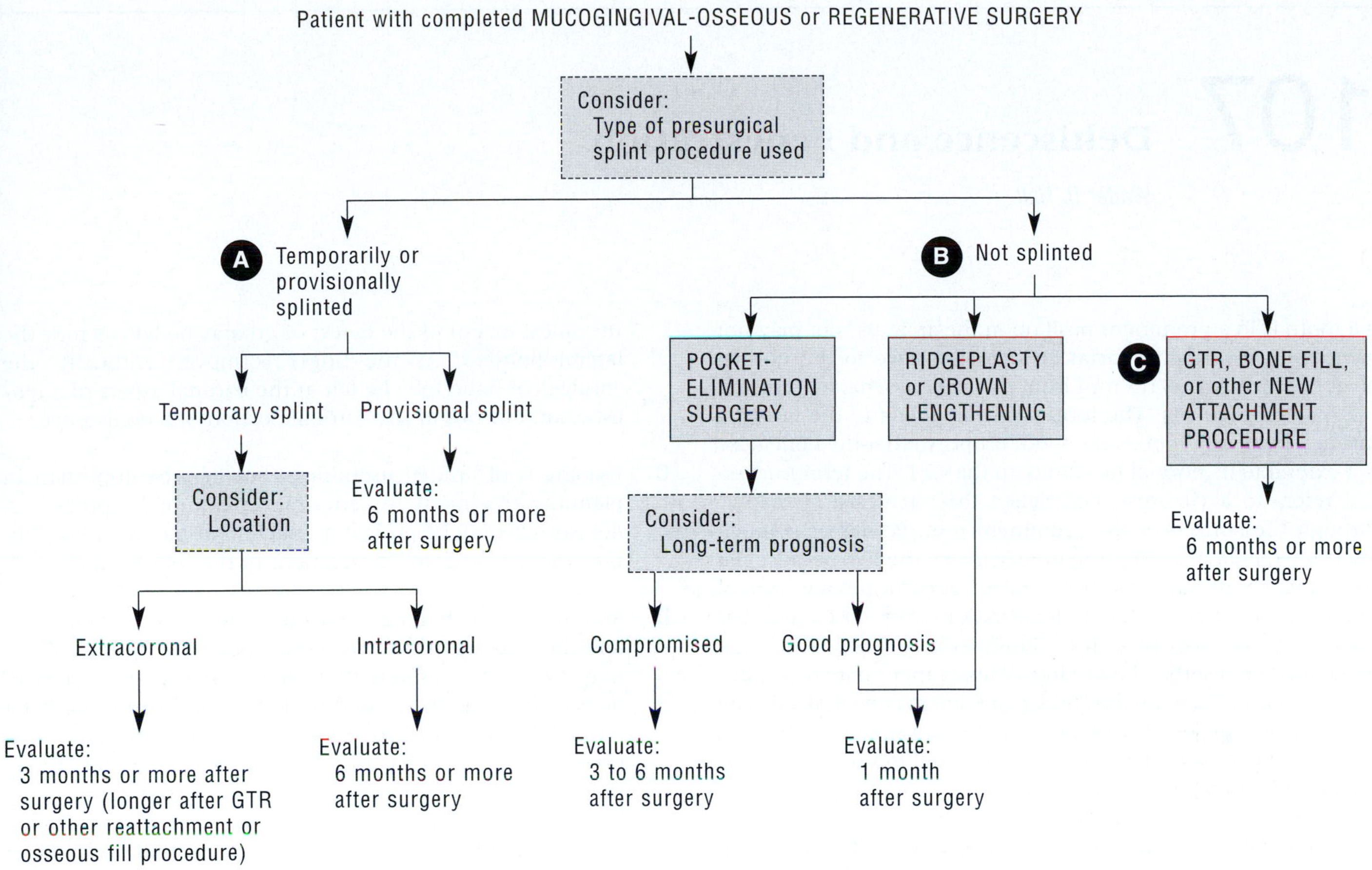

Patient with completed MUCOGINGIVAL-OSSEOUS or REGENERATIVE SURGERY

Consider:
Type of presurgical
splint procedure used

A Temporarily or
provisionally
splinted

B Not splinted

Temporary splint

Provisional splint

POCKET-
ELIMINATION
SURGERY

RIDGEPLASTY
or CROWN
LENGTHENING

C GTR, BONE FILL,
or other NEW
ATTACHMENT
PROCEDURE

Consider:
Location

Evaluate:
6 months or more
after surgery

Consider:
Long-term prognosis

Evaluate:
6 months or more
after surgery

Extracoronal

Intracoronal

Compromised

Good prognosis

Evaluate:
3 months or more after
surgery (longer after GTR
or other reattachment or
osseous fill procedure)

Evaluate:
6 months or more
after surgery

Evaluate:
3 to 6 months
after surgery

Evaluate:
1 month
after surgery

107 Dehiscence and Fenestration

Walter B. Hall

If a tooth is in a prominent position in the arch, its root may not have bone covering its facial or lingual surface to the normal height, which is 1 to 1.5 mm from the cementoenamel junction (CEJ) (Figure 107-1). The term *dehiscence* refers to the bursting through of bone of a root as the tooth erupts so that the bone does not extend to its normal proximity to the CEJ. The term *fenestration* refers to a circumscribed defect that creates a "window" through the bone over the prominent root. Perhaps too much effort is expended in differentiating between the two because the consequences of having a thin "bridge" of cortical bone coronal to the circumscribed defect (a fenestration) and not having that bone (a dehiscence) is of little clinical consequence. True, that bone must be resorbed before loss of attachment may occur, but the ease with which the thin bridge of bone may be destroyed by inflammation makes its existence of little consequence. Various tests may be used to determine which condition is present and the possible therapeutic implications.

A Radiographs are not useful in detecting or differentiating between these two bone defects. Because the defect overlies the root in the radiograph, it cannot be seen on typical films.

B The simplest test, but one that requires considerable experience, is to run a finger over the prominent root in apicocoronal and mesiodistal directions. The crest of the bone at the apical extent of the defect often may be felt, as may the lateral borders. As the finger is moved coronally, the "bridge" of bone may be felt at the coronal aspect of a fenestration but not in the coronal portion of a dehiscence.

C Probing is of limited usefulness, but may be important in planning treatment. A fenestration cannot be probed. A dehiscence may be probed if attachment has been lost, but it cannot be probed if attachment to the root is intact.

D Sounding, which means pushing the probe through the anesthetized soft tissue over the root (see Figure 107-1), may be used to differentiate between the two types of defects. If an apparent fenestration or dehiscence has been located digitally, the probe is positioned over the defect and pressed into contact with the tooth. The sensation transmitted to the dentist on touching the tooth rather than bone is a "quick," "sharp," or "solid" one, whereas bone gives a mushy or softer sensation. If the sensation is one of touching the tooth, the probe is moved halfway to the free margin and is pressed through the soft tissue. If bone is touched, the defect is a fenestration; if not, it probably will prove to be a dehiscence.

E The clinical importance of these determinations relates to the consequences of raising a flap or preparing a receptor bed for a gingival graft. If the defect is a fenestration, soft tissue is capable of "reattaching" to the exposed surface with high predictability. If the defect is a dehiscence, reattachment to the level of the most apical aspect of the pocket or crevice depth also is likely to be successful. If the root has been exposed by inflammatory periodontal disease, only a new attachment may occur where attachment has been lost.

Additional Readings

Elliott JR, Bowers GM. Alveolar dehiscence and fenestration. Periodontics 1963;1:245.

Gartrell JR, Mathews DP. Gingival recession: the condition, process and treatment. Dent Clin North Am 1976;20:199.

Hall WB. Present status of soft-tissue grafting. J Periodontol 1977;48:587.

Hall WB. Pure mucogingival problems. Berlin: Quintessence Publishing; 1984. p. 36.

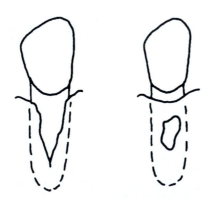

Figure 107-1 A dehiscence is a bursting through of bone of the tooth root, whereas a fenestration is a window in the bone.

Patient's tooth with a PROMINENT ROOT AND SOME MISSING BONE OVER IT

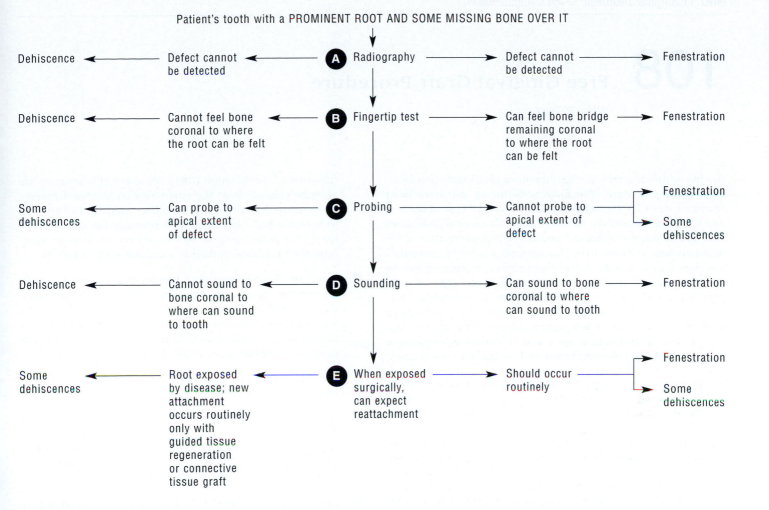

Dehiscence ← Defect cannot be detected ← **A** Radiography → Defect cannot be detected → Fenestration

Dehiscence ← Cannot feel bone coronal to where the root can be felt ← **B** Fingertip test → Can feel bone bridge remaining coronal to where the root can be felt → Fenestration

Some dehiscences ← Can probe to apical extent of defect ← **C** Probing → Cannot probe to apical extent of defect → Fenestration / Some dehiscences

Dehiscence ← Cannot sound to bone coronal to where can sound to tooth ← **D** Sounding → Can sound to bone coronal to where can sound to tooth → Fenestration

Some dehiscences ← Root exposed by disease; new attachment occurs routinely only with guided tissue regeneration or connective tissue graft ← **E** When exposed surgically, can expect reattachment → Should occur routinely → Fenestration / Some dehiscences

108 Free Gingival Graft Procedure

Walter B. Hall

The free gingival graft is perhaps the most predictable periodontal surgical procedure. The indications for its use have been described (see Chapters 44 and 45). The relative ease of mastering this technique and the mystique of plastic surgical procedures have led to more widespread use of the procedure than some clinicians believe is merited. This surgical procedure, nevertheless, has many important uses: to prevent or control loss of attachment (LOA) resulting from recession, to prevent or control esthetic problems, and to permit restorative or orthodontic treatment without iatrogenic root exposure (LOA). If a patient has a problem of minimal attached gingiva, with or without recession, and the dentist and patient agree that treatment is indicated, a series of decisions is needed before proceeding with this surgery.

A Whether root coverage is a goal determines the way the receptor site is prepared. If root exposure has not occurred, the technique is performed one way. If root exposure has occurred, root coverage may become the goal if there are esthetic or restorative indications. Both a connective tissue graft (see Chapter 109) and guided tissue regeneration (see Chapter 88) are better means of successfully covering exposed roots, but some minimal recession may be managed with a free gingival graft. Most often these indications are present in maxillary anterior and maxillary premolar areas. Some teeth need more attached gingiva, whereas adjacent teeth may require root coverage. Modify the surgical procedure to meet these individual needs.

B If root coverage is to be attempted, remove all sulcus epithelium and skim the superficial epithelium and connective tissue from adjacent papillae to the level of the

cementoenamel junction (CEJ). More apically, separate the alveolar mucosa from the gingiva by an incision immediately coronal to the CEJ and reflect apically to expose a 5- to 6-mm bed. Should the root coverage fail, an adequate band of attached gingiva will have been created to minimize the likelihood of further recession (Figure 108-1).

C If root coverage is not a goal, prepare the receptor bed with an incision slightly coronal to the mucogingival junction. Expose a bed 5 to 6 mm in height by reflecting the alveolar mucosa with a periosteal elevator. Make a periosteal fenestration at the apical extent of the bed to ensure that the graft is not mobile (Figure 108-2).

D A combination approach may be indicated if only a singular tooth with a segment to be grafted requires root coverage.

E If root coverage is to be performed, reduce the prominent root with a back-action chisel so that hemorrhage does not pool peripherally. Reduce the root to keep the dentin free of bacteria and endotoxin. The reduced dimension of the root makes new attachment more likely to occur.

F After the graft is taken, if root coverage is the goal, suture the graft, stretching tightly between the de-epitheliated papillae with interrupted or single-sling sutures. If root coverage is not going to be attempted, use single, interrupted sutures in the area of each papilla to stabilize the graft.

G After the graft is placed, apply pressure with wet gauze for 3 to 4 minutes, place a Stomahesive bandage, and instruct on ways to avoid disturbing the graft.

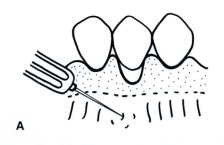
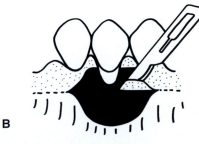
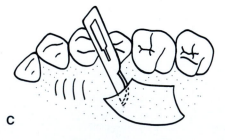
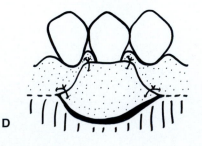
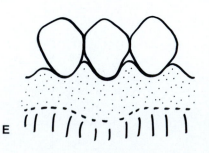

Figure 108-1 *A,* Obtaining anesthesia in an area in which a free gingival graft is used with root coverage as a goal. *B,* Preparation of the receptor site. *C,* Obtaining donor tissue from the palate. *D,* Free gingival graft sutured with root coverage as the goal. *E,* Healed free gingival graft for root coverage.

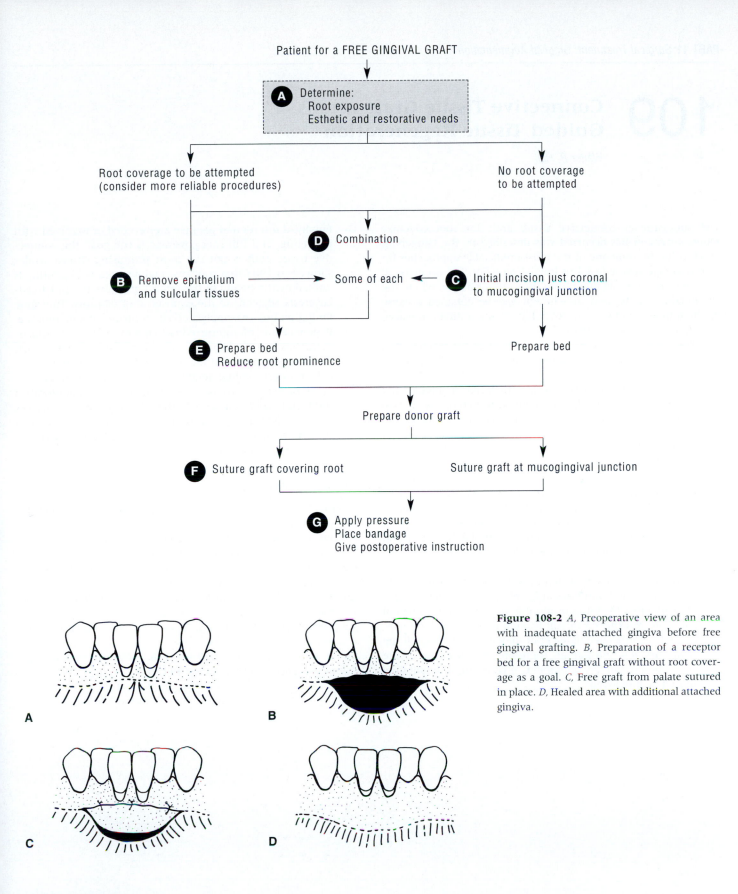

Patient for a FREE GINGIVAL GRAFT

A Determine:
Root exposure
Esthetic and restorative needs

Root coverage to be attempted
(consider more reliable procedures)

No root coverage
to be attempted

D Combination

B Remove epithelium
and sulcular tissues → Some of each ← **C** Initial incision just coronal
to mucogingival junction

E Prepare bed
Reduce root prominence

Prepare bed

Prepare donor graft

F Suture graft covering root

Suture graft at mucogingival junction

G Apply pressure
Place bandage
Give postoperative instruction

A

B

C

D

Figure 108-2 *A,* Preoperative view of an area with inadequate attached gingiva before free gingival grafting. *B,* Preparation of a receptor bed for a free gingival graft without root coverage as a goal. *C,* Free graft from palate sutured in place. *D,* Healed area with additional attached gingiva.

Additional Readings

Carranza FA Jr, Newman MG. Clinical periodontology. 8th ed. Philadelphia: WB Saunders; 1996. p. 653.

Hall WB, Lundergan W. Free gingival grafts—current indications and technique. Dent Clin North Am 1993;37:227.

Hall WB et al. Aktueller Stand der Anwendung freier Gingivatransplantate. Phillip J Restaurative Zahnmed 1995;12:457.

Rateitschak KH et al. Color atlas of periodontology. Stuttgart: Thieme-Verlag; 1985. p. 230.

Sato N. Periodontal surgery: a clinical atlas. Tokyo: Quintessence Publishing; 2000. p. 82, 356.

Schluger et al. Periodontal diseases. 2nd ed. Philadelphia: Lea & Febiger; 1990. p. 567.

109 Connective Tissue Graft versus Guided Tissue Regeneration

Walter B. Hall

The subepithelial connective tissue graft for root coverage where recession has occurred was described by the Langers in 1985. It has become one of the most predictable approaches for root coverage where facial or lingual recession has occurred. If the donor tissue is obtained from the anterior palate, where the submucosa is fatty, new attachment *may* be obtained because epithelium does not grow to cover fatty tissue until it is replaced with fibrous connective tissue.

The connective tissue graft has been used for regeneration in Class II furcation involvements, as described by Han (1992).

A If a patient has a single tooth with facial or lingual root exposure or several adjacent teeth with such recession, two approaches to predictable root coverage are available: the connective tissue graft and guided tissue regeneration (GTR). Because the connective tissue graft uses the patient's own tissue and therefore is much less expensive (although more difficult to do), it should be considered first. An adequate donor site of fatty connective tissue must be present. Its presence may be evaluated by repetitive, gentle finger pressure to the area of the rugae and sagitally to it. If the area feels spongy, the submucosa probably is fatty and usable for a connective tissue graft.

B A connective tissue graft requires the lifting of a superficial flap that is 1 or 2 mm thick at its thinnest point. If the rugae are very gross (3–4 mm or more in height), raising a flap of adequate thickness and still leaving tissue for a fatty subepithelial connective tissue graft may not be possible. If the rugae are too substantial, therefore, a connective tissue graft should not be attempted. GTR using a membrane should be employed.

C Finally, if interdental papillae are receded or involved with pocketing, and full root coverage is the goal, the connective tissue graft is not the most promising choice. Miller showed in 1985 that root coverage by means of grafting is limited by the height of the interdental papillae and alveolar crests adjacent to the exposed root or roots. The same limitation does *not* apply to GTR by means of a membrane. Regeneration of interproximal tissues with new attachment has been predictably achievable since 1989, when the first interproximal membranes for GTR became available. If interproximal height can be gained to increase coverage of exposed roots, GTR by means of a membrane is the technique of choice whether facial or lingual surfaces (with or without furcation involvements) are present in the area to be treated. This technique has limited success at this time, but its promise is great.

Additional Readings

Carranza FA Jr, Newman MG. Clinical periodontology. 8th ed. Philadelphia: WB Saunders; 1996. p. 664.

Hall WB et al. Aktueller Stand der Anwendung freier Gingivatransplante. Phillip J Restaurative Zahnmed 1995;12:457.

Han TJ. Connective tissue membrane: treating grade II furcation involvements. J Calif Dent Assoc 1992;20:47.

Langer B, Langer L. Subepithelial connective tissue graft technique for root coverage. J Periodontol 1985;56:715.

Miller PD. A classification of marginal tissue recession. Int J Periodontics Restorative Dent 1985;2:8.

Sato N. Periodontal surgery: a clinical atlas. Tokyo: Quintessence Publishing; 2000. p. 113, 185, 338, 390.

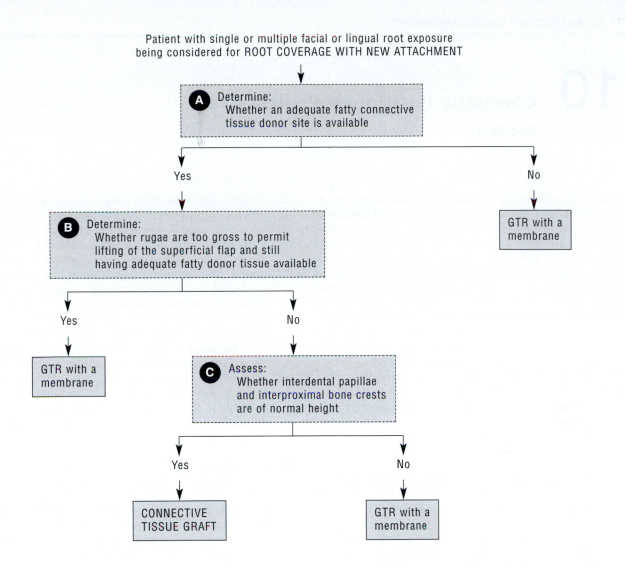

Patient with single or multiple facial or lingual root exposure being considered for ROOT COVERAGE WITH NEW ATTACHMENT

A Determine:
Whether an adequate fatty connective tissue donor site is available

Yes

No

B Determine:
Whether rugae are too gross to permit lifting of the superficial flap and still having adequate fatty donor tissue available

GTR with a membrane

Yes

No

GTR with a membrane

C Assess:
Whether interdental papillae and interproximal bone crests are of normal height

Yes

No

CONNECTIVE TISSUE GRAFT

GTR with a membrane

110 Coronally Positioned Pedicle Graft

Craig Gainza

The coronally positioned flap technique was popularized in the 1970s by Bernimoulin. The indications for it have diminished in recent years owing to the success of single-stage root coverage procedures, but the coronally positioned flap continues to remain a popular therapy. The advantage to this procedure (similar to that for the pedicle graft) is maintenance of a continuous supply of blood during healing. Frequently, this procedure is combined with root conditioning to expose dentinal collagen, detoxify endotoxin, and encourage new tissue attachment. Adequate attached gingiva is necessary for successful coronal positioning of the flap. This procedure requires 3 to 5 mm of keratinized tissue apicocoronally. The tissue should be 1.5 mm in thickness (Figure 110-1).

After determining the adequacy of attached gingiva, address the esthetic needs of the patient. A simple evaluation of the lip posture at rest and during a relaxed smile provides adequate exposure of recessed tissue. The patient's comments and own perception of esthetics are crucial in determining the next stage of treatment planning.

A If no esthetic needs are evident and adequate attached gingiva exists, implement restorative therapy as needed and place the patient on a maintenance program.

B If esthetic concerns are evident and adequate attached tissue is present, a coronally positioned flap provides tissue reattachment to cover the exposed root surfaces. If Class V caries or sensitivity is present, a coronally positioned flap with root conditioning (root planing and citric acid) may resolve the recession and dental pathology without a restoration.

C Patients who have inadequate attached gingiva and request esthetic improvement require evaluation for root caries (and their removal if present) and determination of sufficient or insufficient adjacent donor tissue. If insufficient donor tissue is available, free graft procedures are suggested. Miller, using free soft-tissue autografts, has been successful at complete coverage of wide and deep wide recession. The predictability of free graft procedures has further improved with the interpositional approach to soft-tissue grafting, as described by Langer. The advantage of both techniques is that they involve only a single surgical procedure. Occasionally, complete root coverage cannot be achieved by the free graft procedure alone; however, adequate attached tissue may exist. If incomplete coverage has occurred in the presence of adequate attached gingiva, the coronally positioned flap may be employed as a second-stage surgical procedure.

D If inadequate gingiva is available and no esthetic requirements are evident, as occurs frequently in the premolar and molar regions, a simple free gingival graft may create an adequate band of attached gingiva. If shallow root caries or sensitivity are present, a Class V restoration may be placed and the patient placed on maintenance. To avoid a Class V restoration altogether and correct the gingival recession, a subepithelial connective tissue graft, a large free gingival graft, or a two-stage free graft or coronally positioned flap may be employed.

Figure 110-1 *A,* Flap design for root coverage with a coronally positioned pedicle graft. *B,* Pedicle graft reflected; side flaps removed. *C,* Pedicle graft coronally positioned with a single-sling suture. *D,* Root coverage completed.

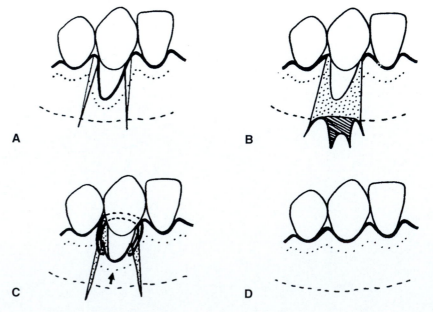

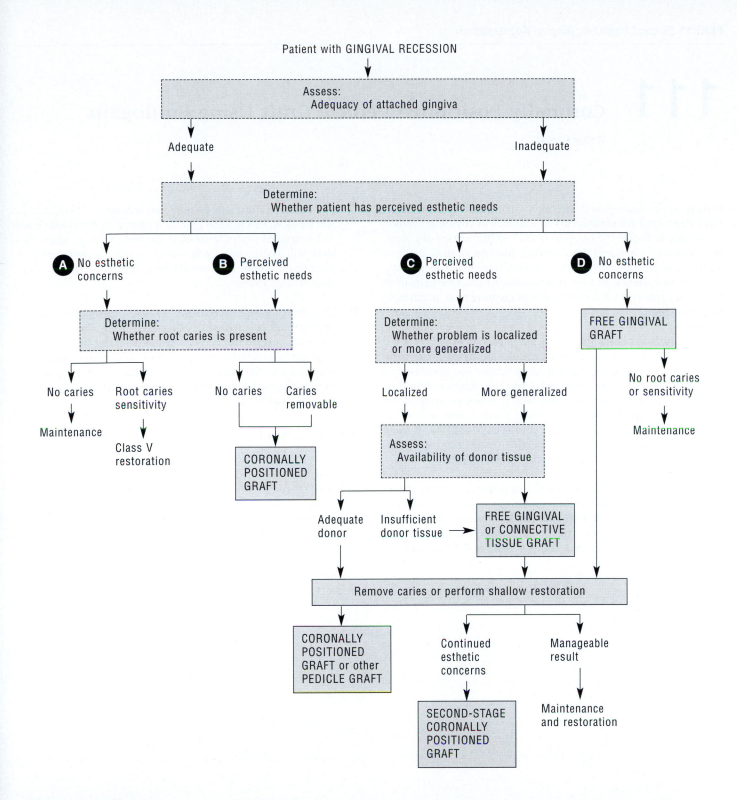

Patient with GINGIVAL RECESSION

Assess:
Adequacy of attached gingiva

Adequate — Inadequate

Determine:
Whether patient has perceived esthetic needs

A No esthetic concerns   **B** Perceived esthetic needs   **C** Perceived esthetic needs   **D** No esthetic concerns

Determine:
Whether root caries is present

No caries — Root caries sensitivity

Maintenance

Class V restoration

No caries — Caries removable

CORONALLY POSITIONED GRAFT

Determine:
Whether problem is localized or more generalized

Localized — More generalized

Assess:
Availability of donor tissue

Adequate donor — Insufficient donor tissue → FREE GINGIVAL or CONNECTIVE TISSUE GRAFT

FREE GINGIVAL GRAFT

No root caries or sensitivity

Maintenance

Remove caries or perform shallow restoration

CORONALLY POSITIONED GRAFT or other PEDICLE GRAFT

Continued esthetic concerns

Manageable result

SECOND-STAGE CORONALLY POSITIONED GRAFT

Maintenance and restoration

Additional Readings

Allen EP. Use of mucogingival surgical procedures to enhance esthetics. Dent Clin North Am 1988;32:2.

Bernimoulin OJ, Luscher B, Muhleman HR. Coronally repositioned flap: clinical evaluation after one year. J Clin Periodontol 1975;2:1.

Carranza FA Jr, Newman MG. Clinical periodontology. 8th ed. Philadelphia: WB Saunders; 1996. p. 663.

Langer B, Calagna L. The subepithelial connective tissue graft. J Prosthet Dent 1980;44:363.

Miller PD. Root coverage using a free soft-tissue autograft following citric acid application. I. Technique. Int J Periodontics Restorative Dent 1982;2:65.

Miller PD. Root coverage using the free soft-tissue autograft following citric acid application. III. A successful and predictable procedure in areas of deep-wide recession. Int J Periodontics Restorative Dent 1985;5:15.

111

Coronally Positioned Pedicle Graft Using Emdogain

Walter B. Hall

Pedicle grafts—positioned laterally, obliquely, or coronally—have been used for many years as a means of covering exposed roots. This is despite the comparatively low percentage of success achieved with them and the lingering question of their mode of attachment to the root. Emdogain was introduced in the late 1990s as an enhancer of new attachment growth. One of its most promising applications is as a means of creating new attachment of pedicle graft.

A Ascertain whether there is a site adjacent to the exposed root where there is sufficient gingiva for an adequate band of attachment thick enough to minimize the likelihood of future recession. For a pedicle graft, the gingiva should be 2 to 3 mm or more in height, and 0.5 mm or more in the thickness, with sufficient width to cover 1 mm or more of connective tissue on each side of the exposed root. If these criteria cannot be met, a connective tissue graft (see Chapter 109) would be a better means of treatment.

B If the adjacent pedicle donor site appears acceptable, determine whether a flap can be mobilized so that it covers the exposed root without being under tension that would compromise its blood supply. The criteria to consider are the vestibular depth and the potential pull from adjacent frenum bands.

C A shallow vestibule or an adjacent frenum pull could limit the freedom of a pedicle graft to a degree that it would have to be sutured under tension at the receptor site. Such tension will compromise the success of the pedicle graft. A connective tissue graft would be a better treatment selection in such cases.

D The site that will receive the coronally positioned pedicle graft should be prepared as described in an earlier chapter. Once the pedicle has been prepared, coat the freshly planed exposed root with Emdogain, and suture—covering both the flap and the root. Wait 6 months, and then probe to determine the level of attachment obtained; this should not be done earlier.

Additional Readings

Carranza FA Jr, Newman MG. Clinical periodontology. 8th ed. Philadelphia: WB Saunders; 1996. p. 663.

Pini-Prato GP et al. Periodontal regeneration therapy with coverage of previously restored root surfaces: a two case report. Int J Periodontics Restorative Dent 1992;12:451.

Sato N. Periodontal surgery. Tokyo: Quintessence Publishing; 2000. p. 336–42.

Patient with a LOCALIZED ROOT EXPOSURE

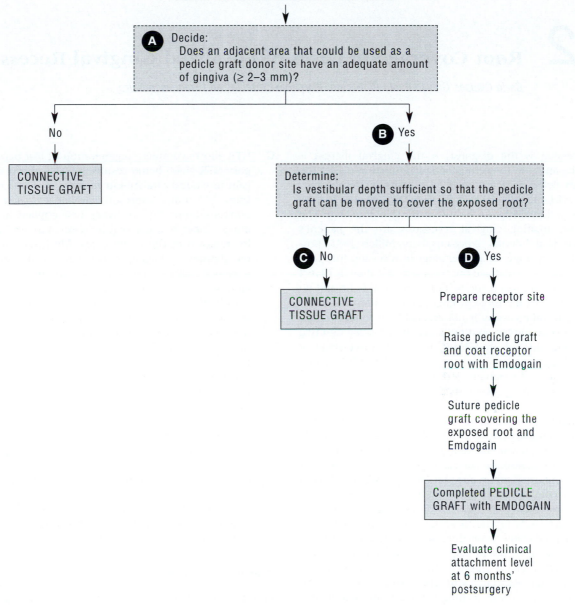

A Decide:
Does an adjacent area that could be used as a pedicle graft donor site have an adequate amount of gingiva (≥ 2–3 mm)?

No

CONNECTIVE TISSUE GRAFT

B Yes

Determine:
Is vestibular depth sufficient so that the pedicle graft can be moved to cover the exposed root?

C No

CONNECTIVE TISSUE GRAFT

D Yes

Prepare receptor site

Raise pedicle graft and coat receptor root with Emdogain

Suture pedicle graft covering the exposed root and Emdogain

Completed PEDICLE GRAFT with EMDOGAIN

Evaluate clinical attachment level at 6 months' postsurgery

112 Root Coverage in Cases of Localized Gingival Recession

Carlo Clauser, Giovan Paolo Pini-Prato, Pierpaolo Cortellini, and Francesco Cairo

Gingival recession is the diagnosis if the gingival margin is observed to be apical to the cementoenamel junction (CEJ). The extent of this defect is determined by measuring the distance between the CEJ and gingival margin. Gingival recession may be caused by periodontal disease or traumatic toothbrushing. The indications for treating gingival recessions are the patient's esthetic concerns and dental hypersensitivity. Miller (1985) proposed a clinical typology separating gingival recession into four classes. Complete root coverage can be obtained if there is Class I or Class II gingival recession (no loss of interdental bone and no loss of soft tissue). Partial root coverage can be achieved in Class III. Class IV gingival recession is not amenable to root coverage. Procedures for covering exposed roots may be classified into two groups: (1) mucogingival procedures (pedicle and free-standing soft tissue grafts) and (2) guided tissue regeneration (GTR). Long-term studies confirm the stability of the clinical outcomes obtainable using root coverage procedures.

A Mucogingival procedures are indicated in cases where gingival recessions are localized and shallow (< 5 mm). An assessment of the residual keratinized tissue (KT) should be performed to choose the correct surgical approach. A pedicle flap is indicated when adequate KT is available adjacent or apical to the recession. A coronally advanced flap (CAF), laterally positioned flap (LPF), or double papilla flap (DPF) may be performed to minimize the gingival recession. The CAF is a predictable procedure to treat shallow gingival recessions. A trapezoidal flap design with a large base allows sufficient blood supply to the pedicle flap. Flap thickness > 0.8 mm is associated with 100% root coverage. Contraindications for these techniques are frenum pull or a shallow vestibule.

B Free-standing soft tissue grafts are indicated in cases of gingival recession with inadequate KT present apically or laterally to the exposed root surface. Epithelium free-standing gingival grafts (EFGGs, epithelium plus connective tissue) may be harvested from the palate and secured to the surgical bed to completely or partially cover the root surface. A two-step surgical technique may be used with the coronal positioning of the previously placed graft. Grafts using connective tissue only (CTGs) are more frequent in clinical practice. CTGs result in more predictable root coverage and a more satisfying esthetic result (eg, better color match).

C GTR allows complete regeneration of lost periodontal support. GTR yields better results in terms of root coverage and gain in clinical attachment in cases of deep gingival recessions (> 5 mm). Nonresorbable barriers such as expanded polytetrafluoroethylene were first applied in GTR procedures. These barriers require a second surgical procedure for removal of the membranes. More recently, resorbable membranes (collagen, polyglycolic acid, polylactic acid) have been introduced to reduce patient discomfort. Similar amounts of root coverage have been obtained using resorbable and nonresorbable membranes. The GTR approach requires the raising of a trapezoidal, full-thickness, large flap to uncover the alveolar bone crest. The membrane is secured at the CEJ to completely cover the root surface. Different approaches may be used to create and maintain sufficient space for regeneration (heavy root planing, reinforced barriers, resorbable materials under the membrane). The flap is then coronally placed to completely cover the membrane. An EFGG may be used before the GTR technique if the amount of KT is inadequate to cover the membrane.

D Class III gingival recession associated with interdental bone loss may be reduced using an EFGG after the periodontitis has been successfully treated. An attempt to regenerate the interdental bone and reduce the recession may be performed using a GTR technique.

Additional Readings

Allen EP, Miller PD. Coronal positioning of existing gingiva: short-term results in the treatment of shallow marginal tissue recession. J Periodontol 1989;60:316.

Borghetti A, Louise F. Controlled clinical evaluation of the subpedicle connective tissue graft for the coverage of the gingival recession. J Periodontol 1994;65:1107.

Miller PD. A classification of the marginal tissue recession. Int J Periodontics Restorative Dent 1985;5:9.

Pini-Prato G, Clauser C, Cortellini P, et al. Guided tissue regeneration versus mucogingival surgery in the treatment of human buccal gingival recessions: a 4-year follow-up study. J Periodontol 1996;67:1216.

Roccuzzo M, Lungo M, Corrente G, Gandolfo S. Comparative study of a bioresorbable and a non-resorbable membrane in the treatment of human buccal gingival recessions. J Periodontol 1996;67:7.

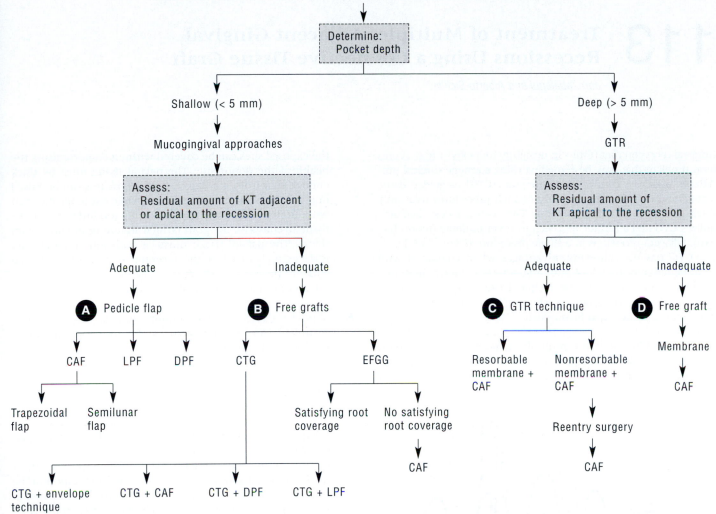

Patient with CLASS I, II, or III RECESSION after treatment of PERIODONTAL DISEASE

Determine: Pocket depth

Shallow (< 5 mm) → Mucogingival approaches

Assess: Residual amount of KT adjacent or apical to the recession

- Adequate
  - **A** Pedicle flap
    - CAF
      - Trapezoidal flap
      - Semilunar flap
    - LPF
    - DPF
- Inadequate
  - **B** Free grafts
    - CTG
      - CTG + envelope technique
      - CTG + CAF
      - CTG + DPF
      - CTG + LPF
    - EFGG
      - Satisfying root coverage
      - No satisfying root coverage → CAF

Deep (> 5 mm) → GTR

Assess: Residual amount of KT apical to the recession

- Adequate
  - **C** GTR technique
    - Resorbable membrane + CAF
    - Nonresorbable membrane + CAF → Reentry surgery → CAF
- Inadequate
  - **D** Free graft → Membrane → CAF

225

113 Treatment of Multiple, Adjacent Gingival Recessions Using a Connective Tissue Graft

Jon Zabalegui and Alberto Sicillia

Gingival recession that results in unsightly root exposure is a common problem that may be remedied using cosmetic surgical procedures such as a connective tissue graft (CTG) or guided tissue regeneration (GTR). The majority of such procedures treat only single or double, adjacent recessions. The treatment described here utilizes CTG and a tunnel approach to cover multiple (more than two), adjacent recessions in a single procedure (Figure 113-1).

CTG has the following advantages when compared with GTR: better color match of graft and adjacent gingiva, high rate of clinical success—with few recipient-site sloughings, greater gain in keratinized tissue, greater gain in attachment, but no donor surgical site—and lower cost.

A To use CTG to cover multiple, adjacent, exposed roots, there must be an adequate donor site where the palatal tissue is thick enough, long enough, and wide enough that

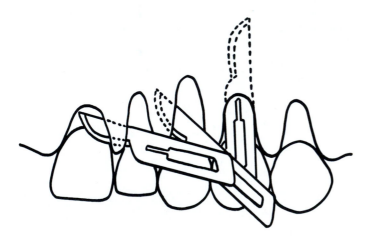

Figure 113-1 A distal furcation involvement on the first molar with apparent second molar root proximity.

the exposed sites can be covered without compromising the health of the donor site. The palatal tissue must be thick enough that from it a flap of 1 mm thickness can be raised in order to obtain underlying connective tissue for the graft without perforating the flap or leaving too little connective tissue to comprise the graft (which should be at least 1 mm thick). The palatal tissue must be both long enough and wide enough to cover the receptor area without causing adjacent palatal root structure to be exposed or damage to the anterior palatal nerve and vessel complex.

B Should no such adequate donor site exist, an alternative treatment can be used, such as one (or more) multiple-tooth GTR procedure.

C If there is an adequate donor site, decide how many teeth can be treated at one time. Then prepare the tunnel receptor site (see Figure 113-1), and freshen all exposed dentine in the areas of recession. Obtain graft material sufficient to fill the tunnel. Cover the exposed roots, and extend the graft site slightly coronally to the cementoenamel junction (CEJ) on each of the teeth being treated. Place two sutures, one at the most mesial and the other at the most distal aspect of the tunnel (Figures 113-2 and 113-3), entering from beneath the tunnel flap and exiting through the most central area of gingival recession. Pick up the most-distal and -mesial ends of the graft material using vertical mattress sutures (Figure 113-4). Pull and push the graft material using the sutures, together with a dull instrument, until it is positioned in such a way that it covers the exposed roots for several millimeters apically to the bone margin and coronally to the CEJs. Fix the graft with sutures at its distal and mesial ends (Figure 113-5). Press in position for 5 minutes using damp gauze and a dull instrument. Remove the gauze.

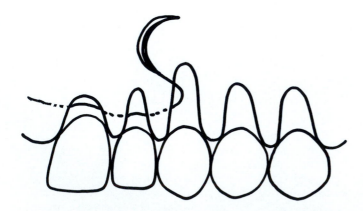

Figure 113-2 Suture placed within tunnel from mesial aspect.

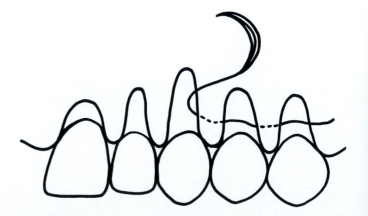

Figure 113-3 Suture placed within tunnel from distal aspect.

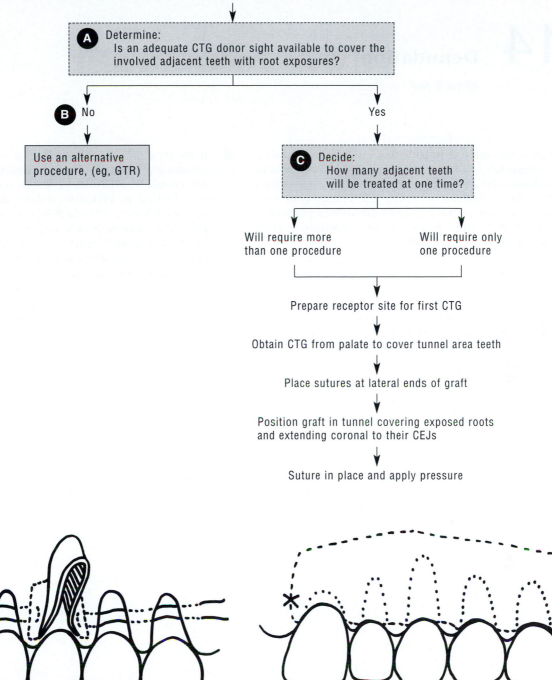

Patient with MULTIPLE, ADJACENT RECESSIONS for treatment with a CONNECTIVE TISSUE GRAFT

A Determine:
Is an adequate CTG donor sight available to cover the involved adjacent teeth with root exposures?

B No

Use an alternative procedure, (eg, GTR)

Yes

C Decide:
How many adjacent teeth will be treated at one time?

Will require more than one procedure

Will require only one procedure

Prepare receptor site for first CTG

Obtain CTG from palate to cover tunnel area teeth

Place sutures at lateral ends of graft

Position graft in tunnel covering exposed roots and extending coronal to their CEJs

Suture in place and apply pressure

Figure 113-4 Connective tissue graft positioned over the mid-most tooth with mesial and distal sutures grasping its mesial and distal ends.

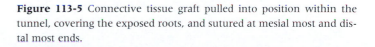

Figure 113-5 Connective tissue graft pulled into position within the tunnel, covering the exposed roots, and sutured at mesial most and distal most ends.

The patient should be advised not to disturb the surgical sites for several weeks. The sites should not be probed for 6 months.

Additional Readings

Allen A. Use of the supraperiosteal envelope in soft tissue grafting for root coverage. II. Clinical results. Int J Periodontics Restorative Dent 1994;14:303.

Langer B, Langer L. Subepithelian connective tissue graft technique for root coverage. J Periodontol 1985;56:715.

Pini-Prato G, Glauser C, Cortellini P, et al. Guided tissue regeneration versus mucogingival surgery in the treatment of human buccal recession: a 4-year follow-up study. J Periodontol 1996;67:1216.

Zabalegui I, Sicilia A, Cambra J, et al. Treatment of multiple adjacent gingival recessions with the tunnel subepithelial connective tissue graft: a clinical report. Int J Periodontics Restortive Dent 1999;19:199.

114 Denudation

Walter B. Hall

Denudation is the exposure of bone that is left nude to heal by secondary intention as additional gingiva. The procedure is of limited usefulness because of its reputation as being uncomfortable and associated with slow healing and further bone loss. Nevertheless, denudation has a place in the armamentarium of any accomplished therapist as a means of predictably creating more attached gingiva, if used judiciously.

A   If a patient has a pure mucogingival problem, a problem of inadequate attached gingiva that is not associated with pocket formation and bone loss (periodontitis), the locale of the problem determines whether gingival grafting or denudation is the appropriate surgical approach. If the problem is on the facial aspect of a mandibular second or third molar, denudation is a logical approach. In this area the vestibule often is shallow and the facial cortical plate is thick. In such cases, gingival grafting is unlikely to be successful. If the vestibule is shallow and the cortical plate is dense, more gingiva may be created by deepening the vestibule with osseous recontouring and apical positioning of the soft tissue so that 4 to 5 mm of bone is left nude to heal by secondary intention as a broader band of attached gingiva. If the vestibule is sufficiently deep already, the soft tissue may be displaced 4 to 5 mm apically and the bone left to heal by secondary intention as a broader band of attached gingiva.

B   If the pure mucogingival problem is in the same area as a mucogingival-osseous problem (periodontitis), two approaches are possible. The flap may be apically positioned after osseous recontouring to eliminate osseous defects; enough bone must be left exposed to heal by secondary intention as gingiva. Alternatively, a two-surgery approach may be used; place a free gingival graft first and then apically position it after osseous recontouring, or apically position the flap and place a free gingival graft later. For most patients, a single-surgery approach involving denudation is preferable to a two-surgery approach that includes free gingival grafting and apical positioning of a flap at separate visits.

Additional Readings

Bohannon HM. Studies in the alterations in vestibular depth: complete denudation. J Periodontol 1962;33:120.

Carranza FA Jr, Newman MG. Clinical periodontology. 8th ed. Philadelphia: WB Saunders; 1996. p. 890.

Hall WB. Pure mucogingival problems. Berlin: Quintessence Publishing; 1984. p. 161.

Lindhe J. Textbook of clinical periodontology. 2nd ed. Copenhagen: Munksgaard; 1989. p. 433.

Schluger S et al. Periodontal diseases. 2nd ed. Philadelphia: Lea & Febiger; 1990. p. 563.

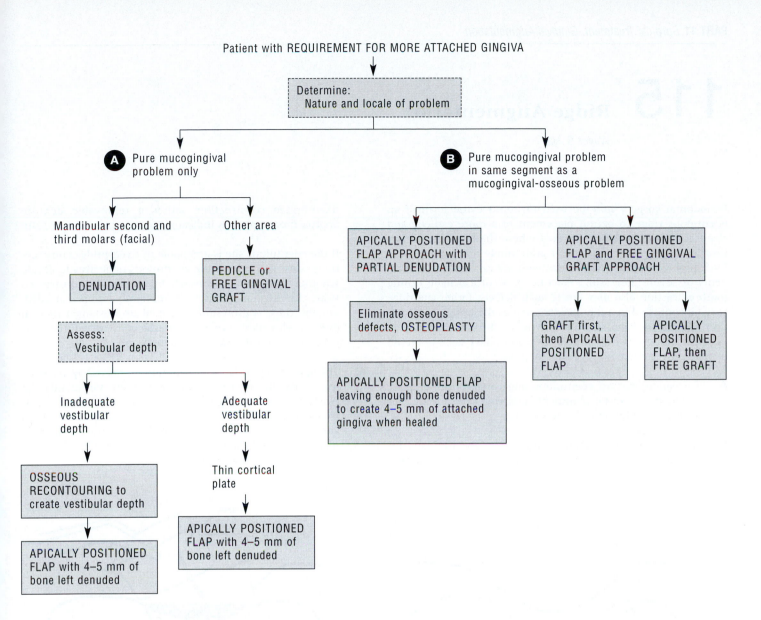

Patient with REQUIREMENT FOR MORE ATTACHED GINGIVA

Determine:
Nature and locale of problem

A Pure mucogingival problem only

B Pure mucogingival problem in same segment as a mucogingival-osseous problem

Mandibular second and third molars (facial)

Other area

DENUDATION

PEDICLE or FREE GINGIVAL GRAFT

Assess:
Vestibular depth

Inadequate vestibular depth

Adequate vestibular depth

OSSEOUS RECONTOURING to create vestibular depth

Thin cortical plate

APICALLY POSITIONED FLAP with 4–5 mm of bone left denuded

APICALLY POSITIONED FLAP with 4–5 mm of bone left denuded

APICALLY POSITIONED FLAP APPROACH with PARTIAL DENUDATION

Eliminate osseous defects, OSTEOPLASTY

APICALLY POSITIONED FLAP leaving enough bone denuded to create 4–5 mm of attached gingiva when healed

APICALLY POSITIONED FLAP and FREE GINGIVAL GRAFT APPROACH

GRAFT first, then APICALLY POSITIONED FLAP

APICALLY POSITIONED FLAP, then FREE GRAFT

115 Ridge Augmentation

Walter B. Hall

Periodontal surgery may be used to improve the form of an edentulous ridge to permit placement of a more esthetic and cleansable fixed bridge on an area where the loss of teeth has resulted in a grossly deficient or grotesquely malformed ridge. Such problems often occur when teeth are lost because of accidents or severe abscessing. Fracture of a cortical plate during tooth extraction also may create such defects. Either the ridge may be contorted in a manner that makes the bridge construction difficult to clean, and unesthetic, or the ridge may be so deficient that excessively long, ugly pontics have been or would be placed in the fixed-bridge construction.

A If a patient has an edentulous ridge area, both adequate proximal and distal abutment teeth must be present for ridge augmentation to be necessary.

B Determine the amenability of the site for fixed-bridge construction. If the edentulous area is too lengthy to permit

fixed-bridge construction, either a removable denture approach or implant is indicated (see Chapter 68 and 120).

C If the edentulous site is amenable to fixed-bridge construction, assess the form of the edentulous ridge area to decide whether an esthetic, cleansable bridge may be constructed using the ridge as it exists. If no augmentation is needed, but the ridge is grotesquely formed or so shaped that an esthetic, cleansable bridge cannot be constructed, the dentist should consider ridge augmentation.

D The approach to ridge augmentation is selected by assessing the availability of a soft-tissue donor site for an inlay or overlay approach (Figure 115-1). If a good donor site is available, that approach may be offered to the patient. If no adequate donor site is available, only the grinded bone augmentation (GBA) approach or use of a synthetic bone fill material may be presented to the patient.

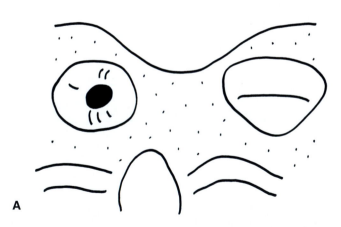

A

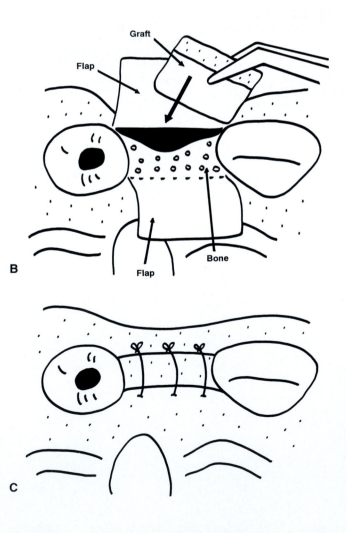

B

C

Figure 115-1 *A,* An incisal view of a disfigured ridge caused by a loss of its facial cortical plate in an accident. *B,* Flaps have been raised, exposing the deficient ridge. A subepithelial connective tissue graft from the palate is being placed into the defect. *C,* The connective tissue graft has been sutured to fill the defect, plumping the ridge to create an esthetically pleasing base for a pontic.

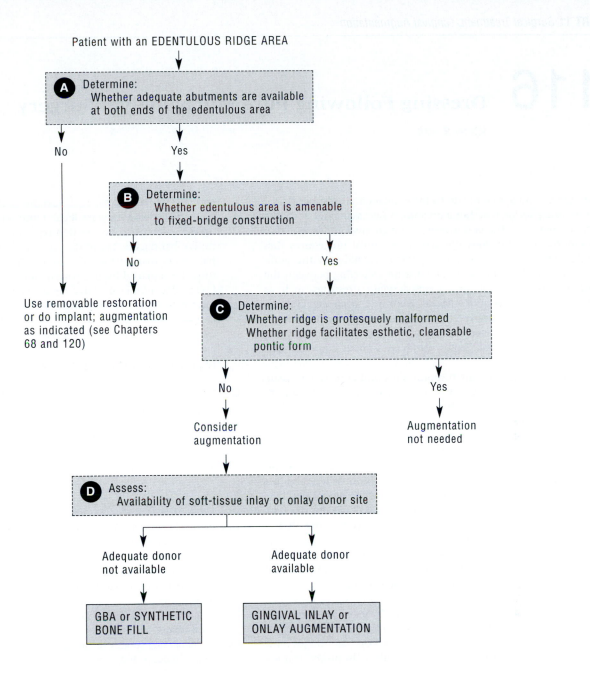

Patient with an EDENTULOUS RIDGE AREA

A Determine:
Whether adequate abutments are available
at both ends of the edentulous area

No → Yes

B Determine:
Whether edentulous area is amenable
to fixed-bridge construction

No → Yes

Use removable restoration
or do implant; augmentation
as indicated (see Chapters
68 and 120)

C Determine:
Whether ridge is grotesquely malformed
Whether ridge facilitates esthetic, cleansable
pontic form

No → Yes

Consider
augmentation

Augmentation
not needed

D Assess:
Availability of soft-tissue inlay or onlay donor site

Adequate donor
not available

Adequate donor
available

GBA or SYNTHETIC
BONE FILL

GINGIVAL INLAY or
ONLAY AUGMENTATION

Additional Readings

Abrams L. Augmentation of the deformed residual edentulous ridge for fixed prosthesis. Compend Cont Educ Dent 1980;1:205.

Genco RJ, Goldman HM, Cohen DW. Contemporary periodontics. St. Louis: Mosby; 1990. p. 643.

Sato N. Periodontal surgery: a clinical atlas. Tokyo: Quintessence Publishing; 2000. p. 422.

Schluger S et al. Periodontal diseases. 2nd ed. Philadelphia: Lea & Febiger; 1990. p. 632.

Seibert J. Reconstruction of the deformed partially edentulous ridges using full-thickness overlay grafts. Parts 1 and 2. Compend Cont Educ Dent 1983;4:437.

116 Dressing Following Pure Mucogingival Surgery

Walter B. Hall

The dentist who has completed a pure mucogingival surgical procedure must decide whether a dressing is necessary and, if so, the proper one to use. The best dressing for a gingival graft is one that does not move and does not require removal procedures that would tug on sutures. It should provide stability for the graft, minimize bleeding, and keep blood from collecting between the graft and the receptor site. Cyanoacrylate dressings such as isobutyl cyanoacrylate or trifluor isopropyl cyanoacrylate are excellent for these purposes, but they are not approved for use in the United States. In some other countries, however, they are available and work well. Donor sites have similar requirements.

A For, free gingival graft receptor sites and connective tissue sites, a dressing may not be necessary; however, Stomahesive bandage has the advantages of maintaining the adaptation of the graft to the receptor bed and minimizing bleeding or blood pooling. The simplicity of placement of a Stomahesive bandage and its gradual dissolvability make it the dressing of choice. Coe Pak or an alternative has the disadvantages of difficulty of stabilization when papillae completely fill interproximal spaces and the probability that movement of the pack during healing will disrupt the tenuous, developing union of graft and receptor site. If the pure mucogingival procedure is part of a mucogingival-osseous procedure, Coe Pak or an alternative becomes the dressing of choice because the opening of interproximal spaces permits solid, stable pack application.

B The donor site for a free gingival graft or connective tissue graft also may need to have a dressing placed to minimize bleeding and protect the donor area from the tongue and food. Isobutyl cyanoacrylate and trifluor isopropyl cyano-

acrylate work well for this purpose and should be used in countries where they are legal. Otherwise the selection of a dressing seems to be the dentist's choice. Use of a Stomahesive bandage is favored; it lasts only 6 to 8 hours in the palate because of tongue activity. In the first few days it must be replaced by the patient several times. Others may favor placement of Colycote or Surgicel, both of which minimize bleeding, although not as well as Stomahesive bandage does. Still others may favor placing Coe Pak and suturing it in place; this is a tedious process that results in poorer control of bleeding, but the Coe Pak does not require replacement. A palatal stent is favored by others.

C If denudation is used to produce a broader band of attached gingiva, it is usually as part of a mucogingival-osseous procedure for pocket elimination. Coe Pak or an alternative is the dressing of choice in such cases. The pack may have to be replaced for a second week because of the slowness of healing when bone is left nude.

Additional Readings

Carranza FA Jr, Newman MG. Clinical periodontology. 8th ed. Philadelphia: WB Saunders; 1996. p. 571.

Coslet JG, Rosenberg ES, Tisot R. The free autogenous gingival graft. Dent Clin North Am 1980;24:675.

Hall WB. Pure mucogingival problems. Berlin: Quintessence Publishing; 1984. p. 107.

Lindhe J. Textbook of clinical periodontology. 2nd ed. Copenhagen: Munksgaard; 1989. p. 418.

Sato N. Periodontal surgery: a clinical atlas. Tokyo: Quintessence Publishing; 2000. p. 362, 378.

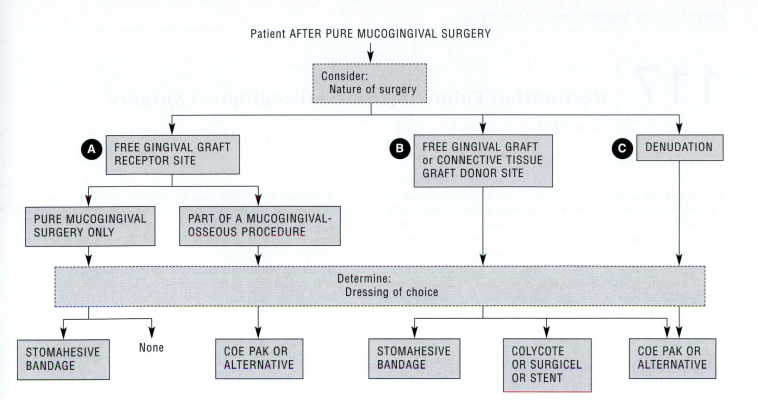

Patient AFTER PURE MUCOGINGIVAL SURGERY

Consider:
Nature of surgery

A FREE GINGIVAL GRAFT RECEPTOR SITE

B FREE GINGIVAL GRAFT or CONNECTIVE TISSUE GRAFT DONOR SITE

C DENUDATION

PURE MUCOGINGIVAL SURGERY ONLY

PART OF A MUCOGINGIVAL-OSSEOUS PROCEDURE

Determine:
Dressing of choice

STOMAHESIVE BANDAGE

None

COE PAK OR ALTERNATIVE

STOMAHESIVE BANDAGE

COLYCOTE OR SURGICEL OR STENT

COE PAK OR ALTERNATIVE

117 Restoration Following Pure Mucogingival Surgery

Walter B. Hall

The timing of a restorative procedure after a pure mucogingival surgical procedure is crucial to maintaining a successful graft. The timing depends on the restorative procedures to be done and the objectives of the graft used (root coverage or only a broader band of attached gingiva to prevent further recession).

A If a supragingival restoration is planned, it may be performed as soon as the success of the graft has been ensured (usually no sooner than 2 weeks postsurgically). If waiting longer presents no great difficulty, a longer period for healing before the supragingival restoration is placed is desirable.

B If a rest-proximal plate I bar type of removable partial denture (RPI) or an overdenture is planned, root coverage is not an objective of pure mucogingival surgery. Grafts are performed to create an adequate band of attached gingiva to underlay a "I bar" for the partial or provide 2 to 5 mm of attached gingiva on the overdenture teeth; nevertheless, allow a month or more before taking impressions to prepare the RPI removable denture or overdenture.

C If a restoration is to be placed close to the free margin of the gingiva or subgingivally after pure mucogingival surgery, the objective of the graft procedure influences when the restorative procedure may be performed. If root coverage has not been attempted, the restoration may be placed 2 weeks or more after the surgical procedure, although a longer period of healing is desirable. If root coverage is the objective of the gingival grafting procedure, allow a longer period for healing before preparing a restoration close to the new free margin of the gingiva or subgingivally. Regardless of whether the graft is a free gingival type or a connective tissue one, disturbance of the new marginal gingiva too soon after surgery may result in graft retraction or failure. Allow several months before restorative preparation. A much longer period is desirable to encourage the development of a more stable attachment of the grafted tissue and root.

Additional Readings

Carranza FA Jr, Newman MG. Clinical periodontology. 8th ed. Philadelphia: WB Saunders; 1996. p. 720.

Lange DE, Bernimoulin JP. Exfoliative cytological studies in evaluation of free gingival graft healing. J Clin Periodontol 1974;1:89.

McFall WT. The laterally repositioned flap: criteria for success. Periodontics 1968;5:89.

Wilderman MR, Wentz FM. Repair of a dentogingival defect with a pedicle flap. J Periodontol 1965;36:218.

Patient with GINGIVAL GRAFT PLACED AND REQUIRING RESTORATION OF TOOTH

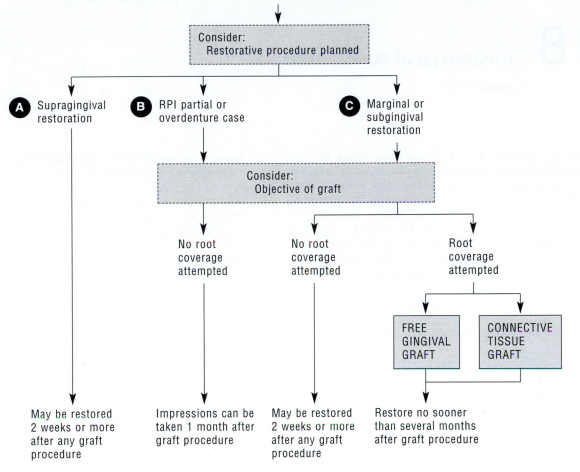

118 Postsurgical Reevaluation

Walter B. Hall

After a patient's periodontal surgery has been completed, the dentist must decide when to evaluate the success of the surgery. The term usually applied to this examination is *reevaluation,* which includes visual examination and charting. Radiographic evaluation is not advisable at this time because little may be learned from the films (insurance companies should be told so if they request films), and the additional radiation exposure cannot be justified. The timing of postsurgical reevaluation depends on the surgical procedures that have been used. Generally, the longer the period before reevaluation, the more accurate the prediction; however, the patient and dentist may have valid reasons to wish to proceed as soon as reasonable (eg, splinting with fixed bridges may improve patient function and comfort).

A After pocket-elimination surgery (apically positioned flap and osseous recontouring, gingivoplasty), reevaluate 1 month after the final surgery. Because no new attachment has been attempted, probing will not endanger the success of the procedure.

B New attachment procedures depend on the development of a new connective tissue attachment to new cementum (cementoid). The success of these procedures may be less predictable. Early probing may disturb a newly developing attachment and result in a less desirable "long epithelial attachment." Allow at least 6 months before the new attachment area is probed. Such areas include all bone regeneration sites, connective tissue grafts in which root coverage has been attempted, and second molar roots exposed in relation to the removal of an impacted or partially erupted third molar.

C *Reattachment* is the term used to describe the healing together of a gingival flap and root surface that have been separated by surgery rather than by disease. The viable root surface and flap routinely heal together. If such an approach has been used (eg, when the retraction of a flap exposes a dehiscence or fenestration), allow 1 month or more after the surgery before performing reevaluation with probing. Such a long wait is not necessary if new attachment has been attempted.

D If gingival grafting procedures are used to broaden the band of attached gingiva and no root coverage is attempted, reevaluation may be performed at 1 month (or possibly earlier).

Additional Readings

Carranza FA Jr, Newman MG. Clinical periodontology. 8th ed. Philadelphia: WB Saunders; 1996. p. 574.

Grant DA, Stern IB, Listgarten MA. Periodontics. 6th ed. St. Louis: Mosby; 1988. p. 1095.

Lindhe J. Textbook of clinical periodontology. 2nd ed. Copenhagen: Munksgaard; 1989. p. 439.

Pihlstrom BL, Ortiz-Campos C, McHugh RB. A randomized four-year study of periodontal therapy. J Periodontol 1981;52:227.

Wilson TG, Kornman KS. Fundamentals of periodontics. Chicago: Quintessence Publishing; 1996. p. 385.

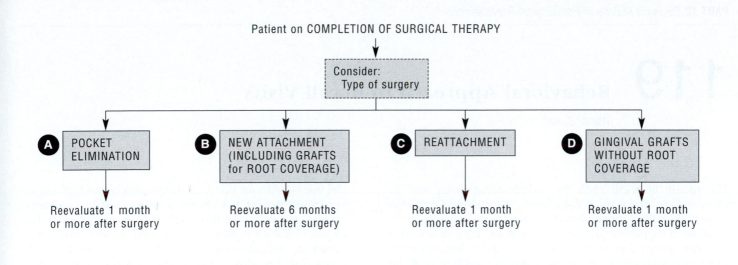

119 Behavioral Approach to Recall Visits

Walter B. Hall

The timing of recall visits for periodontal patients may be planned in several ways. Some dentists, citing long-term studies of periodontal treatment based on a uniform recall interval, recall all their patients at 3-month intervals. They believe that they can predict their success rates with various forms of treatment more accurately on this basis, but the problem with this approach is the patient's response. For years, many dentists recalled their patients twice a year, because studies indicated that with such recalls caries would not develop rapidly enough to endanger many teeth. In behavioral terms, however, many patients learned that they had to return to the dentist every 6 months whether they needed it or not (ie, whether they had made a good effort at oral hygiene or not). Patients understood this message long before dentists did, and oral hygiene and the incidence of caries improved little during that era. An approach that uses long-term study concepts in a more behaviorally sound way is the "rewarding" of patients depending on the adequacy of their home care efforts between visits; thus if a patient is doing well (based on assessments of plaque, inflammation, and pocket depth), the time before the next recall is extended, which offers a direct reward for individual efforts and reinforces desirable behavior. Within a large group of patients, the average recall time is likely to be 3 months; however, no individual patient is likely to be recalled regularly at 3-month intervals.

The greatest advantage of the behavioral approach to the timing of recall visits is that patients are given an immediate reinforcement for good or poor effort. The patients see either that their efforts have paid off or that lack of effort has brought an appropriate response. In the fixed-interval (every 3 months) approach, praise or scolding is the only reward or punishment available to the dentist. The more tangible reward of less cost (in time, money, and discomfort) is much more likely to prove successful. Additionally, the dentist can demonstrate the way the treatment was altered to respond to patient behavior between visits, and patients accept responsibility for their progress and its costs.

A   When a patient's first recall visit is to be scheduled, information on which to base the recall interval is not clearly defined. The patient may have remaining areas of compromise such as individual teeth for which definitive treatment is impossible (because these teeth already had lost too much attachment), or a less definitive treatment may have been selected for financial reasons. Some patients are compromised by the status of their health. Others may be compromised by less-than-ideal restorative work or tooth alignment. If the patient has areas of compromise, they should be annotated and the recall interval decreased. If a compromised patient has shown little motivation to develop home care skills, the first recall visit should be set at 1 to 2 months; with evidence of good oral hygiene, skill development, and motivation, however, the first recall may be set at 2 to 3 months. If the patient has no areas of compromise remaining, evidence of oral hygiene skill and motivation may be used to set the first recall interval. If the patient's efforts have been minimally successful, the first recall visit may be set at 2 to 3 months; with greater success the interval may be increased to 3 months or more.

B   Further recall visits are easier to schedule in a behaviorally successful manner. At each recall visit, evaluate plaque control, the status of gingival inflammation, and the depth of pockets and use this measure of the patient's "success" to determine the next recall interval. Patient behavior over the years is rarely consistent. Many factors in patients' lives influence their efforts at oral hygiene. Periods of stress or illness affect the ability to deal with plaque. If plaque control has been inadequate, shorten the recall interval. If much inflammation is present or if pocket depths are increasing, shorten the intervals even further. If the patient's efforts do not improve, alternative approaches (even extraction of poor-risk teeth that may endanger adjacent abutments) may be necessary. If efforts improve after several recall visits, an increase in the time between recalls is an appropriate reward. Maintain a patient whose efforts are fair or adequate at the current recall intervals. Reward a patient whose efforts have given excellent results by increasing the time between recalls.

Additional Readings

Chace R. The maintenance phase of periodontal therapy. J Periodontol 1951;22:23.

Lindhe I. Textbook of clinical periodontology. 2nd ed. Copenhagen: Munksgaard; 1989. p. 615.

Parr RW. Periodontal maintenance therapy. Berkeley (CA): Praxis; 1974. p. 1.

Ramfjord SP et al. Longitudinal study of periodontal therapy. J Periodontol 1973;44:66.

Ramfjord SP et al. Oral hygiene and maintenance of periodontal support. J Periodontol 1982;53:26.

Schluger S et al. Periodontal diseases. 2nd ed. Philadelphia: Lea & Febiger; 1990. p. 732.

Patient with CURRENT PERIODONTAL TREATMENT COMPLETED

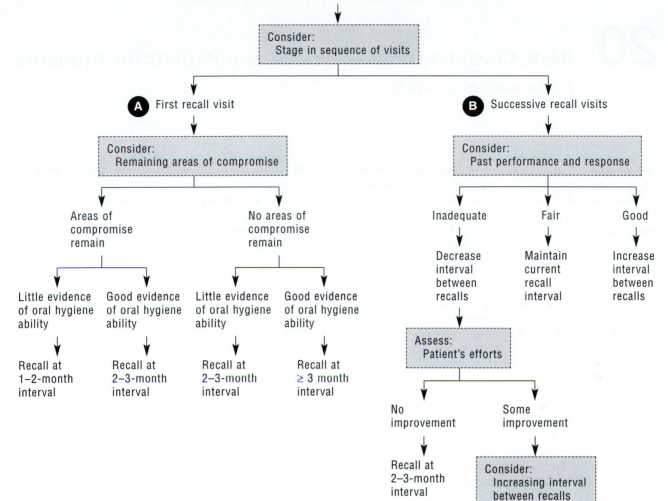

Consider:
Stage in sequence of visits

A First recall visit

Consider:
Remaining areas of compromise

Areas of compromise remain

No areas of compromise remain

Little evidence of oral hygiene ability

Good evidence of oral hygiene ability

Little evidence of oral hygiene ability

Good evidence of oral hygiene ability

Recall at 1–2-month interval

Recall at 2–3-month interval

Recall at 2–3-month interval

Recall at ≥ 3 month interval

B Successive recall visits

Consider:
Past performance and response

Inadequate

Fair

Good

Decrease interval between recalls

Maintain current recall interval

Increase interval between recalls

Assess:
Patient's efforts

No improvement

Some improvement

Recall at 2–3-month interval

Consider:
Increasing interval between recalls

120 Basic Considerations in Selecting a Patient for Implants

E. Robert Stultz Jr and William Grippo

A patient considering an implant approach to an edentulous or partially dentulous condition may seek information from a general dentist or specialist. In each case, a series of decisions is made to determine whether the patient is a reasonable candidate for implant therapy. The initial decisions involve medical and psychologic qualification for implant therapy. After these considerations are met successfully, the dental indications and contraindications may be evaluated.

A A medical evaluation is made from a questionnaire, a patient interview, and any medical consultations necessitated by the history. Conditions that make surgery dangerous or adversely affect healing must be considered. Examples of absolute contraindications are recurrent myocardial infarction, acquired immunodeficiency syndrome, debilitating or transmissible hepatitis, pregnancy, granulocytopenia, poorly controlled diabetes, and drug or alcohol dependency. Other conditions (eg, prolonged corticosteroid use, blood dyscrasias, collagen diseases, malignancies, heavy smoking) make implants a questionable alternative. If any significant medical contraindication exists and cannot be resolved promptly, implants are not indicated and alternative approaches are required.

B If no medical contraindications are detected, the psychologic status of the patient and the reasonableness of patient expectations are evaluated. If the patient is psychologically unstable or has unrealistic expectations of implant therapy, alternative approaches should be considered.

C If the patient is psychologically well adjusted and does not expect "miracles" in esthetics or functional benefits from an implant approach, the consequences of the totally edentulous or partially dentulous condition should be considered next. The status of teeth to be retained is a complicating factor in this decision process. The position of these teeth and their periodontal status and restorability must be considered.

D To determine whether adequate support exists for implants, the quantity of bone available at implant sites must be evaluated. If the height or width of the recipient ridge areas is inadequate or the trajectory is unsatisfactory, an implant may not be feasible. Bony undercuts also present problems, as do the positions of anatomic features such as the mental foramen. These factors may be examined using simple dental radiographs, Panorex films, tomographic or cephalometric film, or computerized tomographic scan imaging. If the ridge is inadequate for any reason, an implant is inappropriate, and alternatives should be considered.

E If bone quantity is satisfactory, bone quality should be considered next. The most ideal alveolar bone is the dense cortical bone of the mandibular anterior ridge; the least desirable is the thin cortical loose trabecular bone typically found in the maxillary posterior region. Bone quality may be classified as follows:

> Class I: Dense cortical bone
> Class II: Dense cortical bone with dense trabecular bone
> Class III: Moderate cortical and trabecular bone
> Class IV: Thin cortical bone with poor trabecular bone

Patients with Class I or Class II bone are good candidates for osseointegrated implants. Those with Class III or Class IV bone require bone augmentation before osseointegrated implants or a subperiosteal approach.

Additional Readings

Branemark PI, Zarb G, Albrecktson T. Tissue integrated prosthesis: osseointegration in clinical dentistry. Chicago: Quintessence Publishing; 1985. p. 1.

Golec TS. Implants, what and when. Calif Dent Assoc J 1987;15:49.

Jensen O. Site classification for the osseointegrated implant. J Prosthet Dent 1989;61:228.

Misch C, Judy K. Classification of partially edentulous arches for implant dentistry. Int J Periodontics Restorative Dent 1986;12:688.

Stambaugh R. Surgical management of the complicated periodontal-prosthesis patient. J Calif Dent Assoc 1989;17:31.

Patient who is EDENTULOUS OR PARTIALLY DENTULOUS AND CONSIDERING IMPLANTS

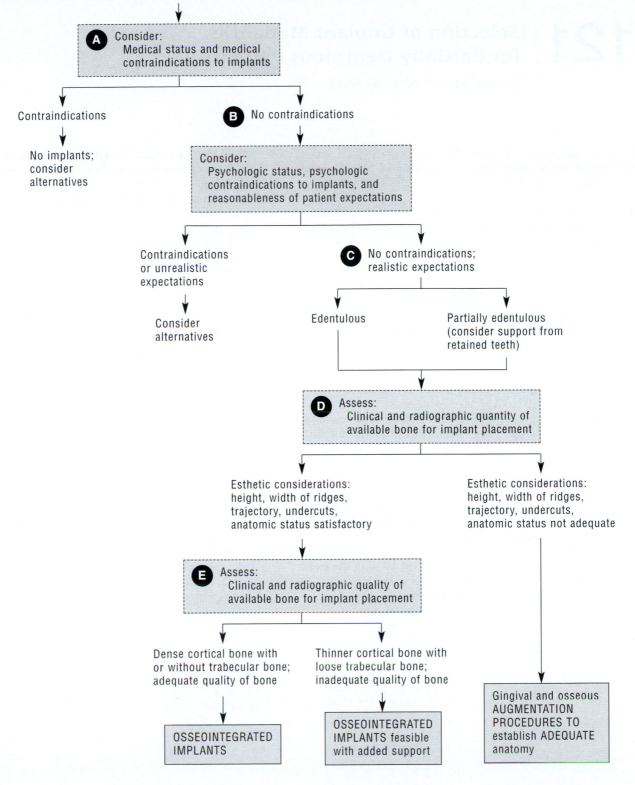

A Consider:
Medical status and medical contraindications to implants

Contraindications

No implants; consider alternatives

B No contraindications

Consider:
Psychologic status, psychologic contraindications to implants, and reasonableness of patient expectations

Contraindications or unrealistic expectations

Consider alternatives

C No contraindications; realistic expectations

Edentulous

Partially edentulous (consider support from retained teeth)

D Assess:
Clinical and radiographic quantity of available bone for implant placement

Esthetic considerations: height, width of ridges, trajectory, undercuts, anatomic status satisfactory

Esthetic considerations: height, width of ridges, trajectory, undercuts, anatomic status not adequate

E Assess:
Clinical and radiographic quality of available bone for implant placement

Dense cortical bone with or without trabecular bone; adequate quality of bone

Thinner cortical bone with loose trabecular bone; inadequate quality of bone

OSSEOINTEGRATED IMPLANTS

OSSEOINTEGRATED IMPLANTS feasible with added support

Gingival and osseous AUGMENTATION PROCEDURES TO establish ADEQUATE anatomy

121 Selection of Implant Modalities for Partially Dentulous Patients

E. Robert Stultz Jr and William Grippo

After the basic factors that determine the eligibility of a patient for implant therapy have been met (see Chapter 120), the periodontal status of teeth to be retained must be determined.

A If the remaining teeth are healthy periodontally, an implant approach to therapy for the partially dentulous patient becomes feasible.

B If significant periodontal problems are detected (eg, deep pockets, furcation involvement, poor crown-to-root ratio), the likelihood of treatment making affected teeth useful in the overall treatment plan must be assessed. The ability of the patient to perform adequate plaque control may be evaluated during the periodontal treatment phase. If the periodontal problems are refractory (response is poor) or good plaque control is not demonstrated, implants are not likely to be helpful, and alternatives should be explored.

C If periodontal problems appear resolvable, their resolution must be established after treatment. Unsuccessful cases should not receive implant therapy. Implant therapy is feasible in successful cases.

D Available bone support is considered next. If alveolar bone height is greater than 10 mm, its width greater than 6 mm, and the trajectory less than 25°, endosseous cylinder implants are the best approach.

E If the available bone height is less than 10 mm, the width only 4 to 6 mm, and the trajectory greater than 25°, endosseous blade implants are indicated.

F If inadequate bone height or width is present for endosseous root form implants, various procedures such as membrane-assisted hard tissue grafts, monocortical onlay grafts from the chin or ascending ramus, ridge expansion techniques, and sinus elevation procedures in the maxilla may be employed to create an adequate ridge.

If these procedures succeed, the adequacy of the available bone may be reassessed. In some cases, guided bone augmentation may be employed at the time of placement of the cylinder implant into an extraction socket.

G In selected cases in which the alveolar ridge is deficient in height but adequate in width (> 6 mm), a subperiosteal implant may be the treatment of choice. This choice is most useful in the posterior mandible, where monocortical onlay grafting or nerve lateralization is not recommended.

Additional Readings

Branemark Pl, Zarb G, Albrektson T. Tissue integrated prosthesis: osseointegration in clinical dentistry. Chicago: Quintessence Publishing; 1985. p. 1.

Golec TS. Implants, what and when. Calif Dent Assoc J 1987;15:49.

Jensen O. Site classification for the osseointegrated implant. J Prosthet Dent 1989;61:228.

Misch C, Judy K. Classification of partially edentulous arches for implant dentistry. Int J Periodontics Restorative Dent 1986;12:688.

Meffert RM, Block MS, Kent JN. What is osseointegration? Int J Periodontics Restorative Dent 1987;11:135.

Smiler DG. Evaluation and treatment planning. Calif Dent Assoc J 1987;15:35.

Patient for IMPLANT THERAPY: EVALUATION OF PERIODONTAL STATUS

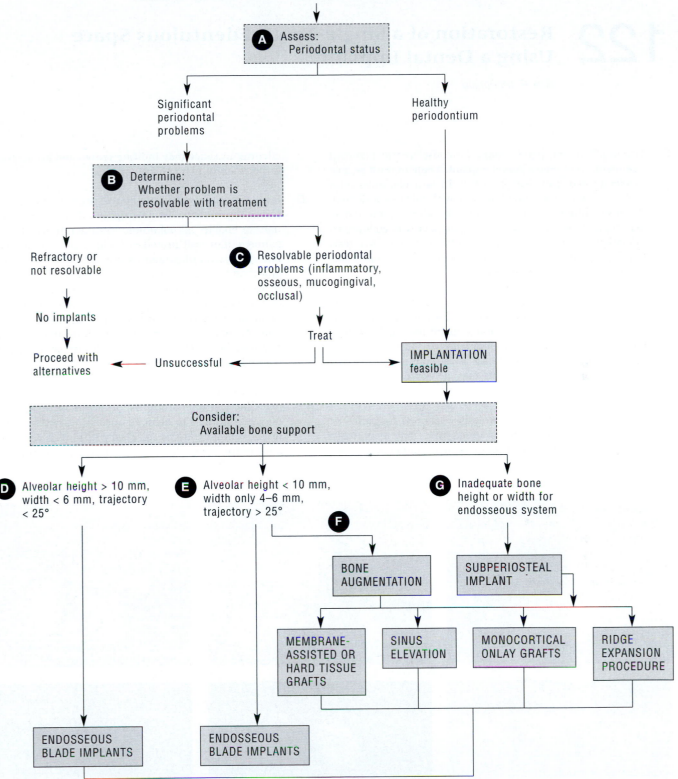

A Assess: Periodontal status

Significant periodontal problems

Healthy periodontium

B Determine: Whether problem is resolvable with treatment

Refractory or not resolvable

C Resolvable periodontal problems (inflammatory, osseous, mucogingival, occlusal)

No implants

Treat

Proceed with alternatives ← Unsuccessful ←

IMPLANTATION feasible

Consider: Available bone support

D Alveolar height > 10 mm, width < 6 mm, trajectory < 25°

E Alveolar height < 10 mm, width only 4–6 mm, trajectory > 25°

G Inadequate bone height or width for endosseous system

F

BONE AUGMENTATION

SUBPERIOSTEAL IMPLANT

MEMBRANE-ASSISTED OR HARD TISSUE GRAFTS

SINUS ELEVATION

MONOCORTICAL ONLAY GRAFTS

RIDGE EXPANSION PROCEDURE

ENDOSSEOUS BLADE IMPLANTS

ENDOSSEOUS BLADE IMPLANTS

122 Restoration of a Single-Tooth Edentulous Space Using a Dental Implant

Alex R. McDonald

A The health of the patient must be considered in planning treatment. To receive a dental implant, a patient must be able to tolerate an oral surgical procedure. In particular, any health problems interfering with blood supply should be considered. Blood supply and wound healing can be adversely affected by diabetes and smoking. Bone density in older women is a consideration. However, recent data demonstrate a positive relationship between maxillary implant success and women taking hormone replacement therapy.

B Potential lateral occlusal forces on dental implant restorations should be minimized to ensure long-term success. If it is not possible to fully manage parafunctional occlusal habits, then alternatives to implant treatment should be considered. Occlusal overload is a common cause of implant failure; however, this may be decreased by fabricating an occlusal splint.

C Adjacent teeth should be carefully examined for caries or the presence of large restorations that may eventually require crowns. The need for crowns on either side of an

edentulous space may indicate crown and bridge treatment rather than implant treatment.

D Both quantitative and qualitative aspects of bone in edentulous regions must be determined. Radiographs are essential to enable all anatomic considerations. Typically, a panorex film will provide excellent osseous information, but additional radiographic studies may be required. Tomograms and computerized tomographic scans are often used to assess the mandible to avoid injuries to the inferior alveolar nerve. Soft tissue should be examined, and the amount of keratinized tissue should be determined prior to an implant placement. Soft-tissue grafting may be necessary and may be initiated either prior to implant placement or before final restorations are placed.

E Even when bone and soft tissue are ideal for implant placement, small amounts of orthodontic intervention may be required to achieve optimal esthetics. Orthodontic movement may be necessary if there is a size discrepancy of the edentulous space relative to the other teeth in

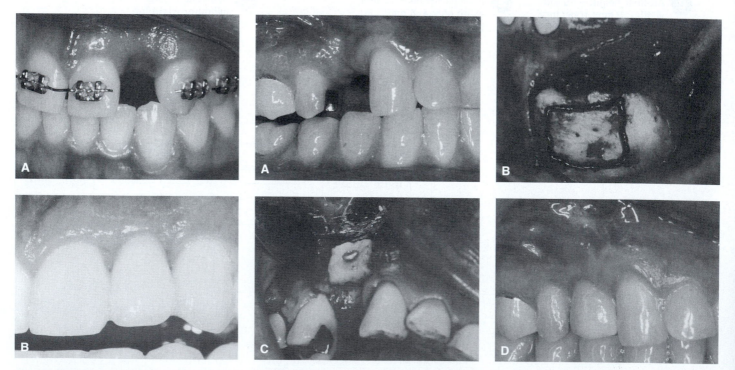

Figure 122-1 *A,* Congenitally missing lateral incisor space is idealized with orthodontic appliances to improve width and root angulation. *B,* The final implant-supported restoration in place. The soft-tissue architecture is now ideal.

Figure 122-2 *A,* Patient with a large buccal defect in the area of tooth 5. Note very consevative restoration on tooth 4. *B,* Chin site providing cortical autogenous bone graft. *C,* Veneer graft rigidly fixed in the intended implant site. *D,* Final restoration with good emergence profile.

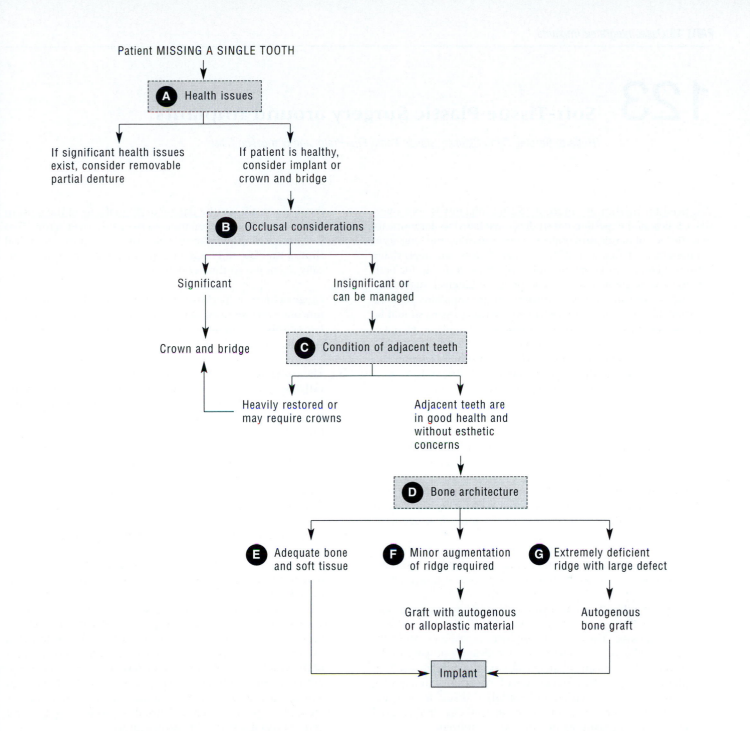

Patient MISSING A SINGLE TOOTH

A Health issues

If significant health issues exist, consider removable partial denture

If patient is healthy, consider implant or crown and bridge

B Occlusal considerations

Significant

Insignificant or can be managed

Crown and bridge

C Condition of adjacent teeth

Heavily restored or may require crowns

Adjacent teeth are in good health and without esthetic concerns

D Bone architecture

E Adequate bone and soft tissue

F Minor augmentation of ridge required

G Extremely deficient ridge with large defect

Graft with autogenous or alloplastic material

Autogenous bone graft

Implant

the area. Often orthodontic treatment is required to improve root angulations prior to implant placement (Figure 122-1).

F Small augmentations can be achieved using alloplastic material such as demineralized freeze-dried bone. Recently available bioactive peptides show great promise in directing bone growth in deficient areas.

G When large bone defects exist, it is essential to replace missing bone to permit placing the implant in an ideal position. The most predictable treatment for larger defects is to harvest and place autogenous bone. Typically sites include the chin and ramus. Bone removed from a donor site vascularizes in the recipient site for 3 months prior to implant place-

ment. It is important to rigidly fix such bone grafts to ensure optimal healing (Figure 122-2).

Additional Readings

August M, Chung K, Chang Y, Glowacki J. Influence of estrogen status on endosseous implant osteointegration. J Oral Maxillofac Surg 2001;11:1285.

Loos L, McDonald A. Treatment planning dental implants in the partially edentulous patient. J Calif Dental Assoc 1997;25:852.

Yukna R, Callan D, Krauser J, et al. Multi-center evaluation of combination anorganic bovine-derived hydroxyapatite matrix (ABM)/cell binding peptide (P–15) as a bone replacement graft material in human periodontal osseous defects: 6-month results. J Periodontol 1998;69:655.

123 Soft-Tissue Plastic Surgery around Implants

Roberto Barone, Carlo Clauser, Giovan Paolo Pini-Prato, and Francesco Cairo

The need for masticatory mucosa around implants is controversial. Clinical and experimental studies have failed to demonstrate that the lack of masticatory mucosa may jeopardize the long-term maintenance of dental implants. Nevertheless, an appreciable band of keratinized tissue around implants is desirable for both esthetic and hygienic reasons. The need for gingival augmentation (to restore masticatory mucosa) around implants remains questionable, and, therefore, soft-tissue plastic surgery should be used infrequently. Where there is a submerged implant, adequate masticatory mucosa may be obtained in the second surgical session (implant exposure). Before placing a nonsubmerged implant, however, ensure that there is adequate masticatory mucosa necessary to allow complete soft-tissue closure.

A   The evaluation of the masticatory mucosa at the implant site is the first step in planning soft-tissue plastic surgery. It might be necessary to augment the amount of available keratinized tissue as determined by clinical requirements such as esthetics, easier restorative manipulation, less gingival recession, and easier plaque control. Correct planning of soft-tissue management becomes a critical factor for the success of single-tooth implants in the maxilla anterior segment.

B   In the maxillary arch, soft-tissue plastic surgery to enhance masticatory mucosa should be performed at phase 2 surgery so as not to increase the number of surgical sessions.

C   In the mandibular arch, augmentation before implant placement might be necessary to obtain a sufficient band of keratinized tissue. The choice to augment is related to the difficulty of obtaining an increase of masticatory mucosa in the lower arch by means of an apically positioned flap (APF) at phase 2 surgery. Two millimeters of masticatory mucosa are considered as a minimum of keratinized tissue. If the existing tissue allows less than 2 mm, an epithelial-free gingival graft before implant placement may be utilized.

D   To ensure that a significant width of masticatory mucosa is available, use two periodontal probes to measure it after the installation of the implant and before suturing the APF flap. The first probe is aligned horizontally with the mucogingival junction (MGJ) of the adjacent teeth. The second probe measures the vertical distance between the buccal bone margin at the emergence of the implant and the horizontal probe. If the distance is < 3 mm, an APF is planned for the implant exposure. If the distance is > 3 mm, gingivectomy is planned for the phase 2 surgery.

E   The APF may be performed during implant exposure to allow for an increase of the keratinized tissue. A horizontal incision is made on the palatal or lingual side of the crest to preserve the masticatory mucosa over the cover screw. Two vertical incisions in the alveolar mucosa allow the apical shift of the flap and implant exposure. The flap is then apically anchored to the periostium.

F   Gingivectomy is performed by removing the masticatory mucosa over the head of the implant using a circular blade. Use of this technique is indicated in cases where there is a wide flat crest with thick tissue.

G   The thickness of the keratinized tissue is crucial for esthetics, easier restorative manipulation, easier plaque control, and the prevention of the gingival recession. Augmentation of buccal tissue thickness may be performed using a modified Abram's roll technique (MRT). The flap is elevated from the palate. The palatal portion is deepithelialized and then inserted between the buccal flap and the bone crest. Buccal releasing incisions are avoided. This technique is useful in cases of ridges without need of soft-tissue augmentation.

H   Where there is a thin soft-tissue ridge, augmentation may be achieved using a connective tissue graft (CTG) performed at the time of implant exposure. This procedure may be performed in combination with an APF or a repositioned flap (RF).

An attempt to recreate papillae adjacent to a maxillary single-tooth implant may be performed with a modified flap at phase 2 surgery. A palatal U-shaped flap is dissected over the implant. Two vertical incisions in the buccal aspect of the vestibule complete the flap design. After the insertion of the healing abutment, the flap is split—separating mesial and distal pedicles. Then each part of the buccal flap is secured over the deepithelialized adjacent papillae and sutured using a vertical mattress suture.

Additional Readings

Barone R, Clauser C, Grassi R, et al. A protocol for maintaining or increasing the width of masticatory mucosa around submerged implants: a 1-year prospective study on 53 patients. Int J Periodontics Restorative Dent 1998;18:377.

Berglundh T, Lindhe J, Ericsson I, et al. The soft tissue barrier at implants and teeth. Clin Oral Implants Res 1991;2:81.

Nemcovsky CE, Moses O, Artzi Z. Interproximal papillae reconstruction in maxillary implants. J Periodontol 2000;71:308.

Wenströmm J, Bengazi F, Lekholm U. The influence of the masticatory mucosa on the periimplant soft tissue condition. Clin Oral Implants Res 1994;5:1.

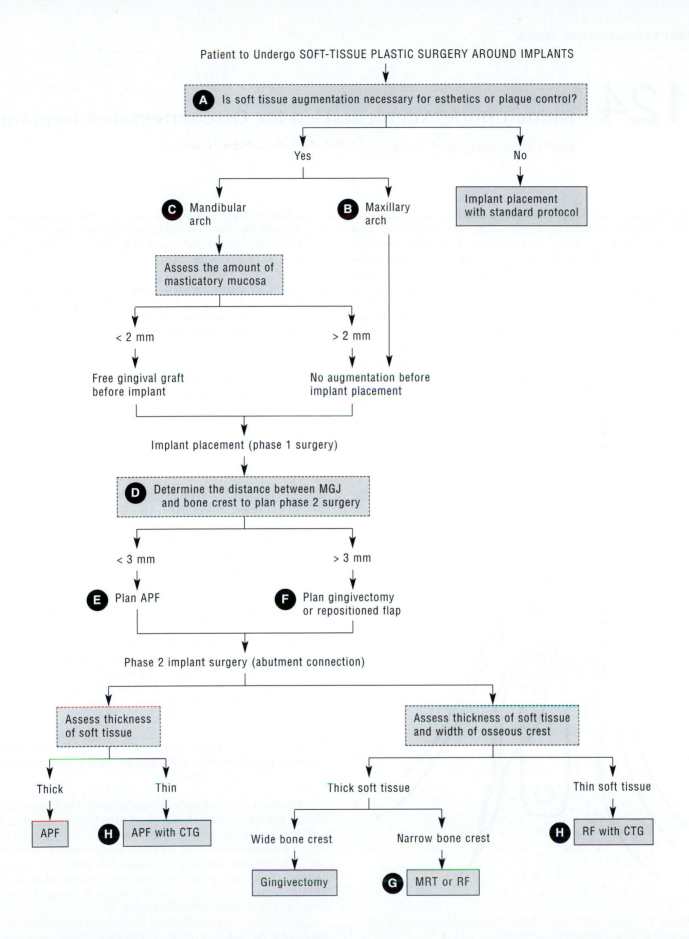

Patient to Undergo SOFT-TISSUE PLASTIC SURGERY AROUND IMPLANTS

A Is soft tissue augmentation necessary for esthetics or plaque control?

Yes

No

Implant placement with standard protocol

C Mandibular arch

B Maxillary arch

Assess the amount of masticatory mucosa

< 2 mm

> 2 mm

Free gingival graft before implant

No augmentation before implant placement

Implant placement (phase 1 surgery)

D Determine the distance between MGJ and bone crest to plan phase 2 surgery

< 3 mm

> 3 mm

E Plan APF

F Plan gingivectomy or repositioned flap

Phase 2 implant surgery (abutment connection)

Assess thickness of soft tissue

Assess thickness of soft tissue and width of osseous crest

Thick

Thin

Thick soft tissue

Thin soft tissue

APF

H APF with CTG

Wide bone crest

Narrow bone crest

H RF with CTG

Gingivectomy

G MRT or RF

124 Guided Bone Augmentation for Osseointegrated Implants

William Becker and Burton E. Becker

The principles of guided tissue regeneration (GTR) that have been used for periodontal regeneration also may be used for root form dental implants. The tissues involved in the healing of an extraction socket are flap connective tissue and bone. Membrane barriers may be used to exclude flap connective tissue from collapsing into an extraction socket that has received an immediately placed implant, thus allowing the cells necessary for bone formation access to the area. The barrier creates a space and protects the clot during the early healing phase, creating an environment for potential bone formation around the portion of the implant that is not fully encompassed by bone. A specially designed expanded polytetrafluoroethylene membrane (Gore-Tex augmentation material) is used for this purpose. The oval-shaped material has a totally occlusive inner portion and a peripheral portion that allows for the ingrowth of connective tissue fibrils. The use of guided bone augmentation (GBA) with osseointegrated implants has been shown successful on a predictable basis.

A Successful use of GBA for implants placed into extraction sockets requires careful case selection. Teeth that have advanced untreatable periodontitis, recurrent endodontic lesions, or fractures that are not exposable by crown lengthening are ideal candidates for extraction accompanied by immediate implant placement. To obtain maximal

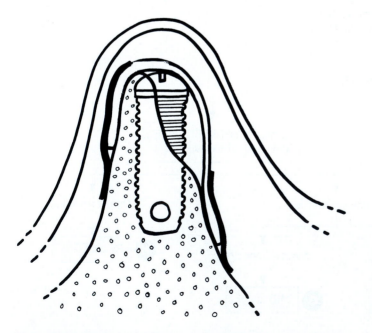

Figure 124-1 An implant with exposed body knurling covered with a membrane for guided bone augmentation.

implant stability, a minimum of 3 to 5 mm of bone apical to the root tip should be available. Implants placed into thin edentulous ridges may result in fenestrations. These defects may be treated with GBA.

B When the site is exposed surgically, the type of defect and site are evaluated and the prospective stability of an implant or its condition after placement is assessed. If a stable implant cannot be placed, alternative restorative plans should be proposed.

C Fenestration defects that result from placing the implant close to the facial surface of the implant may be treated with GBA. The implant must be completely stable. If the fenestration exposes only one or two threads, no barrier is necessary. If a large fenestration is present, exposing three or more threads of the implant, a barrier should be placed over the defect for GBA (Figure 124-1).

D If an implant has been placed into an extraction socket, an intra-alveolar defect may exist. If implants are placed into extremely narrow sockets (as those present on mandibular anterior teeth) or extremely wide bone and leave no exposure of the implant in the adjacent socket, no GTR is necessary. Defects that are less than 3 mm deep and do not expose more than three threads may have a barrier placed. Defects that are more than 3 mm deep and expose more than three threads should be considered for GBA.

E An implant placed into an extraction socket that is missing one or more bony walls may be treated with GBA. If two walls cannot be stabilized, the implant should be removed immediately. Many times, one or two bony walls are partially missing and the implant is stable. This is the ideal defect in which to use GBA.

F If any of the aforementioned defects occur in conjunction with a narrow ridge, GBA may be used to attempt to augment the width of the ridge.

If barriers are used for implant augmentation, complete flap closure over the barrier should be obtained before removal; the barrier occasionally becomes exposed. If a small area becomes exposed before 30 days, the area may be cleansed by the patient with chlorhexidine swabs. If the barrier has a large exposed area and inflammation is present, it should be removed immediately. Ideally the barrier should remain completely covered until its removal 4 to 6 weeks after placement.

Allogenic bone and alloplasts used under membranes act as fillers and do not contribute to osseointegration. Autologous bone is the best graft material for implant or ridge augmentation.

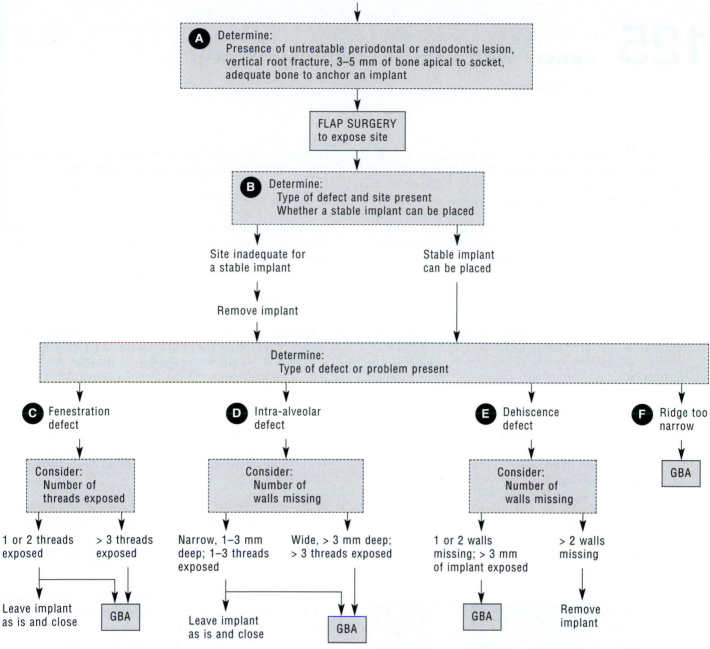

Patient for an OSSEOINTEGRATED IMMEDIATE IMPLANT

A Determine:
Presence of untreatable periodontal or endodontic lesion, vertical root fracture, 3–5 mm of bone apical to socket, adequate bone to anchor an implant

FLAP SURGERY to expose site

B Determine:
Type of defect and site present
Whether a stable implant can be placed

Site inadequate for a stable implant

Remove implant

Stable implant can be placed

Determine:
Type of defect or problem present

C Fenestration defect

Consider:
Number of threads exposed

1 or 2 threads exposed

> 3 threads exposed

Leave implant as is and close

GBA

D Intra-alveolar defect

Consider:
Number of walls missing

Narrow, 1–3 mm deep; 1–3 threads exposed

Wide, > 3 mm deep; > 3 threads exposed

Leave implant as is and close

GBA

E Dehiscence defect

Consider:
Number of walls missing

1 or 2 walls missing; > 3 mm of implant exposed

> 2 walls missing

GBA

Remove implant

F Ridge too narrow

GBA

Additional Readings

Becker W et al. Bone formation at dehisced dental implant sites treated with implant augmentation material: a pilot study in dogs. Int J Periodontics Restorative Dent 1989;9:333.

Becker W et al. Root isolation for new attachment procedures: a surgical and suturing method: three case reports. J Periodontol 1987;58:819.

Dahlin C et al. Generation of new bone around titanium implants using a membrane technique: an experimental study in rabbits. Int J Oral Maxillofac Implants 1989;4:19.

Gottlow J, Nyman S, Lindhe J. New attachment formation as a result of controlled tissue regeneration. J Clin Periodontol 1984;11:494.

Lazzara RJ. Immediate implant placement into extraction sites: surgical and restorative advantages. Int J Periodontics Restorative Dent 1989;9:333.

Nyman S et al. Bone regeneration adjacent to titanium dental implants using guided tissue regeneration: a report of two cases. Int J Oral Maxillofac Implants 1990;5:9.

125 Patient with a Single Edentulous Space

Larry G. Loos

A Healthy or predictably treatable teeth adjacent to a single edentulous space are more important to long-term implant success than is the edentulous site itself. Adjacent teeth must be capable of carrying a greater incisal-occlusal load during function and parafunction to prevent implant overload. Crown-to-root ratio, root morphology, tooth mobility, and sulcus depths are important periodontal considerations. The amount of parafunctional tooth wear must be correlated with patient age. Endodontically treated teeth with short dowels or large-diameter cast dowels must be evaluated for their potential for root fracture.

B If one or both of the teeth adjacent to the space are compromised or not predictably treatable to carry a share of loading, will splinting to the adjacent tooth or teeth create adequate multiple abutments for a four- or five-unit fixed partial denture? Periodontal health, control of tooth mobility, and Ante's law should be satisfied. If double-abutting does not provide predictable abutment teeth adjacent to the space, selective tooth extraction should be considered.

C Determine the result of extracting one or both teeth adjacent to the edentulous space. The new edentulous space will be larger. The new potential abutment teeth must be evaluated for their ability to sustain incisal-occlusal loading for each of the three treatment choices. The quantity of the edentulous ridge must be evaluated for the vastly different requirements of a long-span, tooth-supported fixed partial denture (FPD), a

removable partial denture, or multiple dental implants. The risk/benefit assessments will be different for each.

D When both teeth adjacent to the single space have sound clinical crowns with small or no existing restorations, a single implant should be evaluated as the potential treatment of choice. If one or both adjacent teeth may benefit from a full-coverage cast restoration, a three-unit FPD solves both the missing tooth problem and the restorative needs of the abutment teeth. Full-coverage cast restorations may improve tooth esthetics, function, and strength.

E The single edentulous space must be evaluated for the maximum length of an implant that it can safely accept. This is the most important feature of restored implant predictability. A 10 mm implant is the absolute minimum length, a 13 mm length is better, and longer than 13 mm is best. If 10 mm of bone is not present and cannot be obtained by guided tissue regeneration or augmentation, a three-unit FPD should be fabricated. The edentulous space must have adequate width to accommodate the desired implant diameter. Ridge augmentation may be used to create the acceptable width.

F Bone quality affects dental implant success. Type II quality is ideal for single-tooth implants. Type I and type III are frequently acceptable if the implant has good length. Type IV bone is of poor quality and not recommended for single teeth. A three-unit FPD is more predictable.

G Evaluation of single-tooth implant loading is more crucial than is loading of four to six splinted implants. An implant placed in posterior segments receives greater forces than does an identical implant in the anterior segment. Different functional positions and contours of the restored implant and its opposing teeth produce variations in loading. Faciolingual forces created by steep occlusal morphology on posterior teeth are problematic. A single implant protected from parafunctional loading has a better future than one that is overloaded. Implants do not have the overload safety feature provided by a periodontal ligament, so they are more susceptible to overload than are teeth. Minimal loading of single-tooth implants is highly recommended. Moderate-to-extensive loading may compromise success, so a tooth-supported FPD would be more predictable (Figure 125-1).

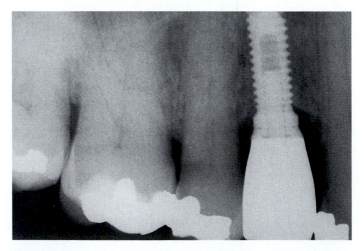

Figure 125-1 A single tooth implant in place. It has no periodontal ligament as teeth do.

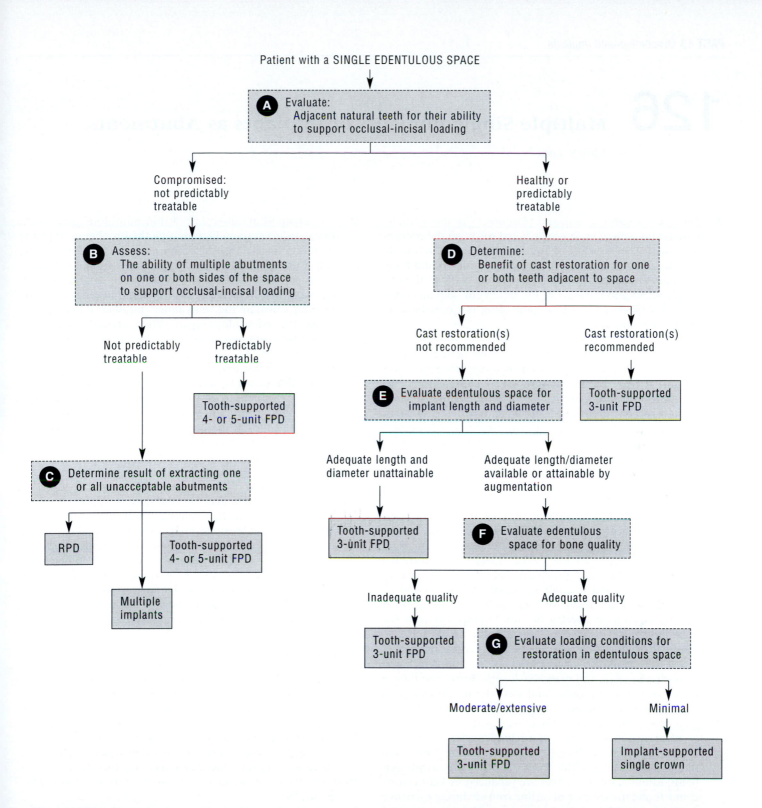

Patient with a SINGLE EDENTULOUS SPACE

A Evaluate:
Adjacent natural teeth for their ability
to support occlusal-incisal loading

Compromised:
not predictably
treatable

Healthy or
predictably
treatable

B Assess:
The ability of multiple abutments
on one or both sides of the space
to support occlusal-incisal loading

D Determine:
Benefit of cast restoration for one
or both teeth adjacent to space

Not predictably
treatable

Predictably
treatable

Cast restoration(s)
not recommended

Cast restoration(s)
recommended

Tooth-supported
4- or 5-unit FPD

E Evaluate edentulous space for
implant length and diameter

Tooth-supported
3-unit FPD

C Determine result of extracting one
or all unacceptable abutments

Adequate length and
diameter unattainable

Adequate length/diameter
available or attainable by
augmentation

RPD

Tooth-supported
4- or 5-unit FPD

Tooth-supported
3-unit FPD

F Evaluate edentulous
space for bone quality

Multiple
implants

Inadequate quality

Adequate quality

Tooth-supported
3-unit FPD

G Evaluate loading conditions for
restoration in edentulous space

Moderate/extensive

Minimal

Tooth-supported
3-unit FPD

Implant-supported
single crown

Additional Readings

Branemark PI, Zarb GA, Albrektsson T. Tissue-integrated prostheses. Chicago: Quintessence Publishing; 1985. p. 201.

Engelman MJ. Clinical decision making and treatment planning in osseointegration. Chicago: Quintessence Publishing; 1996. p. 169.

Jemt T, Lekholm U, Grondahl A. A 3-year follow-up study of early single implant restorations ad modum Branemark. Int J Periodontics Restorative Dent 1990;10:341.

Misch CE. Contemporary implant dentistry. St. Louis: Mosby; 1993. p. 164, 175, 575.

Shillingburg HT et al. Fundamentals of fixed prosthodontics. 3rd ed. Chicago: Quintessence Publishing; 1996. p. 85.

126 Multiple Single Implants or Implants as Abutments

Larry G. Loos

A Decisions regarding implant placement in the partially edentulous patient must not be based solely on the edentulous site. The location, condition, and function of the remaining natural teeth are important in determining the fixed prosthodontic treatment plan. Problematic teeth must be identified and included in the treatment. The mentality of "see a space, place an implant" does not contribute to predictable long-term success.

B The periodontal status of the remaining natural teeth is important whether consideration is being given to tooth-supported fixed partial denture (FPD) abutments, teeth-opposing implants, teeth adjacent to implants, or teeth located remote distances from implants in the same or opposing arch. Remaining teeth contribute directly or indirectly to the forces delivered to the implant(s). Crown-to-root ratio, root morphology, tooth mobility, and wear are necessary determinants for present restorative design and future prognosis.

C Functional incisal loading may be categorized by the static anterior tooth position in maximal intercuspation and its contact relationship during right lateral, left lateral, and protrusive mandibular excursions. Ideally the functional horizontal overlap (ie, the distance between the maxillary lingual surface and mandibular facial surface) should be less than 1 mm. Facial or lingual loading forces then depend on vertical overlap (ie, the distance between the maxillary incisal surface and mandibular incisal surface). Minimal loading forces are created by vertical overlap of 0 to 2 mm. Moderate loading forces result from 3 to 5 mm of vertical overlap, and extensive loading forces result from 6 mm or greater overlap. Parafunctional incisal loading is potentially more damaging because the amount of force is greater and the duration of load is longer.

Parafunctional loading of occlusal surfaces has even greater significance because maximal biting forces are much greater on posterior teeth than they are on anterior teeth. Minimal loading forces are produced by light centric contacts and the absence of incline contact during excursive movements. Solid centric contacts and the presence of incline contact on shallow occlusal morphology produce moderate loading forces. Extensive loading forces are created by heavy centric contacts and the presence of incline contact on steep occlusal morphology.

D The mesiodistal dimension of the edentulous space is the first consideration in determining the number of implants. A minimum distance of 2 mm must exist between adjacent restored implants as they emerge through soft tissue for predictable soft-tissue health to be maintained. By knowing the diameter of each restored implant, the dentist may calculate the "maximum" number of implants for a specific edentulous span. The "actual" number of implants recommended for the space may be determined by evaluating implant length and diameter, bone quality, and implant loading. Implant length is the single most predictable factor in success rates. Larger implant diameters may compensate for shorter implants. Bone quality is determined from radiographs and surgical assessment. Type I and type II are good quality, type III is mediocre, and type IV is poor quality. Implant loading is affected by the anteroposterior location of the restoration, functional contours of the restoration with its opposing surfaces, and the degree and duration of parafunction. A thorough evaluation of these loading conditions produces categories of loading described as minimal, moderate, or extensive. *Unfavorable conditions* for implants include short length implants (less than 10 mm), poor bone quality (type IV), and extensive loading. *Neutral conditions* for implants are average length (10 to 13 mm), average bone quality (type III), and moderate loading. *Favorable conditions* include long implants (15 mm or longer), good quality bone (type I or II), and minimal loading.

Additional Readings

Branemark PI, Zarb GA, Albrektsson T. Tissue-integrated prostheses. Chicago: Quintessence Publishing; 1985. p. 201.

Engelman MJ. Clinical decision making and treatment planning in osseointegration. Chicago: Quintessence Publishing; 1996. p. 169.

Kaukinen JA, Edge MJ, Lang BR. The influence of occlusal design on simulated masticatory forces transferred to implant-retained prostheses and supporting bone. J Prosthet Dent 1996;76:50.

Misch CE. Contemporary implant dentistry. St. Louis: Mosby; 1993. p. 164, 705.

Swanberg DF, Henry MD. Avoiding implant overload. Implant Society 1995;6(1):12–4.

Weinberg LA, Krugar B. Biomechanical considerations when combining tooth-supported and implant-supported prostheses. Oral Surg Oral Med Oral Pathol 1994;78(1):622–7.

Patient with MULTIPLE SINGLE IMPLANTS OR IMPLANTS AS ABUTMENTS

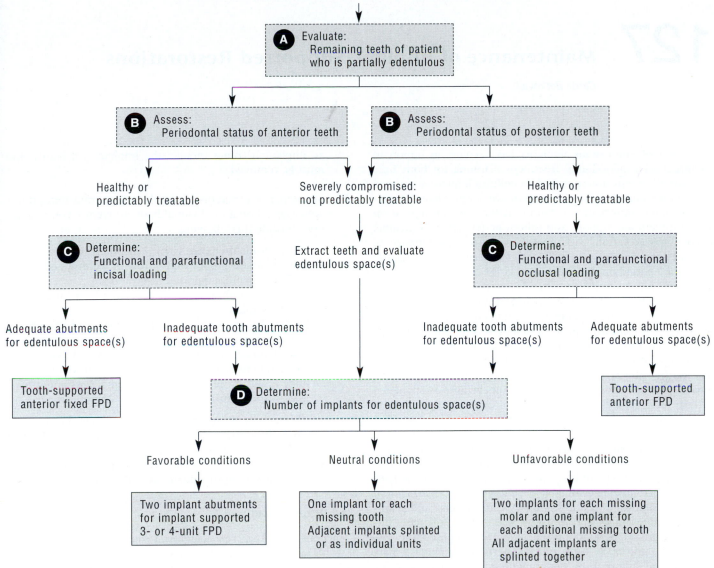

127 Maintenance of Implant-Supported Restorations

Carrie Berkovich

Placement of endosseous implants has become an option in comprehensive periodontal treatment planning for both fully and partially edentulous patients. Benefits of implant-supported restorations include ease of maintenance (unlike fixed bridgework), more conservative restorations that do not depend on adjacent teeth for support, and (often) better esthetic outcome. Following restoration with dental implants, maintenance of implant-supported prosthesis becomes a necessary and regular part of the periodontal maintenance visit.

There are several types of endosseous dental implant systems currently available. They include a range of sizes, shapes, coatings, and prosthetic components. Implant shape is usually a screw-type or cylindrical press-fit design. A threaded screw-type implant may provide additional surface for bonding, and therefore increased support, than a press-fit implant. The implant surface further affects the long-term fixation and stability of the implant. Surface modifications of implants include a roughened surface (acid-etched or grit-blasted), microgrooved or plasma-sprayed titanium, and hydroxyapatite coatings.

A   Just as natural teeth may be affected by periodontal disease, dental implants may develop *periimplantitis*, which is caused by the same type of bacteria as periodontitis. Patients with implants must be evaluated at regular visits for periodontal maintenance procedures and any clinical signs, and symptoms of periimplantitis must be recorded and treated. Clinical signs of periodontitis include radiographic bone loss around implant fixture, inflamed periimplant gingival margin, and suppuration. Periimplantitis can be treated using both surgical and nonsurgical techniques. However, when an implant becomes mobile, the implant is a failure and must be removed.

B   Maintenance programs for implant-supported restorations are designed on an individual basis. Current recommendations include the following:

- Frequent maintenance visits (3–4 times/yr)
- Use of plastic probes and curets or gold-tipped curets around implant-supported restorations
- Avoidance of ultrasonic and steel curet instrumentations around implants
- Rubber-cup polishing using a fine abrasive paste or polishing using air-powdered abrasives
- Patient home care procedures that may include topical chemotherapeutic agents (Listerine, chlorhexidine, or fluoride mouth rinses), dental tape, dental floss, interproximal brushes (proxi-brushes), and end-tuft brushes

Although it is presumed that application of chemical agents such as citric acid and antibiotics can reduce adsorbed bacteria, the clinical significance of these procedures has not yet been determined. These procedures may require a surgical access based on the judgment of the clinician.

Additional Readings

American Academy of Periodontology. Dental implants in periodontal therapy. J Periodontol 2000;71:1934.

Klokkevold PR, Newman MG. Current status of dental implants: a periodontal perspective. Int J Oral Maxillofac Implants 2000;15:56.

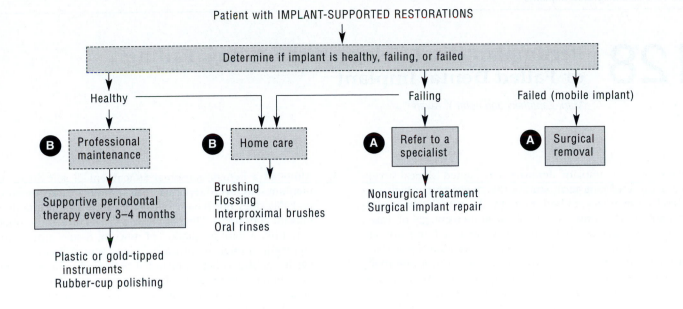

Patient with IMPLANT-SUPPORTED RESTORATIONS

Determine if implant is healthy, failing, or failed

Healthy

Failing

Failed (mobile implant)

B Professional maintenance

B Home care

A Refer to a specialist

A Surgical removal

Supportive periodontal therapy every 3–4 months

Brushing
Flossing
Interproximal brushes
Oral rinses

Nonsurgical treatment
Surgical implant repair

Plastic or gold-tipped instruments
Rubber-cup polishing

128

Periimplantitis: Etiology of the Ailing, Failing, or Failed Dental Implant

Mark Zablotsky and John Y. Kwan

The discipline of implant dentistry has gained clinical acceptance because of long-term studies that suggest very high success and survival rates in both partially and completely edentulous applications; however, in a small percentage of cases, implant failure and morbidity have been reported. Implant failure as a result of surgical overheating of bone has been minimized with the advent of slow-speed, high-torque internally (and often externally) irrigated drilling systems. After integration (either biointegration or osseointegration) has taken place, the major cause of implant failure is thought to be the biomechanics (ie, overload, heavy lateral interferences, lack of a passive prosthesis fit) or infection (plaque induced).

Complications may be eliminated or minimized if clinicians plan treatment adequately. Mounted study models with diagnostic wax-ups or tooth set-ups are mandatory to evaluate ridge relationships, occlusal schemes, and restorative goals. Using adequate radiographs and clinical examination, the implant team (restoring dentist, surgeon, and laboratory technician) can adequately plan for the location, number, and trajectory of implants to ensure the most healthy esthetic and functional prosthesis. Often additional implants may be proposed to satisfy the implant team and patient requirements (eg, fixed versus removable prostheses). The final restoration should be one that is esthetic, is adequately engineered (enough implants of sufficient length in sufficient quality and quantity of supporting bone), and gives the patient accessibility for adequate home care. When evaluating the ailing or failing implant, often one or more of the aforementioned criteria have not been met.

A In referring to a dental implant as ailing, failing, or failed, the dentist really is referring to the status of the periimplant supporting tissues (unless the implant is fractured). An ailing implant displays progressive bone loss and pocketing, but no clinical mobility. A failing implant displays features similar to the ailing implant, but is refractory to therapy and continues to become worse. This implant also is immobile. The term *ailing* suggests a somewhat more favorable prognosis than the term *failing*.

A failed implant is one that is fractured, has been totally refractory to all methods of treatment, or demonstrates clinical mobility or circumferential periimplant radiolucency. These implants must be removed immediately, because progressive destruction of surrounding osseous tissues may occur.

B The etiology of periimplant disease often is multifactorial. Many times the clinician must do detective work to discover the etiology. Meffert (1996) has coined the terms *traditional* and *retrograde* pathways in differentiating bacterial versus biomechanic etiologies.

C Although a hemidesmosomal attachment of soft tissues to titanium has been reported, this histologic phenomenon probably does not have clinical relevance around titanium implant abutments. The periimplant seal is thought to originate from a tight adaptation of mucosal tissues around the abutment through an intricate arrangement of circular gingival fibers and a tight junctional epithelium. Because this "attachment" is tenuous at best, a plaque-induced (traditional pathway) periimplant gingivitis may not truly exist and plaque-induced inflammation of periimplant tissues may directly extend to the underlying supporting osseous tissues.

The periodontal ligament acts as a "shock absorber" around the natural tooth when excessive occlusal or orthodontic forces are present. In the absence of bacterial plaque, occlusal trauma does not cause a loss of attachment to teeth; however, because implants lack a periodontal ligament, force may be transmitted to the implant or bone interface. If significant enough, microfractures of this interface may occur and allow for an ingress of soft tissues and secondary bacterial infection.

In fixed bridgework that does not fit passively and is cemented on natural teeth, orthodontic movement of abutments occurs because of the presence of the periodontal ligament. In this scenario, little if any damage occurs around abutments because of this orthodontic movement. If this same phenomenon occurs on dental implant abutments (either screw retained or cemented), one of a few complications may result. The restoration may become loose as a result of cement failure, screws backing out, or fracture. Abutments may loosen or fracture, or the implant body may fracture or have bone loss because of progressive microfractures at the interface (retrograde pathway); therefore, frameworks must fit precisely. Lateral interferences or excessive off-axis loading have led to greater stresses on components and the implant-bone interface and should be minimized. Bruxism may be extremely destructive and should be addressed by modifying occlusal schemes to eliminate lateral contacts in function or parafunction; alternatively the patient should commit to permanent splint or night guard treatment before placement of the implant. In some instances, a removable prosthesis may be fashioned to address this concern.

Clinical signs of periimplant problems in the ailing or failing implant include increased probing depths, bleeding on probing, suppuration, erythema and flaccidity of tissues, and radiographically evident bone loss. Pain may be present, but usually it is a late symptom. If plaque is absent with minimally inflamed tissues, the dentist must suspect occlusal etiology. Often this may be confirmed with culture and sensitivity testing. If bacteria associated

Patient with INCREASING PROBING DEPTHS AND BONE LOSS

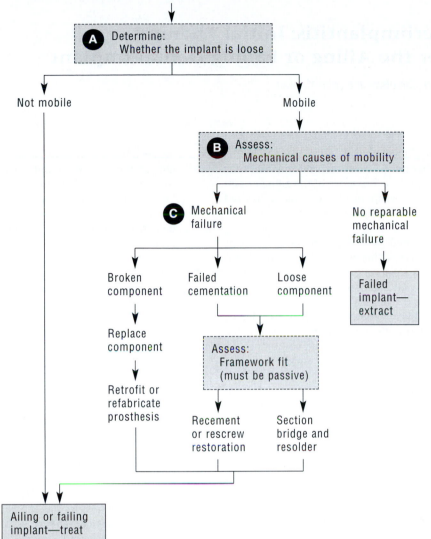

with gingival health are present (eg, *Streptococcus* sp or *Actinomyces* sp), an occlusal component is strongly suggested. If, however, periodontal pathogens (eg, *P. gingivalis*, *P. intermedius*) are present, the dentist should have a high suspicion for periimplant infection. This is not to say that an occlusal component may not also be present. Inspect restorations for fit. A loose restoration is always bad news. Remove and evaluate each component until the loose or failed component is found. If the implant is loose, it is a failure and should be removed immediately. It will never reintegrate and be functional. Replacement implants may be placed either at the time of implant removal or within 6 months of implant removal, and various regenerative techniques may be contemplated to maintain alveolar height and width.

Additional Readings

Meffert R. Periodontitis vs peri-implantitis. The same disease? The same treatment? Br Rev Oral Biol Med 1996;7:278.

Meffert R, Block M, Kent J. What is osseointegration? Int J Periodontics Restorative Dent 1987;11(2):88.

Newman M, Fleming T. Periodontal considerations of implants and implant associated microbiota. J Dent Educ 1988;52:737.

Rosenberg E, Torosian J, Slots J. Microbial differences in 2 distinct types of failures of osseointegrated implants. Clin Oral Implant Res 1991;2:135.

129 Periimplantitis: Initial Therapy for the Ailing or Failing Dental Implant

Mark Zablotsky and John Y. Kwan

A differential diagnosis should be made as early as possible in the initial stages of implant therapy because such information may be crucial in the follow-up and maintenance of the ailing or failing implant. If an accurate assessment of the etiology has not been established, interceptive therapy may be compromised.

A Effective patient-performed plaque control is mandatory, and the patient must accept this responsibility. The therapist should customize a hygiene regimen for each implant patient. The use of conventional oral hygiene aids (ie, brush, floss) may be augmented with any number of instruments (eg, Superfloss, yarn, plastic-coated proxibrushes, electric toothbrushes). If the patient's oral hygiene is suspect, the addition of a topical application of chemotherapeutics (eg, chlorhexidine), either by rinsing or applying locally (using a dipping brush), may be beneficial in maintenance. The restorative dentist must give the patient access to implant abutments circumferentially to ensure hygiene.

B Evaluate occlusion and eliminate centric and lateral prematurities and interferences with occlusal adjustment. Initiate night guard or splint therapy if parafunctional activity is suspected. Often the clinician can remove the prosthesis and place healing cuffs on the implants in hopes of getting a positive response by reducing the load if occlusal etiology is suspected. Single implants that are attached to mobile natural teeth may be overloaded as a result of compression and subsequent relative cantilevering of the prosthesis from the implant. If occlusal etiology is suspected in this case, contemplate the attachment of more implants to the existing weakened implant to support the cantilever of periodontally weak teeth. If the dentist suspects bacterial etiology, initial conservative treatment may consist of subgingival irrigation with a blunt-tipped, side-port irrigating needle. Chlorhexidine is the irrigant of choice. Local application of tetracycline using monolithic fibers may be an effective adjunct.

C Perform culture and sensitivity testing to guide therapy if a course of systemic antibiotics is planned. Consider débridement of hyperplastic periimplant tissues using hand or ultrasonic plastic (if the implant or abutment is going to be touched) instrumentation.

D Ideally the implant abutment should emerge through attached keratinized mucosa. This gives the patient an ideal mucosa. It also gives the patient an ideal environment to perform home care because movable alveolar mucosal margins may be irritating and cause difficulty in effecting oral hygiene. Increased failures of implants and morbidity have been associated with areas deficient in attached keratinized gingival tissues. Soft-tissue augmentation procedures may be performed either before implant placement, during integration, at uncovering (stage 2), or for repair procedures.

E Consider reevaluation of periimplant tissues 2 to 4 weeks after initial therapy. Probing depths should be reduced, and no bleeding or suppuration should occur on probing. The clinician must decide whether the improvement in clinical indices is a predictable long-term end point. The dentist also must remember that the success of periodontal therapy depends on the therapist's ability to remove plaque, calculus, and other bacterial products from radicular surfaces. Because root planing the implant surfaces is neither possible nor recommended (because of the detrimental effects of conventional curets and ultrasonics), the dentist must consider that the titanium abutment or hydroxyapatite-coated titanium implant surface is contaminated with bacteria and their products (ie, endotoxins). Therefore, the dentist must conclude that the implant and periimplant tissues will benefit from surgical intervention.

If the therapist feels that a successful end point has been attained, close maintenance with monitoring of clinical, radiographic, and microbiologic parameters is imperative. If problems recur promptly, the dentist must question either the initial diagnosis (incorrect etiology) or the predictability of more conservative nonsurgical therapy. In this instance, the clinician should strive to stabilize or arrest the active disease process nonsurgically, then reevaluate to determine a clinical end point. Commonly, cases that are refractory to nonsurgical therapy do well after surgical intervention because the contaminated implant surface may be addressed more adequately during surgery.

Additional Readings

Gammage D, Bowman A, Meffert R. Clinical management of failing dental implants: four case reports. J Oral Implants 1989;15:124.

Kwan J. Implant maintenance. J Calif Dent Assoc 1991;19(12):45.

Kwan J, Zablotsky M. The ailing implant. J Calif Dent Assoc 1991;19(12):51.

Orton G, Steele D, Wolinsky L. The dental professional's role in monitoring and maintenance of tissue-integrated prostheses. Int J Oral Maxillofac Implants 1989;4:305.

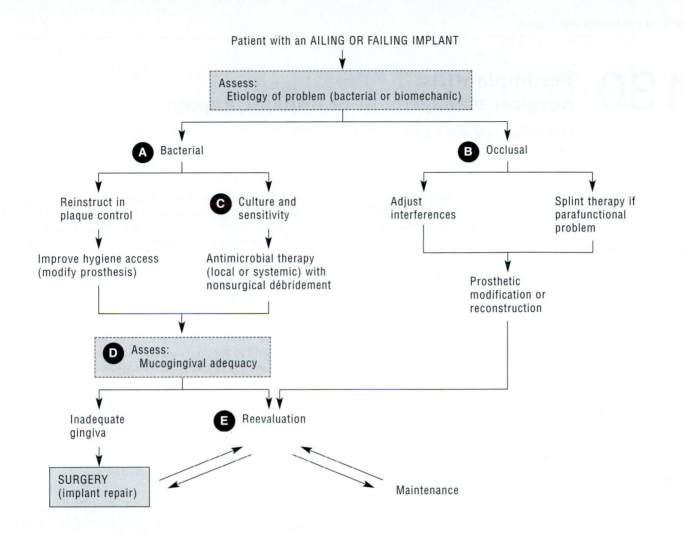

130 Periimplantitis: Surgical Management of Implant Repair

Mark Zablotsky and John Y. Kwan

The surgical repair of the ailing or failing implant depends on an accurate diagnosis and effective nonsurgical intervention to stabilize or arrest the progression of the active periimplant lesion.

A   The dentist must assess the mucogingival status of periimplant tissues before repair surgery. If mucogingival defects exist only around the ailing or failing implant, subsequent osseous repair surgery may not be necessary if soft-tissue augmentation is performed around the ailing or failing implant. If indicated, osseous repair surgery on keratinized tissues is less technically demanding.

B   Modifications of periodontal surgical procedures, either resective or regenerative, have been reported with some success. After making the initial incisions and degranulating the osseous defect (open débridement), the dentist must evaluate the defect before selecting the appropriate surgical modality.

C   Periimplant osseous defects that are predominantly horizontal in nature respond most predictably to resective procedures (ie, definitive osseous surgery) with or without fixture modification.

D   Fixture modification is performed to remove macroscopic or microscopic features that interfere with subsequent plaque control in the supracrestal aspect of the defect. Fixture modification consists of smoothing with a series of rotary instruments in descending grit (ie, fine diamond, white stone, rubber points) and using copious irrigation because these instruments may generate significant heat. Some clinicians concerned about contaminating implant surfaces or periimplant tissues with rotary instruments have reported a healthy soft-tissue response against hydroxyapatite-coated or plasma-sprayed titanium implant surfaces. If the patient's oral hygiene is suspect, consider fixture modification for these microscopically rough surfaces.

E   Regenerative procedures—bone grafting with or without guided tissue regeneration (GTR)—have been reported for the repair of the ailing or failing implant. Regenerative procedures are most appropriate if the adjacent osseous crest is close to the rim of the implant (ie, narrow two- or three-walled moat, dehiscence or fenestration defects) (Figures 130-1 through 130-3). If the dentist is considering these procedures, fixture modification is not recommended.

F   Detoxification procedures to treat the infected implant surface are recommended before regenerative modalities. A 30-second to 1-minute application of a supersaturated solution of citric acid (pH 1) burnished with a cotton pledget may be beneficial in detoxifying the infected hydroxyapatite-coated implant surface. If the coating appears pitted and altered, however, the coating should be removed either with ultrasonic or air/powder abrasives. A short application of an air/powder abrasive detoxifies the titanium implant surface. Extreme caution is recommended if the defect to be treated with the air/powder abrasive is a narrow intrabony

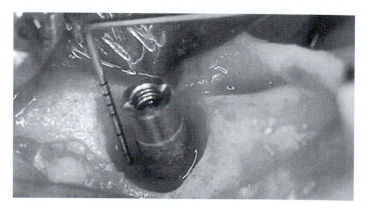

Figure 130-2 The defect surgically exposed prior to ePTFE membrane placement.

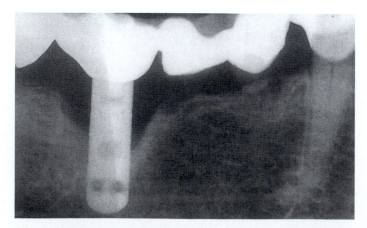

Figure 130-1 Preoperative radiograph of an "ailing" implant prior to guided bone augmentation repair.

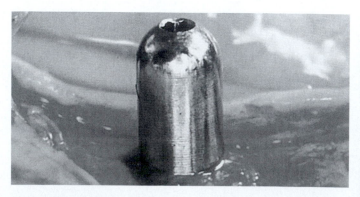

Figure 130-3 Six months after guided bone augmentation, the defect is filled with hard tissue.

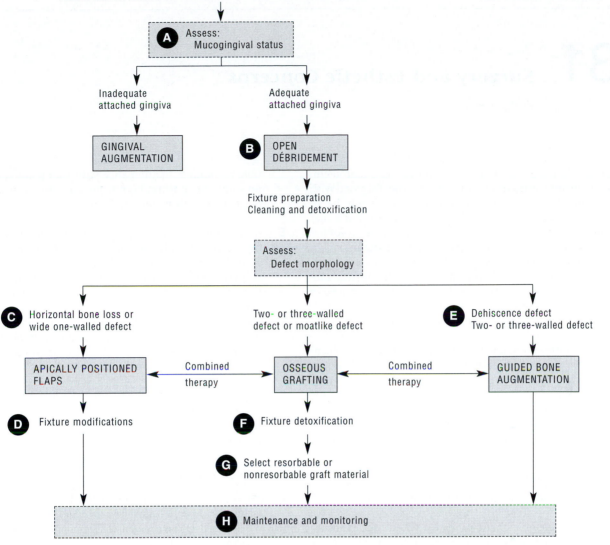

Patient with an AILING OR FAILING IMPLANT AND SURGERY INDICATED

A Assess: Mucogingival status

- Inadequate attached gingiva → GINGIVAL AUGMENTATION
- Adequate attached gingiva → **B** OPEN DÉBRIDEMENT

Fixture preparation
Cleaning and detoxification

Assess: Defect morphology

C Horizontal bone loss or wide one-walled defect → APICALLY POSITIONED FLAPS

Two- or three-walled defect or moatlike defect → OSSEOUS GRAFTING

E Dehiscence defect Two- or three-walled defect → GUIDED BONE AUGMENTATION

Combined therapy

D Fixture modifications

F Fixture detoxification

G Select resorbable or nonresorbable graft material

H Maintenance and monitoring

defect because pressurized air may enter the marrow spaces and produce a risk of embolism.

G The choice of bone-grafting materials should be based on the clinician's level of certainty that the site to be grafted is free of bacterial contaminants. If the clinician is certain that the defect is not contaminated, resorbable materials such as autogenous bone, detoxified freeze-dried bone allograph, resorbable hydroxyapatite, or GTR materials may be considered. If the surface of the implant is suspect, nonresorbable materials, for example, dense nonresorbable hydroxyapatite) should be considered. Use nonresorbable bone-grafting materials to obturate apical vents and basket holes because osseous regeneration probably will not occur in these anatomically contaminated environments.

Contemplate combined therapies whenever defect combinations include horizontal bone loss and dehiscence or intrabony defects. Postoperative care is much like that for periodontal surgical procedures, with close follow-up and reevaluation before the patient is placed back on a supportive maintenance schedule.

H The goals of periimplant surgical and nonsurgical therapies are to reestablish a healthy perimucosal seal and regenerate a soft- or hard-tissue attachment to the implant and abutment. This requires a definitive diagnosis, comprehensive therapy,

and effective maintenance. At this time, no prospective or retrospective studies exist examining the short- or long-term results attained through implant repair procedures; therefore close follow-up for recurrence of disease is warranted. Although the goals of therapy are clear, the clinician must be willing to accept and recognize failure if it occurs. The dental implant that is refractory to all attempts at treatment is a failure and should be removed as soon as this diagnosis is made.

Additional Readings

Lozada J et al. Surgical repair of peri-implant defects. J Oral Implant 1990;16:42.

Meffert R. How to treat ailing and failing implants. Implant Dent 1992;1:25.

Meffert R. Periodontitis vs peri-implantitis: the same disease? The same treatment? Br Rev Oral Biol Med 1996;7:278.

Zablotsky M. The surgical management of osseous defects associated with endosteal hydroxylapatite-coated and titanium dental implants. Dent Clin North Am 1992;36(1):117.

Zablotsky M, Diedrich D, Meffert R. The ability of various chemotherapeutic agents to detoxify the endotoxin-contaminated titanium implant surface. Implant Dent. [In press]

Zablotsky M et al. The ability of various chemotherapeutic agents to detoxify the endotoxin infected HA-coated implant surface. Int J Oral Maxillofac Implants 1991;8(2):45.

131 Surgery and Esthetic Concerns

Walter B. Hall

Before undertaking a surgical solution to a periodontal problem, two types of ensuing esthetic concerns need to be discussed with the patient: one is, in certain areas, root exposure might be an unsightly consequence of periodontal surgery; the second is that ridge resorption after tooth extraction may create a grotesque form. These problems are most likely to occur in the maxillary anterior, premolar, and, occasionally, first molar areas. A surgical procedure in these areas therefore may be a therapeutic success but an esthetic disaster. This result may not be acceptable to the patient, and so discussion to obtain informed (even if unwritten) consent prior to treatment is necessary.

A What the dentist considers to be a potential esthetic problem may not be a problem to the patient. If an informed patient is not bothered by potential esthetic problems, the dentist should select the best procedure to accomplish therapeutic goals without the restrictions that esthetic concerns entail (eg, pocket elimination may be the objective with no concomitant concern for the unsightliness of exposed roots).

B If the patient does perceive esthetics to be an important concern, the dentist must select a treatment approach that will yield both an esthetic and a therapeutic result.

C Surgery may create esthetic problems when root exposure is the result in readily visible areas of the mouth. Ridge inadequacy may be created by extracting a tooth. Both the problem of root exposure and the problem of ridge inadequacy can be remedied.

D If the roots of the teeth in the surgical segment are round, and the pocket depths are not large enough to be inacces-

sible to planing, maintenance with root planing alone (and no surgical exposure) best meets the esthetic and therapeutic goals of both patient and dentist.

E If the roots of the teeth in the surgical segment contain flutings or furcation involvements, or the pockets are so deep as to be inaccessible for planing, the type of surgery to employ depends on the nature of the osseous defects. If there is only horizontal bone loss and it is not severe, or if vertical defects (but not bone loss) are present, guided tissue regeneration (GTR) provides a reasonable approach with which to meet the esthetic and therapeutic goals of the patient and the dentist. If horizontal bone loss is great, extractions followed by implants should be considered.

F If the esthetic problem is one of ridge inadequacy that would compromise the esthetics of a planned restoration, ridge augmentation is an option that should be offered to the patient (see Chapter 115).

Additional Readings

Allen EP et al. Improved technique for localized ridge augmentation: a report of 21 cases. J Periodontol 1985;56:195.

Hall WB. Periodontal preparation of the mouth for restoration. Dent Clin North Am 1980;24:204.

Schluger S et al. Periodontal diseases. 2nd ed. Philadelphia: Lea & Febiger; 1989. p. 500.

Seibert J. Reconstruction of deformed partially edentulous ridges using full-thickness grafts: technique and wound healing. Compend Cont Educ Dent 1983;4:437.

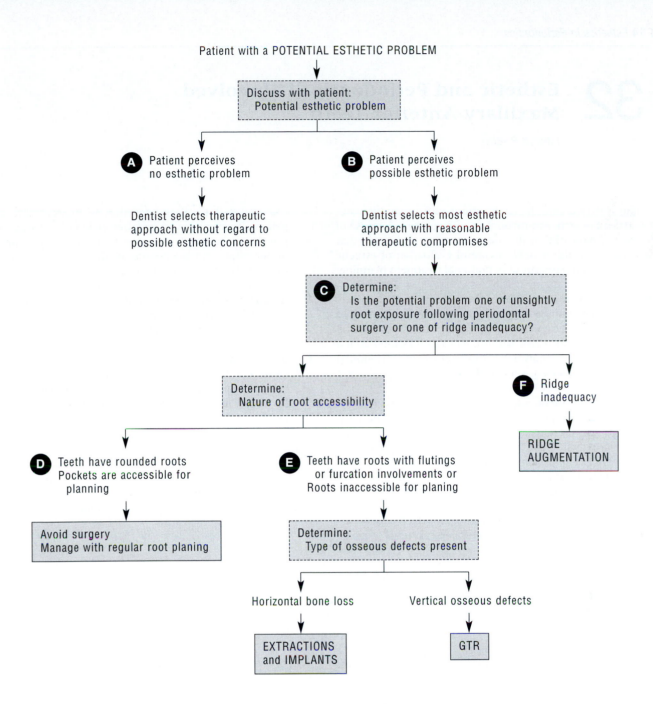

Patient with a POTENTIAL ESTHETIC PROBLEM

Discuss with patient:
Potential esthetic problem

A Patient perceives
no esthetic problem

B Patient perceives
possible esthetic problem

Dentist selects therapeutic
approach without regard to
possible esthetic concerns

Dentist selects most esthetic
approach with reasonable
therapeutic compromises

C Determine:
Is the potential problem one of unsightly
root exposure following periodontal
surgery or one of ridge inadequacy?

Determine:
Nature of root accessibility

F Ridge
inadequacy

RIDGE
AUGMENTATION

D Teeth have rounded roots
Pockets are accessible for
planing

E Teeth have roots with flutings
or furcation involvements or
Roots inaccessible for planing

Avoid surgery
Manage with regular root planing

Determine:
Type of osseous defects present

Horizontal bone loss

Vertical osseous defects

EXTRACTIONS
and IMPLANTS

GTR

132 Esthetic and Periodontically Involved Maxillary Anterior Teeth

Edward P. Allen

Treatment of periodontal disease in the maxillary anterior segment may lead to esthetic problems in some patients because of the destructive nature of the disease process. To avoid results that are dissatisfying to the patient, a careful evaluation of esthetic considerations should be part of periodontal treatment planning.

A   First, perform an evaluation of the patient's smile to determine whether papillary or marginal gingiva is exposed. If the patient has no gingival exposure, optimal periodontal therapy may be provided without concern for esthetics. If a high lip line with gingival exposure is evident, periodontal therapy may adversely affect esthetics.

B   The potential esthetic impact of periodontal therapy must be discussed with the patient. If the patient is unconcerned with the possible effects, appropriate periodontal therapy may be provided. If the patient is concerned with esthetics, a conservative approach is indicated. This may be accomplished by root débridement through a closed approach followed by an evaluation of response to treatment.

C   Even in moderate-to-severe cases in which disease is controlled by a conservative approach, esthetics may be compromised to an extent that is unacceptable to the patient. Two options to improve esthetics at this point are prosthetic therapy or removal of the teeth with ridge preservation and augmentation therapy, where required, followed by prosthetic therapy.

D   In cases in which closed débridement has controlled the disease, and esthetics are acceptable, the patient may be placed on a systematic maintenance program.

E   If the disease has not been controlled by the initial conservative therapy, a surgical approach, including regenerative therapy, open flap débridement, or pocket-elimination therapy, is indicated. Surgical therapy would be followed by prosthetic evaluation and therapy as needed for esthetics.

Additional Readings

Allen EP. Use of mucogingival surgical procedures to enhance esthetics. Dent Clin North Am 1988;32:307.

Hall WB. Periodontal preparation of the mouth for restoration. Dent Clin North Am 1980;24:204.

Patient with PERIODONTAL DISEASE INVOLVING THE MAXILLARY ANTERIOR TEETH

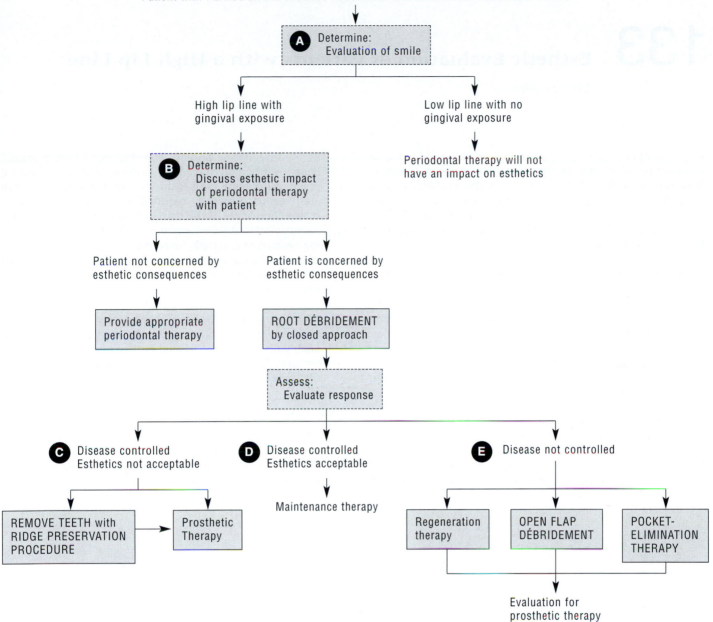

133 Esthetic Evaluation of Patients with a High Lip Line

Edward P. Allen

When a patient comes to the practitioner with an esthetic concern because of a high lip line or "gummy" smile, a careful evaluation is indicated. In many cases this problem can be treated by surgical exposure of more tooth length, as the sole treatment or as a finishing procedure orthognathic therapy. The first step in the esthetic evaluation is a determination of clinical crown length.

A If the clinical crown length is normal, evaluate the patient for possible vertical maxillary excess (VME). If VME is not present, the gummy smile may be caused by excessive muscle activity or a short upper lip, and no treatment is indicated. If VME is present, orthognathic surgery is indicated.

B If the clinical crown length is less than normal, evaluate the patient for VME. If VME is present, evaluate the patient for orthognathic surgery. After this evaluation, or if no VME is evident, determine the length of the anatomic crown by probing for the subgingival location of the cementoenamel junction (CEJ) on the facial aspect of the teeth.

C If the anatomic crown is incompletely exposed, surgical crown lengthening to the level of the CEJ is indicated.

Before surgery, the position and thickness of the marginal bone must be determined by sounding with a periodontal probe. If the bony crest is thick or located at the CEJ, flap and osseous surgery is required to expose the anatomic crown completely. If the margin is thin and approximately 2 mm apical to the CEJ, excision of the marginal tissue during internal or external gingivectomy is indicated, provided adequate dimensions of gingiva remain postsurgically. If the gingival dimensions will still be inadequate, crown lengthening by flap surgery is required.

D In some patients with short clinical crowns, the anatomic crown also is short and may already be completely exposed. Such patients may be treated by flap and osseous surgery for tooth lengthening, but they must then be treated prosthetically to achieve an esthetic result.

Additional Readings

Allen EP. Use of mucogingival surgical procedures to enhance esthetics. Dent Clin North Am 1988;32:307.

Bell WH. Modern practice in orthognathic and reconstructive surgery. Philadelphia: WB Saunders; 1991.

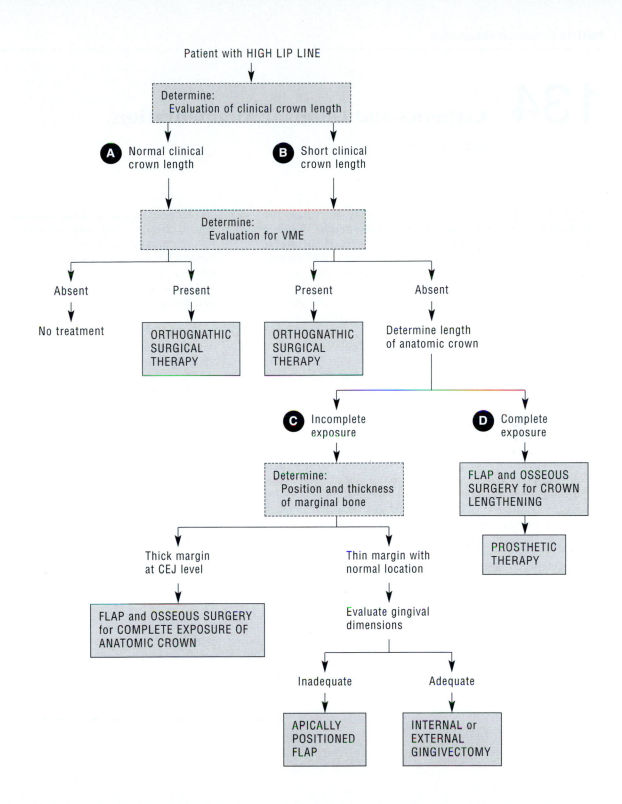

Patient with HIGH LIP LINE

Determine:
Evaluation of clinical crown length

A Normal clinical crown length

B Short clinical crown length

Determine:
Evaluation for VME

Absent

Present

Present

Absent

No treatment

ORTHOGNATHIC SURGICAL THERAPY

ORTHOGNATHIC SURGICAL THERAPY

Determine length of anatomic crown

C Incomplete exposure

D Complete exposure

Determine:
Position and thickness of marginal bone

FLAP and OSSEOUS SURGERY for CROWN LENGTHENING

Thick margin at CEJ level

Thin margin with normal location

PROSTHETIC THERAPY

FLAP and OSSEOUS SURGERY for COMPLETE EXPOSURE OF ANATOMIC CROWN

Evaluate gingival dimensions

Inadequate

Adequate

APICALLY POSITIONED FLAP

INTERNAL or EXTERNAL GINGIVECTOMY

134 Esthetics and Gingival Augmentation

Edward P. Allen

In determining the need for a gingival grafting procedure, the practitioner must evaluate several factors before deciding whether treatment is needed. If treatment is needed, the practitioner must assess whether the procedure selected will be for root coverage or for gingival augmentation without root coverage.

A The practitioner must determine the presence of gingival recession, recording the distance from the gingival margin to the cementoenamel junction and the classification of recession. This decision tree applies to Miller Class I and Class II recession. Complete root coverage is predictable only in these classifications in which no loss of interdental bone or soft tissue occurs.

B The need for certain dimensions of gingiva for the prevention of recession remains controversial. However, the observation of progressive recession is generally accepted as an indication of a need to increase the width and thickness of marginal tissue. Also, in certain clinical situations, including orthodontic therapy and the placement of subgingival restoration margins, a need to increase the gingival dimension to prevent recession may be evident.

C The esthetic impact of recession is most often seen in the maxillary arch and includes the incisors, canines, premolars, and occasionally molars. In patients with high lip lines, recession in the maxillary arch requires root-cover grafting to restore a natural appearance. This is particularly important in patients who are having restorative procedures performed in this area. The normal form of the tooth and proper harmony with adjacent teeth should be corrected by treating the recession before performing the restorative procedures.

D Root sensitivity may be treated in a variety of ways. In sites in which complete root coverage can be achieved, it may be the most desirable procedure. Areas of root exposure with shallow caries and shallow restorations also can be treated using root-cover grafting.

Additional Readings

Miller PD Jr. A classification of marginal tissue recession. Int J Periodontics Restorative Dent 1985;5:9.

Newman MG, Takei HH, Carranza FA. Carranza's clinical periodontology. 9th ed. Philadelphia: WB Saunders; 2002. p. 854–72.

Pini-Prato GP et al. Periodontal regeneration therapy with coverage of previously restored root surfaces: a two case report. Int J Periodontics Restorative Dent 1992;12:451.

Wennström JL et al. Some periodontal tissue reactions to orthodontic tooth movement in monkeys. J Clin Periodontol 1987;14:121.

Patient with PERIODONTAL DISEASE INVOLVING THE MAXILLARY ANTERIOR TEETH

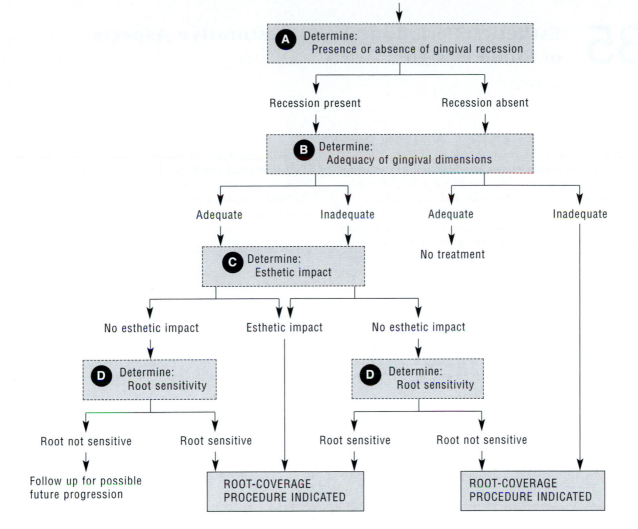

135 Esthetics: Periodontal and Restorative Aspects of Smile Design

Ian Van Zyl

Smile design involves the lips, gingivae, and teeth (Figure 135-1). The lips and the lower teeth can move; this requires a dynamic solution to esthetic problems. Shape design involves the shape of the teeth and gingivae and can be altered by the dentist.

Esthetic smile design is complex, simplified by breaking the problem down into component parts. The teeth are the picture, the gingivae the frame, and the lips the movable curtains. For a pleasing smile, the lips and gingivae need to be in harmony with well-proportioned teeth. Teeth lose their ideal proportion with age. This is due to incisal edges wearing faster than proximal surfaces, so that the ideal length-to-width ratio of 1.6:1 is lost. Ideal proportion can be regained by increasing the length of the crown. This can be done gingivally, incisally, or both.

Planning gingival recontouring is easily performed on accurate stone casts. Changes in height and contour of the free gingival margin can be chiseled and marked on the cast (picture).

By combining this with waxing up the teeth, an accurate model of the final result can be made. Using the technique of simulated shape design, this can be tried in the mouth.

First consider esthetics of the lips, then the free gingival margin shape, and finally tooth proportions.

Additional Readings

Chiche G, Pinault A. Anterior fixed prosthodontics. Chicago: Quintessence Publishing; 1994.

Rufenacht CR. Fundamentals of esthetics. Chicago: Quintessence Publishing; 1990.

Scharer P, Rinn LA, Kopp FR. Esthetic guidelines for restorative dentistry. Chicago: Quintessence Publishing; 1982.

Van Zyl IP, Geissberger M. Simulated shape design: helping patients decide their esthetic ideal. J Am Dent Assoc 2001;132(Aug):1105.

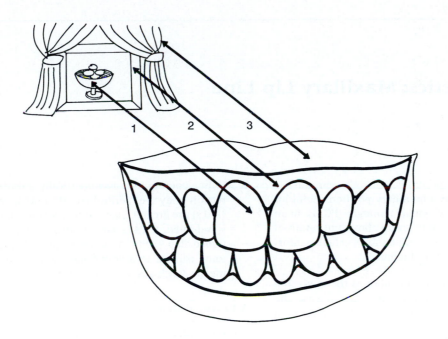

Figure 135-1 Esthetic smile design broken down into component parts. 1. Picture = teeth. 2. Frame = gingivae. 3. Curtain = lips.

136 Esthetics: Maxillary Lip Line

Ian Van Zyl

The upper lip can assume many positions. The only reproducible position is a forced smile. This is a boundary position useful for deciding on the position of the free gingival margin (FGM). In an ideal forced smile, the upper lip rests 1 mm above the zenith of the FGM. Taking a picture of a forced smile shows valuable information usually lost by movement of the lip.

A   If the upper lip covers one-third or more of the teeth in a forced smile, consider frenectomy. This may release the upper lip to move more coronally and display more teeth and FGM (Figure 136-1A and B).

B   If the upper lip rises 2 mm or more beyond the FGM, the shape of the FGM becomes critical, and ideal tooth proportion and gingival position reduce the "gumminess" of the smile. Attention to esthetic details can still produce a pleasing smile (Figure 136-1C).

C   If the upper lip rises asymmetrically, a unilateral surgical correction may be performed. If probing attachment levels (PALs) are greater than 3 mm, recontouring by gingivectomy is indicated. If PALs are less than 3 mm, an apically repositioned flap (APF) must be employed, possibly with ostectomy (similar to a crown-lengthening procedure). By these means, tooth size harmony of the two sides can be created.

Additional Readings

Chiche G, Pinault A. Anterior fixed prosthodontics. Chicago: Quintessence Publishing; 1994.

Rufenacht CR. Fundamentals of esthetics. Chicago: Quintessence Publishing; 1990.

Scharer P, Rinn LA, Kopp FR. Esthetic guidelines for restorative dentistry. Chicago: Quintessence Publishing; 1982.

Van Zyl IP, Geissberger M. Simulated shape design: helping patients decide their esthetic ideal. J Am Dent Assoc 2001;132(Aug):1105.

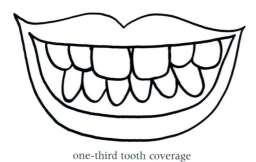

A   one-third tooth coverage

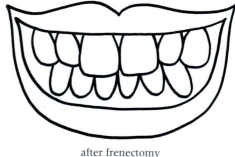

B   after frenectomy

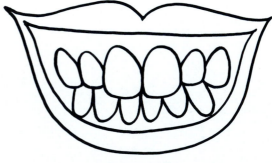

C   gummy smile

Figure 136-1 Considerations in position of maxillary lip line with a forced smile. *A,* Teeth covered by low lip line. *B,* Corrected by means of frenectomy. *C,* "Gummy" smile where considerable gingiva is exposed when smiling broadly.

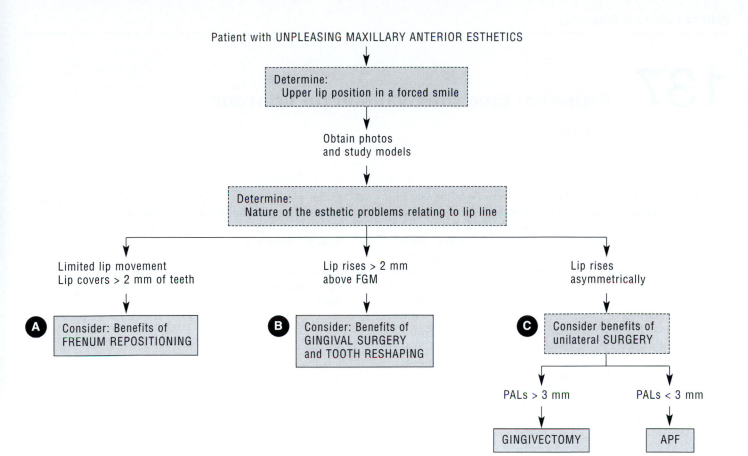

Patient with UNPLEASING MAXILLARY ANTERIOR ESTHETICS

Determine:
Upper lip position in a forced smile

Obtain photos
and study models

Determine:
Nature of the esthetic problems relating to lip line

Limited lip movement
Lip covers > 2 mm of teeth

Lip rises > 2 mm
above FGM

Lip rises
asymmetrically

A Consider: Benefits of
FRENUM REPOSITIONING

B Consider: Benefits of
GINGIVAL SURGERY
and TOOTH RESHAPING

C Consider benefits of
unilateral SURGERY

PALs > 3 mm

PALs < 3 mm

GINGIVECTOMY

APF

137 Esthetics: Free Gingival Margin Contour

Ian Van Zyl

Ideal free gingival margin (FGM) form adds to the dominance of the central incisors. Draw a line through the zenith of the FGM of the centrals and canines. This line should be close to the esthetic plane. The gingival zenith of the lateral incisors are ideally 0.5 to 1 mm short of this line. This makes the lateral incisors appear recessive. Long axes of teeth can be distalized by placing the zenith of the FGM in the distal third. Distalized long axes of the teeth make the smile look broader and the teeth less crowded. The gingival zenith should be positioned in the middle of teeth numbers 7 and 10. Leaning all long axes to the distal will make a broader-looking smile.

A The FGMs of the lateral incisors frequently are at the same level as those of the central incisors. This causes the central incisors to lose dominance. Depending on lip level, this problem can be corrected in three ways. First, lengthen the central incisor to be 1 mm apical to the lateral incisors' zenith, which would be most esthetic in a patient presenting with a high lip line. Second, slow extrusion of the laterals may bring down the height of the FGMs. Finally, consider a graft or augmentation procedure on the lateral incisors. Various combinations of these procedures can be utilized to optimize esthetic results.

B If the teeth have a short length-to-width ratio, consider gingivectomy or modification by flap design to put the gingival zenith in the distal third which makes the smile look broader (long axes lean to the distal) and the teeth longer.

C There may be a step in the undulating line of the FGM, often distal to numbers 5 or 6 and numbers 11 or 12. Consider repositioning the FGM to reestablish radiating symmetry by means of gingivectomy if probing attachment levels (PALs) are greater than 3 mm or by crown lengthening if PALs are less than 3 mm.

Additional Readings

Chiche G, Pinault A. Anterior fixed prosthodontics. Chicago: Quintessence Publishing; 1994.

Rufenacht CR. Fundamentals of esthetics. Chicago: Quintessence Publishing; 1990.

Scharer P, Rinn LA, Kopp FR. Esthetic guidelines for restorative dentistry. Chicago: Quintessence Publishing; 1982.

Van Zyl IP, Geissberger M. Simulated shape design: helping patients decide their esthetic ideal. J Am Dent Assoc 2001;132(Aug):1105.

Patient with an ESTHETIC PROBLEM RELATING TO FREE GINGIVAL MARGIN CONTOURS

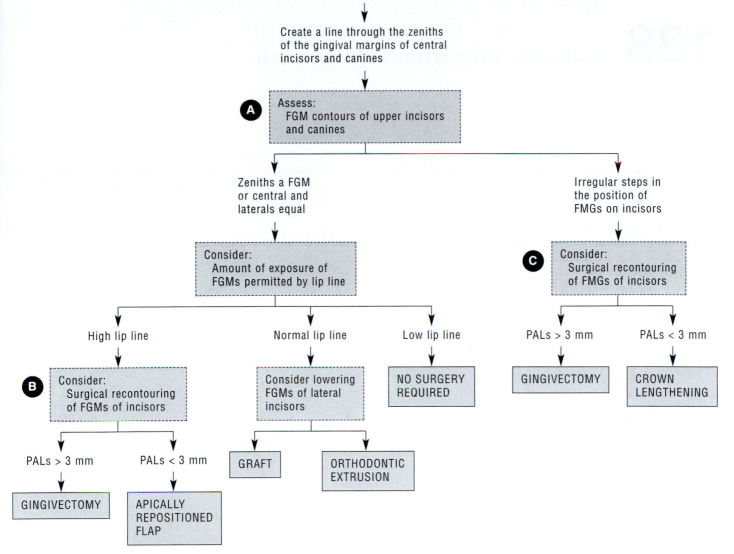

138   Esthetics: Proportions of the Teeth

Ian Van Zyl

Esthetically pleasing teeth make patients look younger. Ideal proportions are close to a length-to-width ratio of 1.6 to 1. Length can be altered in two ways: gingivally or incisally (Figure 138-1).

A   For a length-to-width ratio under 1 to 1 (Figure 138-2A), increase the height of the clinical crown with a gingivectomy or gingival sculpting, if probing attachment levels (PALs) exceed 3 mm. Otherwise, consider an apically positioned flap (APF) procedure to make the gingival zenith of the free gingival margin (FGM) more distal to achieve the ideal length-to-width ratio of 1.6 to 1 (Figure 138-2B).

B   For teeth with a length-to-width ratio greater than 1.8 to 1, consider the upper lip line. If in a forced smile the lip covers the gingival recession, no treatment is necessary for esthetic purposes. For ideal proportion, or high lip line, the FGM needs to be restored at a lower level. Treatment possibilities include slow forced eruption, grafting, or augmentation procedures. It is also possible to use a pink silicone gingival shroud, although this is rarely acceptable to patients (Figure 138-2B).

C   Teeth that are too narrow or too wide may be improved by reshaping their crowns. Those that are too wide may be narrowed by reshaping them using enamel plasty. Those that are too narrow may be reshaped using composite buildups or veneer (Figure 138-2C).

A combination of B and C may be used (Figure 138-2D).

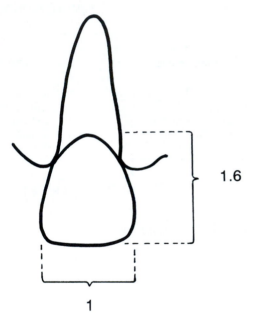

Figure 138-1 Ideal ratio of length of crown to width of crown.

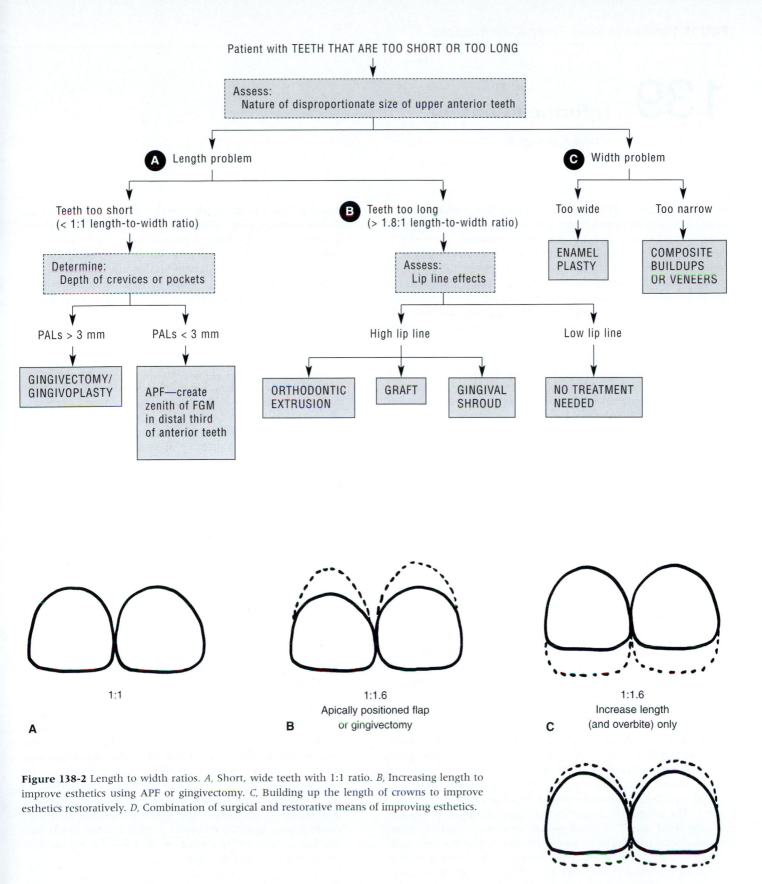

Figure 138-2 Length to width ratios. *A*, Short, wide teeth with 1:1 ratio. *B*, Increasing length to improve esthetics using APF or gingivectomy. *C*, Building up the length of crowns to improve esthetics restoratively. *D*, Combination of surgical and restorative means of improving esthetics.

139 Informed Consent

Charles F. Sumner III

Dentistry has entered into the world of litigation, which demands detailed records and all-inclusive forms. Because most dental procedures are elective, and the risks may outweigh the benefits, dentists have a potential problem of informed consent. Consent need not be written. If the information is complete and conveyed to the patient in understandable language, and if the patient is given the opportunity to ask questions that are then satisfactorily answered, the duty to inform probably has been fulfilled. The courts have held that patients may give valid consent to surgery if disclosure of risks has been made by a nurse assistant and not by the surgeon; however, the legal process tends to create fictions. In the area of informed consent the fiction is that the patient, by signing a form, is provided usable information for a reasoned decision. A wise practitioner should not rely only on a record of having satisfactorily informed the patient of the risk and alternatives of the pending procedure, but also should have in the patient's files a signed and witnessed consent form.

A   Although the purpose of the documented consent is to reduce the dentist's exposure to litigation, it also has value as a practice-building tool. Properly planned, written, and presented, the consent form may allay the patient's normal fears and apprehension and educate regarding the scope and limitations of treatment, thereby avoiding unrealistic expectations. The dentist has no excuse for failing to compose and properly present individual consent forms for general and special procedures.

B   Originally conceived as an offshoot of the law of battery, informed consent is now generally treated under a theory of negligence. The battery theory remains applicable if the treatment or procedure was completely unauthorized, whereas negligence principles apply to more commonly encountered situations in which the treatment was authorized but consent was uninformed. Under negligence theory, a duty of care, a breach of that duty, and injury and proximate or legal causal relationship between the breach and the injury must be established. A patient establishes proximate cause in an informed consent case by proof that a proper disclosure would have resulted in a decision against the proposed treatment or procedure.

The proper disclosure in the majority of jurisdictions is the "traditional" or "professional" view with regard to scope of disclosure. The physician is required to disclose only such risks that a reasonable practitioner of like training would have disclosed in the same or similar circumstances; however, each state has its own standards for informed consent, and these standards are rapidly changing. Some states hold the "material risk and objective" standard. Others take their standard from battery and have a "patient-based" standard. Others require that the patient be advised in great graphic detail of all risks and the alternatives to each procedure. In view of this variability, the dentist should learn the standard currently being followed in the locale before finalizing a consent form in print. A good consent form also is customized to the treatment procedure. Generalized consent forms are less likely to provide usable information for reasoned decisions. The rule is that the dentist performing the procedure, not the referring dentist, has the obligation to explain the procedure to the patient.

C   The courts have held that, as an integral part of the physician's overall obligation to the patient, a duty of reasonable disclosure of available choices with respect to proposed therapy and of the dangers inherently and potentially involved in each choice exists. This holding is based on four postulates that have become the basis of the informed consent laws. First, the knowledge of the patient and the doctor are not in parity. Second, an adult of sound mind exercises control over his or her own body and in exercising this control has the right to determine whether to undergo treatment. Third, the patient's consent to proposed treatment must be an informed one. Fourth, because of the nature of the physician-patient relationship, the physician has an obligation to the patient that transcends arm's-length transactions. Alternative plans must be explained as thoroughly and objectively as is the plan favored by the doctor.

D   If the treatment is cosmetic or if cosmetics plays a large role in the patient's decision to accept therapy, an even greater need exists to communicate and gain acceptance of the limitations of proposed therapy and the alternatives available. Dentistry is both an art and a science. Treatment results are judged by experts from among a dentist's peers. Judgment of cosmetic results is determined by the limitations indicated in the pretreatment agreement.

E   Customized, detailed consent material is recommended for high-risk procedures. The complexity and extent of the description should be in proportion to the complexity and extent of the proposed procedure and the risk to the patient. If the risks are relatively minor, and are known to be of low incidence, the demand for detail in disclosure is diminished. Conversely, if the risks are high but their incidence is low, or if the incidence is high but the risk is low, the fact is material and must be disclosed for a patient to arrive at a reasoned decision.

F   The essence of informed consent is that a patient cannot agree to a treatment without being presented with sufficient facts and time to allow for a reasoned decision. Nevertheless, some discussion and agreement must occur as to the course to be taken when emergencies arise during treatment and time is not sufficient for deliberation and consent.

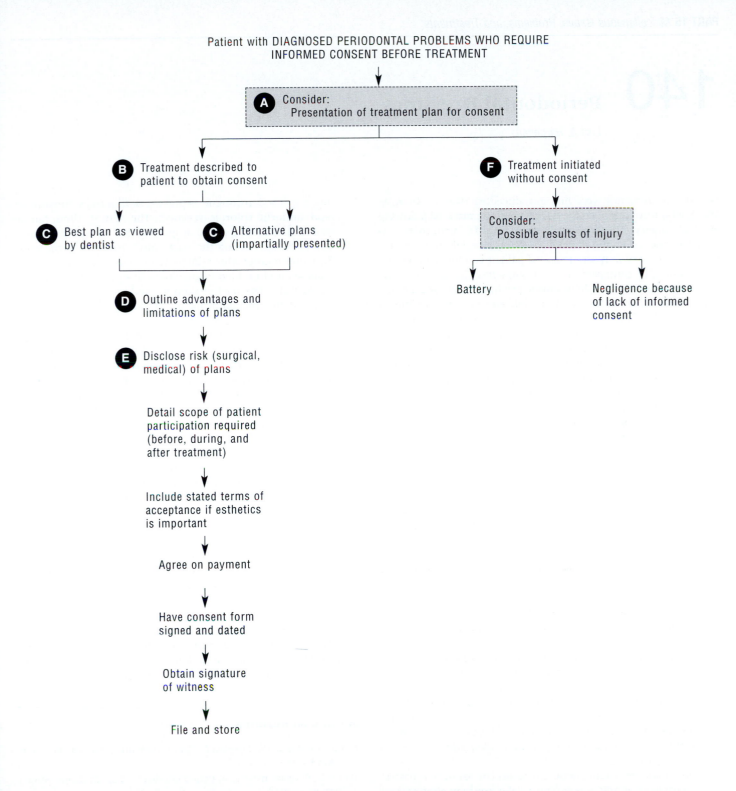

Patient with DIAGNOSED PERIODONTAL PROBLEMS WHO REQUIRE
INFORMED CONSENT BEFORE TREATMENT

A Consider:
Presentation of treatment plan for consent

B Treatment described to
patient to obtain consent

F Treatment initiated
without consent

Consider:
Possible results of injury

C Best plan as viewed
by dentist

C Alternative plans
(impartially presented)

Battery

Negligence because
of lack of informed
consent

D Outline advantages and
limitations of plans

E Disclose risk (surgical,
medical) of plans

Detail scope of patient
participation required
(before, during, and
after treatment)

Include stated terms of
acceptance if esthetics
is important

Agree on payment

Have consent form
signed and dated

Obtain signature
of witness

File and store

Caveat

The most complete, signed, and witnessed consent form does
not excuse responsibility or mitigate against damages if battery
or negligence can be established by the evidence. In the question of "Whose standard is to be followed in informed consent?"
the answer may well be that no matter the standard, members
of a jury must give their verdict, and they will probably use their
personal standards in doing so.

Additional Readings

Canterbury v Spence, 464F2d 354 (D.C. Cir. 1972).

Cobbs v Grant, 502 P2d 1 (1972).

Gaskin v Goldwasser, 520 N.E. 1d 1085 (1988).

Llera v Wisner, 557 P2d 805 (1976).

Moore v Preventive Medicine Medical Group, Inc, 178 Cal. App. 3d 738
(1986).

Mustacchio v Parker 535 So. 2nd 833 (1988).

Professional liability committee—first line of defense in malpractice
claims. J Am Dent Assoc 1974;88:341.

Roybal v Bell, 7878 P2d 108 (1989).

140 Periodontal Dressings

Lisa A. Harpenau

Periodontal dressings were first introduced in 1923 by Dr A.W. Ward, who recommended the use of a packing material following gingival surgery. The dressing material, Ward's Wondrpak, was made of zinc oxide and eugenol, alcohol, pine oil, and asbestos fibers. Its primary purposes included patient comfort and wound protection. The composition of dressings has changed over the years, eliminating potentially caustic products (such as asbestos) and adding others for added retention and healing. Additional benefits of dressings include reduction of hemorrhage and postoperative infection, control of granulation tissue growth, retention of apically positioned flaps by preventing coronal displacement, additional stabilization of a soft-tissue graft, protection of denuded bone during healing, and splinting of postsurgically mobile teeth. One of the most important benefits is the psychological comfort provided to the patient after surgery.

Periodontal dressings are generally divided into the following three categories: (1) those containing zinc oxide and eugenol; (2) those containing zinc oxide without eugenol; and (3) those containing neither zinc oxide nor eugenol.

A Zinc oxide and eugenol dressings are supplied as a liquid containing eugenol and peanut and/or rose oil, and resin and a powder containing zinc oxide, powdered resin, and tannic acid. The two components are mixed together on a waxed paper pad using a wooden tongue depressor. The powder is gradually incorporated into the liquid until a doughlike consistency forms. The dressing may be used immediately or wrapped in aluminum foil and refrigerated for up to 1 week. The advantages of this type of dressing include splinting (since it adheres to the teeth) and the hemostatic effects produced by the tannic acid. The disadvantages include a rough surface on setting that adds to plaque accumulation and bacterial proliferation; a hardsetting consistency that may complicate removal if engaged in an undercut; the inability to adhere to mucosal surfaces; the distinct taste of eugenol while the pack is in place; and possible allergic reaction to eugenol that may produce burning pain and reddening of the treated area.

B Zinc oxide without eugenol dressings consist of two pastes: an accelerator and a base. The accelerator may contain zinc oxide, vegetable and/or mineral oil (for plasticity), and magnesium oxide, and the base may consist of petrolatum and denatured alcohol. The setting action results from the reaction between the metallic oxide and the fatty acids. The accelerator and base are dispensed in tubes. Equal lengths of material are placed on a waxed paper pad and mixed using a wooden tongue depressor until a thick consistency and uniform color is reached. The setting time can be reduced by adding a few drops of warm water during mixing or by immersing the pack into a bowl of warm water just after mixing. Once the paste loses its tackiness, it can be handled and molded using gloves lubricated with water or petrolatum. The pack is then formed into pencil-sized rolls that are then mechanically interlocked in the facial and lingual interproximal areas. Working time is approximately 15 to 20 minutes. The advantages of this dressing include pleasant color and neutral taste; pliability, which facilitates removal from undercut areas; and the absence of eugenol and asbestos. The disadvantages include the inability to adhere to mucosa; premature loss of the packing if it is not firmly locked interproximally; minimal splinting ability due to its soft, rubbery consistency; and the absence of tannic acid in the material.

C Additional hemostasis may be required for palatal donor sites. Surgical absorbable hemostat (Surgicel, Colycote, Avitene) may be applied over the wound bed, over which the periodontal dressing or a palatal stent can then be placed.

D Some surgeons report the use of a Stomahesive bandage when there is a mucosal coverage requirement for a short time (24 to 36 hours). Stomahesive is a gelatinlike material with an adhesive surface protected by a paper coating. After the paper is removed, the product may be placed on mucosal surfaces, and it will adhere if it is slightly warmed by gloved hands and the warmth of the oral environment. The longevity of this bandage is minimal; however, some surgeons find this short time adequate for protecting the donor and recipient sites of a soft-tissue graft or a gingivoplasty procedure.

Additional Readings

Grant DA, Stern IB, Listgarten MA. Periodontics. 6th ed. St. Louis: Mosby; 1988. p. 731–2.

Hall WB. Decision making in periodontology. 3rd ed. St. Louis: Mosby; 1998. p. 254.

Newman MG, Takei H, Carranza FA Jr. Clinical periodontology. 9th ed. Philadelphia: WB Saunders; 2002. p. 729–31.

Sachs HA, Farnoush A, Checchi L, Joseph CE. Current status of periodontal dressings. J Periodontol 1984;55:689.

Watts TL, Combe EC. Periodontal dressing materials. J Clin Periodontol 1979;6:3.

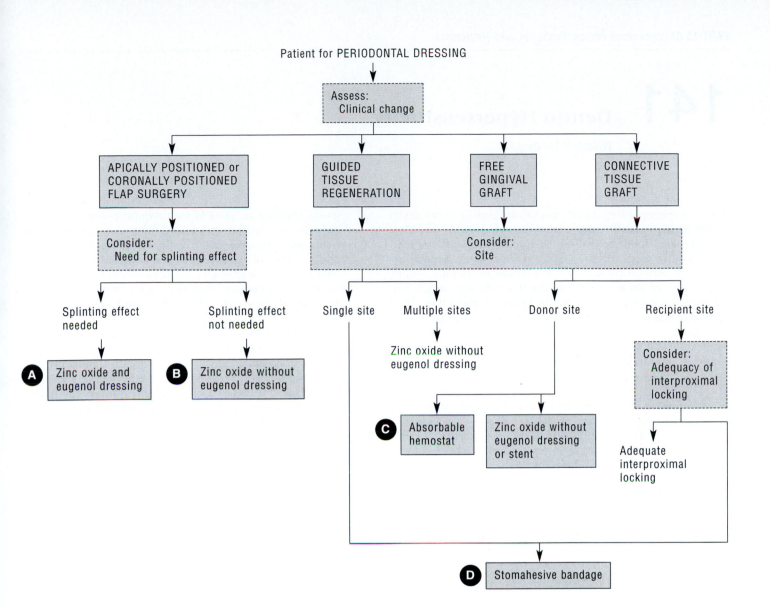

Patient for PERIODONTAL DRESSING

Assess:
Clinical change

APICALLY POSITIONED or
CORONALLY POSITIONED
FLAP SURGERY

GUIDED
TISSUE
REGENERATION

FREE
GINGIVAL
GRAFT

CONNECTIVE
TISSUE
GRAFT

Consider:
Need for splinting effect

Consider:
Site

Splinting effect
needed

Splinting effect
not needed

Single site

Multiple sites

Donor site

Recipient site

Zinc oxide without
eugenol dressing

Consider:
Adequacy of
interproximal
locking

A Zinc oxide and
eugenol dressing

B Zinc oxide without
eugenol dressing

C Absorbable
hemostat

Zinc oxide without
eugenol dressing
or stent

Adequate
interproximal
locking

D Stomahesive bandage

141 Dentin Hypersensitivity

William P. Lundergan

Dentin hypersensitivity affects about one out of every seven dental patients. Furthermore, with the aging of the populace and increased tooth retention, the number of dental patients with sensitive teeth will no doubt increase. Dentin hypersensitivity may occur if fresh dentin is exposed to thermal, tactile, evaporative, or chemical stimuli. The term *root hypersensitivity* is commonly used to describe dentin hypersensitivity associated with gingival recession, abrasion, erosion, root planing, and periodontal flap surgery. Root hypersensitivity may present a perplexing and frustrating problem for both the patient and dentist during definitive periodontal treatment and subsequent maintenance therapy.

A   The first steps in treating dentin hypersensitivity are to identify the sensitive area and establish an etiology. Caries, a fractured tooth or restoration, occlusal trauma, recent restorative therapy, gingival recession, abrasion, erosion, and recent root planing or periodontal flap surgery should be evaluated as possible causes. Treatment should be appropriate for the identified etiology. If an evaluation of tooth vitality shows irreversible pulpal inflammation, endodontic therapy is required. If the tooth is fractured, an endodontic and periodontal evaluation may be required to establish a prognosis. Severe fractures usually require extraction of the tooth.

B   Treatment for root hypersensitivity begins with meticulous plaque control and the use of a desensitizing toothpaste. (Toothpastes containing potassium nitrate or strontium chloride have been shown to be effective desensitizers. Several commercial products have been evaluated and accepted by the American Dental Association's Council on Dental Therapeutics.) Root hypersensitivity associated with severe abrasion or erosion may require restorative procedures in conjunction with instructions on proper brushing technique (abrasion cases) or dietary counseling (erosion cases). If the patient experiences no relief after 2 weeks of meticulous home care with a densensitizing toothpaste or is too sensitive to practice proper plaque control, office procedures should be combined with the home regimen.

C   A multitude of agents and methods have been used in the treatment of root hypersensitivity, but no one therapy has proven universally effective. The dentist should use the most conservative treatment that is effective for a particular patient. Multiple office procedures, often combining more than one method, may be required for best results. In some instances, local anesthesia may be necessary before initiation of the desensitizing procedure. Commonly used agents include fluoride, calcium hydroxide, potassium oxalate, ferric oxalate, restorative resins, and varnishes. Iontophoresis, a method of delivering charged molecules or medicaments through an electric current, has been used successfully with a 1 to 2% sodium fluoride solution. In severe cases that do not respond to more conservative treatment, endodontic therapy may be required.

Additional Readings

Curra FA. Tooth hypersensitivity. Dent Clin North Am 1990;34(3).

Hodosh N, Hodosh S, Hodosh A. About dentinal hypersensitivity. Compendium 1994;151:658.

Newman MG, Takei HH, Carranza FA. Carranza's clinical periodontology. 9th ed. Philadelphia: WB Saunders; 2002. p. 133.

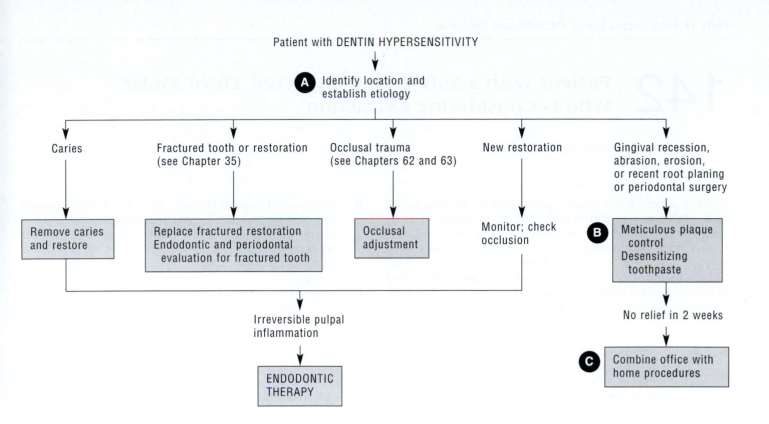

Patient with DENTIN HYPERSENSITIVITY

A Identify location and establish etiology

Caries

Fractured tooth or restoration (see Chapter 35)

Occlusal trauma (see Chapters 62 and 63)

New restoration

Gingival recession, abrasion, erosion, or recent root planing or periodontal surgery

Remove caries and restore

Replace fractured restoration Endodontic and periodontal evaluation for fractured tooth

Occlusal adjustment

Monitor; check occlusion

B Meticulous plaque control Desensitizing toothpaste

Irreversible pulpal inflammation

No relief in 2 weeks

ENDODONTIC THERAPY

C Combine office with home procedures

142

Patient with a Soft-Tissue Impacted Third Molar Who Is Considering Extraction

James Garibaldi

When a patient has a symptomatic soft-tissue impaction, the most likely cause is pericoronitis. The tooth begins to erupt somewhat but because of proximity to the ramus or adjacent second molars, or abnormal eruption pattern, is prevented from erupting fully. The overlying soft-tissue operculum can often become the site for entrapment of food debris and proliferation of microorganisms leading to inflammation. Generally, this phenomenon is very painful, involves the mandibular wisdom teeth, and can progress to a full-blown infection.

A The first thing to assess is whether the patient is symptomatic and if the cause is pericoronitis or not. If so, one should next consider the age of the patient, which generally correlates with the amount of root formation present.

B The ideal time to remove an impacted wisdom tooth is when one-third to two-thirds of the root is formed, which generally corresponds with the middle to late teenage years. If it is removed too early, when no root is formed, the extraction process is difficult because the tooth tends to roll around in its bony crypt. If, on the other hand, the roots are completely formed, the tooth is anchored firmly in place.

C Hence, with *lack of full eruption potential*, symptoms of pericoronitis, which can subside and recur at any time, and one-third to two-thirds of the root formed, the tooth should be extracted. Other factors that also would indicate the need for an extraction include associated pathology, not enough attached gingiva if the wisdom tooth could erupt, or the tooth cannot be kept clean on the distal if it were to erupt fully. The key is to remove a tooth with these factors when the patient is young so the chances of regeneration of periodontal structures on the distal of the second molar are more predictable. The surgery itself is easier compared with later in life, and the recuperation is generally uneventful, with less potential for postoperative complications. If none of these factors are present, the tooth can be left and monitored.

D If the patient is asymptomatic, one should again consider the age of the patient. The ideal time for extraction is when one-third to two-thirds of the root is formed and no pathology is noted, especially if the potential for full eruption is improbable or impossible.

E If the patient is older, the status of the second molar should be considered. If no pathology or periodontal problems are noted, the situation should be monitored. However, if radiographs show that the wisdom tooth is abutted against the distal of the second molars, potentially compromising the distal of the second molar's periodontal structures and (1) there is not enough space for full eruption of the wisdom tooth, (2) there is pathology or inadequate attached gingiva, or (3) the patient is unable to keep it clean if the tooth were to erupt, the tooth should be extracted—even if asymptomatic. Guided tissue regeneration may be considered (see Chapter 146).

Additional Readings

Kugelberg CF, Ahlstrom U, Ericson S, et al. The influence of anatomical, pathophysiological and other factors on periodontal healing after impacted lower third molar surgery. J Clin Periodontol 1991;18:37.

Laskin DM. Indications and contraindications for removal of impacted third molars. Dent Clin North Am 1969;13:919.

Leone SA, Edenfield MJ, Coehn ME. Correlation of acute pericoronitis and the position of the mandibular third molar. Oral Surg Oral Med Oral Pathol 1986;62:245.

Osborne WH, Snyder AJ, Tempen TR. Attachment levels and crevicular depths at the distal aspect of mandibular second molars following removal of adjacent third molars. J Periodontol 1982;53:93.

Pedersen GW. Oral surgery. Philadelphia: WB Saunders; 1988. p. 60.

Robinson PD. The impacted lower wisdom tooth: to remove or to leave alone? Dent Update 1994;21:245.

Tate TE. Impactions: observe or treat? J Calif Dent Assoc 1994;22(6):59.

Patient with SOFT-TISSUE IMPACTED WISDOM TOOTH WHO IS CONSIDERING EXTRACTION

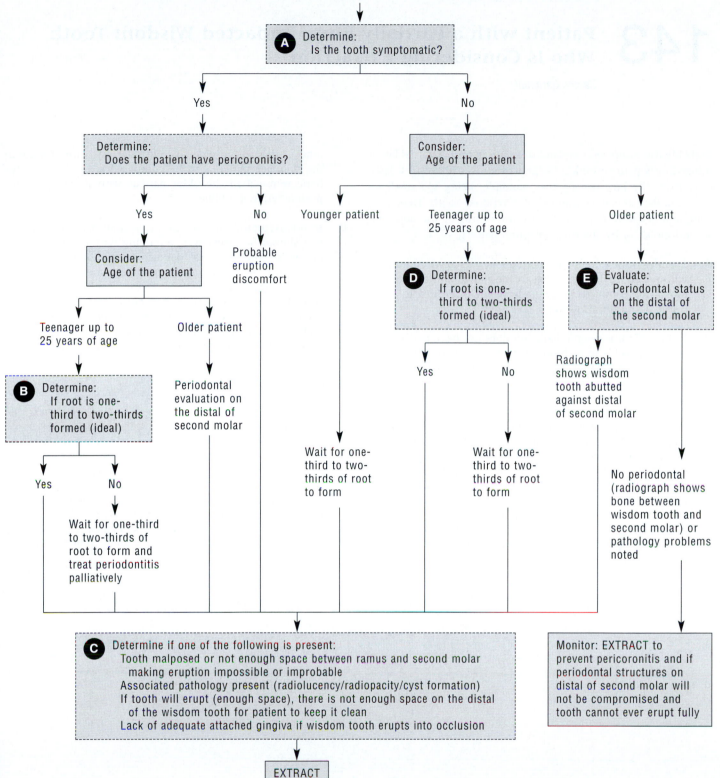

143 Patient with a Partially Bony Impacted Wisdom Tooth Who Is Considering Extraction

James Garibaldi

Probably the common complaint of a patient with a partial bony impaction is pain secondary to pericoronitis. This results basically from the jaw, usually the mandible, being too small to accommodate the full eruption of a wisdom tooth. Hence its complete eruption is prevented by the ramus or the adjacent second molar, or by abnormal eruption pattern.

A The ideal time to remove a partially impacted wisdom tooth without enough space between the ramus and the second molar for complete eruption is when one-third to two-thirds of the root is formed.

B If the patient is symptomatic but does not have pericoronitis, the cause is most probably eruption discomfort. If the tooth possesses pathology or is malposed or impacted under the ramus making complete eruption improbable or impossible, it should be removed.

C When the patient is asymptomatic, but radiographically a partial bony impaction is noted, the patient, especially a teenager with one-third to two-thirds of the root formed, should be evaluated. The reason is if pathology or other factors, such as impossible or improbable eruption of the tooth, are noted, this is the ideal time for removal. The bone is elastic, and the roots are not completely formed to anchor the tooth. The surgery is then met with fewer postoperative complications, and the recovery is generally quicker than in an older patient. The elasticity of bone in the younger patient can be compared with the need for bone removal in the older patient with its potential for postoperative morbidity.

D In the asymptomatic patient, as with all patients, risk factors should be assessed in removing wisdom teeth. Sinus proximity and potential damage to the inferior alveolar nerve must be considered. In the older patient, where bone elasticity decreases, these risk factors can be of more concern than in the teenager. If significant, the status of the distal of the second molar should be evaluated periodically and, if no pathology or periodontal concerns are noted, the tooth should be monitored and followed up closely.

Additional Readings

Braden BE. Deep distal pockets adjacent to terminal teeth. Dent Clin North Am 1969;13:161.

Koerner KR. The removal of impacted third molars: principles, indications and procedures. Dent Clin North Am 1994;38:255.

Laskin DM. Indications and contraindications for removal of impacted third molars. Dent Clin North Am 1969;13:919.

Mercier P, Precious D. Risks and benefits of removal of impacted third molars. Int J Oral Maxillofac Surg 1992;21(1):17.

Peterson IJ, Ellis E, Hupp JR, Tucker MR. Contemporary oral and maxillofacial surgery. 3rd ed. St. Louis: Mosby; 1998. p. 224.

Patient with a PARTIALLY BONY IMPACTED WISDOM TOOTH WHO IS CONSIDERING EXTRACTION

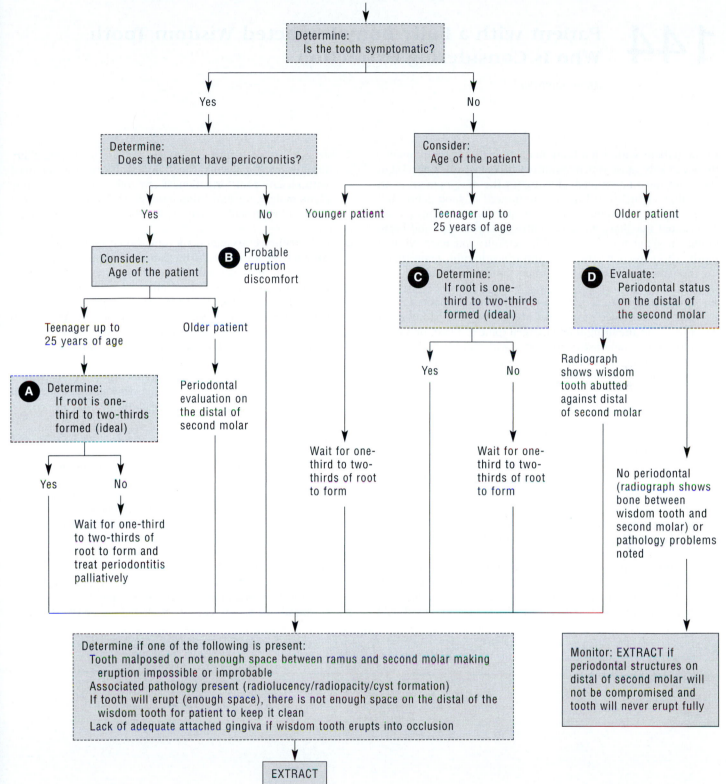

Determine:
Is the tooth symptomatic?

Yes

Determine:
Does the patient have pericoronitis?

No

Consider:
Age of the patient

Yes

Consider:
Age of the patient

No

B Probable
eruption
discomfort

Younger patient

Teenager up to
25 years of age

Older patient

Teenager up to
25 years of age

Older patient

C Determine:
If root is one-
third to two-thirds
formed (ideal)

D Evaluate:
Periodontal status
on the distal of
the second molar

A Determine:
If root is one-
third to two-thirds
formed (ideal)

Periodontal
evaluation on
the distal of
second molar

Yes

No

Radiograph
shows wisdom
tooth abutted
against distal
of second molar

Yes

No

Wait for one-third
to two-thirds of
root to form and
treat periodontitis
palliatively

Wait for one-
third to two-
thirds of root
to form

Wait for one-
third to two-
thirds of root
to form

No periodontal
(radiograph shows
bone between
wisdom tooth and
second molar) or
pathology problems
noted

Determine if one of the following is present:
 Tooth malposed or not enough space between ramus and second molar making
  eruption impossible or improbable
 Associated pathology present (radiolucency/radiopacity/cyst formation)
 If tooth will erupt (enough space), there is not enough space on the distal of the
  wisdom tooth for patient to keep it clean
 Lack of adequate attached gingiva if wisdom tooth erupts into occlusion

Monitor: EXTRACT if
periodontal structures on
distal of second molar will
not be compromised and
tooth will never erupt fully

EXTRACT

144 Patient with a Fully Bony Impacted Wisdom Tooth Who Is Considering Extraction

James Garibaldi

In the patient with a full bony impaction that is symptomatic, the *least* likely cause is pericoronitis. This is because a portion of the tooth must be erupted allowing for the development of an operculum, which can lead to entrapment of food debris and proliferation of micoorganisms. However, there are times when an erupted maxillary wisdom tooth can supererupt and begin biting the gingiva overlying the lower fully impacted wisdom tooth. This can create the same sort of symptoms, hence making the patient with a full bony impaction symptomatic.

A The first thing to consider in the symptomatic patient is age and the presence or absence of pathology. If pathology is present in the form of an enlarged follicle, a cyst, or a radiolucency or radiopacity associated with the tooth, the tooth in question should be removed, and the specimen sent to a pathology laboratory for evaluation. The most common pathology noted with full bony impactions is the dentigerous cyst, which can continue to enlarge over time.

B Neoplasms, such as squamous cell carcinoma, can develop in the epithelial lining of cysts, especially as the patient becomes older. Therefore if a third molar without pathology is left at an early age, the tooth needs to be followed up with periodic radiographs. If it is found that the symptoms are caused by a supererupted maxillary molar biting the gingiva of a full bony mandibular impaction, the supererupted tooth should be removed.

C In the young asymptomatic patient with a full bony impaction, if no pathology is present, one should wait until at least one-third to two-thirds of the root is formed. The reason for this is twofold: (1) usually the wisdom tooth will erupt more with time (ie, not be as close to the maxillary sinus or inferior alveolar canal) and (2) if a tooth is removed without any root formation, if can roll around in its bony crypt, making the extraction more difficult than if some root structure is present to stabilize the tooth during extraction.

D If the patient is asymptomatic, one should again consider the patient's age. Generally, as the patient grows older, the health can decline and may necessitate the use of prescription drugs for such things as high blood pressure, arthritis, or chronic atrial fibrillation. The dentist needs to take into account this information before deciding on an extraction. At times, a medical consultation, laboratory work, or even hospitalization may be required to complete the procedure. If the distal of the second molar is periodontally sound, the wisdom tooth cannot be felt with a periodontal probe, and no pathology is noted in association with the wisdom tooth, it should be monitored with periodic radiographic evaluation.

Additional Readings

Eversole LR. Clinical outline of oral pathology. 3rd ed. Philadelphia: Lea & Febiger; 1992. p. 254.

Main DW. Follicular cysts of mandibular third molar teeth: radiological evaluation of enlargement. Dentomaxillofac Radiol 1989;18:156.

Mercier P, Precious D. Risks and benefits of removal of impacted third molars. Int J Oral Maxillofac Surg 1992;21(1):17.

Robinson PD. The impacted lower wisdom tooth: to remove or to leave alone? Dent Update 1994;21:245.

Stanley HR, Alattar M, Collett WK, et al. Pathological sequelae of "neglected" impacted third molars. J Oral Pathol 1988;17:113.

Tate TE. Impactions: observe or treat? J Calif Dent Assoc 1994;22(6):59.

Patient with a FULLY BONY IMPACTED WISDOM TOOTH WHO IS CONSIDERING EXTRACTION

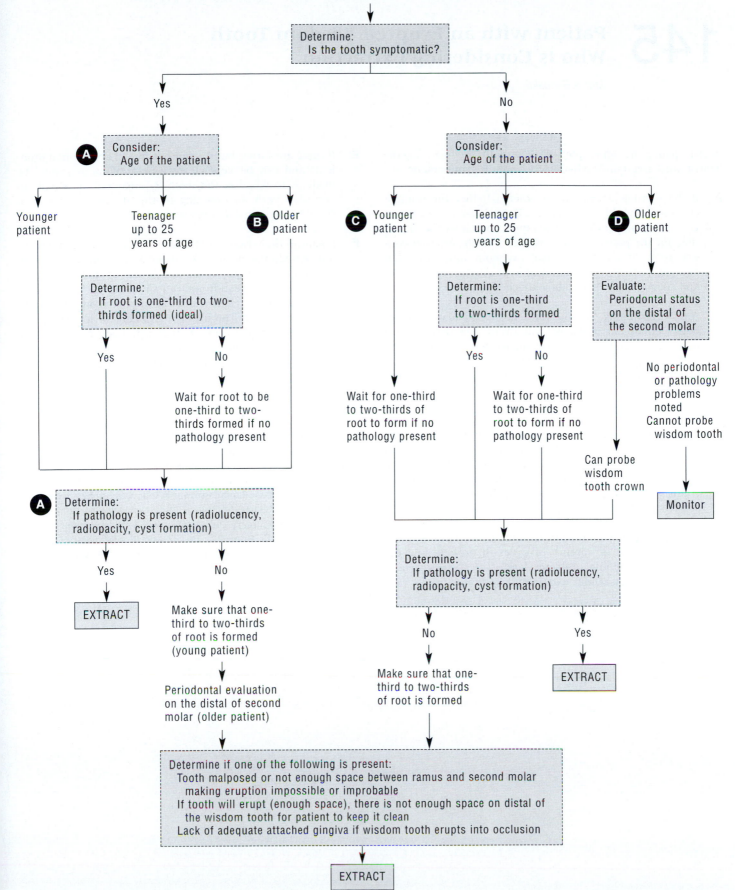

145 Patient with an Erupted Wisdom Tooth Who Is Considering Extraction

James Garibaldi

When a patient has an erupted wisdom tooth, the first thing the dentist must ascertain is whether the tooth is symptomatic.

A If the tooth is asymptomatic, then whether the tooth is cleansable should be considered. If the distal of the wisdom tooth is against or close to the ramus, then it will be impossible for the patient to keep this area clean. Another consideration in an asymptomatic wisdom tooth that has enough space on the distal to be kept clean is the presence and adequacy of surrounding attached gingiva.

B After determining that the tooth is cleansable and free of both periodontal problems and caries, the dentist must make sure that the tooth has erupted into normal occlusion and that it is not in buccal or lingual version. Also, it should be noted whether the tooth has an opposing tooth, allowing it to be functional and preventing possible supereruption.

C However, if the wisdom tooth does not have an opposing tooth but is asymptomatic and periodontally sound, then it is up to the dentist and patient with regard to retention or extraction. The question to answer is if this tooth could ever be used in a future treatment plan or if it could simply supererupt with time and cause problems, such as cheek biting.

D If the patient is symptomatic, then the first item to ascertain is the presence or absence of caries. If present, and the tooth has periodontal problems, lack of attached gingiva, or is up against the ramus, extraction is indicated.

E If there are caries, but the tooth is free of periodontal problems and can be kept clean, a determination should be made as to whether the tooth is functional or not (ie, in occlusion with an opposing tooth). If this is the case it should be restored and maintained.

F Finally, if the wisdom tooth in occlusion is cleansable without periodontal or attached gingiva problems and has no caries (but is symptomatic), the patient should be checked for cracked-tooth syndrome (see Chapter 35). If this can be ruled out, oral hygiene should be improved and symptoms further evaluated. This includes checking for sensitivity secondary to exposed cementum and prematurity in occlusal contact. If symptoms do not resolve after appropriate treatment, the tooth should be extracted if of no value in a future treatment plan.

Additional Readings

Hooley JR, Whitacre RJ. Assessment of and surgery for third molars: a self-instructional guide. 3rd ed. Seattle: Stoma Press; 1983.

Lysell L, Rohlin M. A study of indications used for removal of the mandibular third molar. Int J Oral Maxillofac Surg 1988;17:161.

Meister F Jr et al. Periodontal assessment following surgical removal of erupted mandibular third molars. Gen Dent 1986;14:120.

Pedersen GW. Oral surgery. Philadelphia: WB Saunders; 1988. p. 60.

Peterson IJ, Ellis E, Hupp JR, Tucker MR. Contemporary oral and maxillofacial surgery. 3rd ed. St. Louis: Mosby; 1998. p. 224.

Patient with an ERUPTED WISDOM TOOTH WHO IS CONSIDERING EXTRACTION

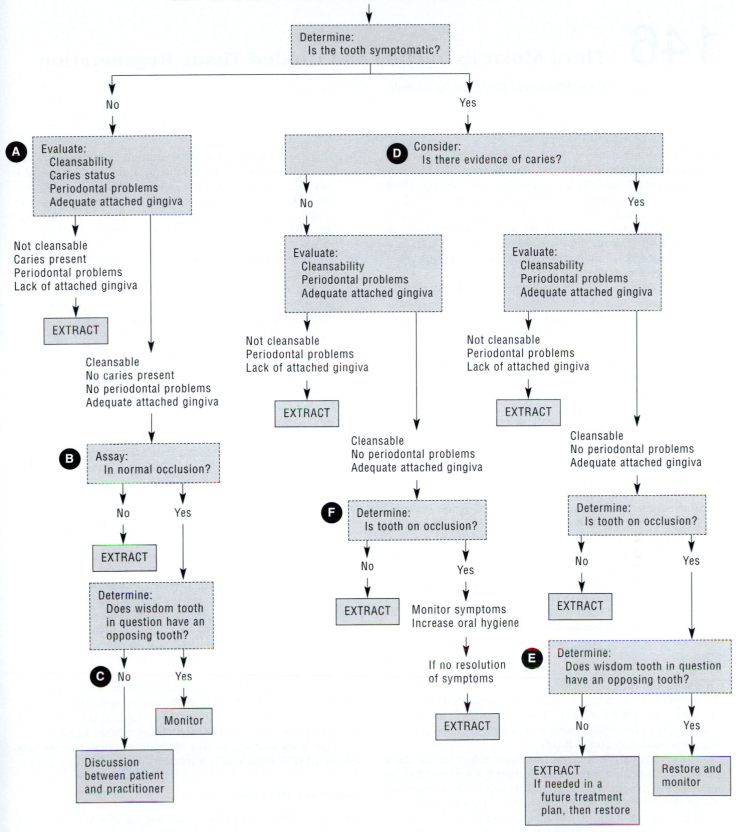

146 Third Molar Extraction and Guided Tissue Regeneration

Daniel Etienne and Mithridade Davarpanah

Guided tissue regeneration (GTR) is an accepted method for treating deep intrabony defects. The principle is based on numerous animal and clinical studies in which barrier membranes were used to isolate periodontal defects from the gingival epithelium and gingival connective tissues, allowing cells from the periodontal ligament to repopulate the detached root surface. To date the majority of studies relating to GTR have used expanded polytetrafluoroethylene (ePTFE) barrier membranes, which are considered the gold standard.

The hoped-for outcome in removing impacted third molars is to do so without injury to the adjacent tooth. Improper surgical technique may cause postoperative pain and result in intrabony defects adjacent to second molars. Partially impacted third molars are frequently accompanied by periodontal breakdown of the adjacent tooth. In a retrospective study, Kugelberg reported that 2 years after impacted third-molar surgery, 43.3% of the cases showed probing depths greater than 7 mm and 32.1% showed intrabony defects greater than 4 mm on the distal surface of the adjacent second molar. Of patients older than 26 years, 44% demonstrated intrabony defects greater than 4 mm distal to second molars. Of patients younger than 25 years, 4% developed defects greater than 4 mm.

GTR is an accepted and appropriate method for treating advanced periodontal defects and diseases associated with horizontally impacted third molars. Pecora and colleagues evaluated the possibilities of using GTR procedures to prevent or treat periodontal lesions after third-molar extractions (the use of ePTFE membranes to regenerate tissue lost as a result of periodontal disease has been well documented).

In this study, periodontal healing of 20 vertical intrabony defects located distally to second molars was monitored for 7 years after impacted third-molar surgery. Data showed that all defects healed with a combination of recession and decreased probing depths. In the test group, the mean decrease in probing depth was 5.7 mm, compared with 4 mm in the control group. A mean gain of probing attachment level of 4.3 mm occurred for the test group, compared with 1.9 mm for the control group. The use of ePTFE membranes significantly enhanced the gain of attachment level in the test sites compared with the control sites ($p < .01$). However, both treatment modalities resulted in a significant reduction in pocket depth.

The proper diagnosis of an intrabony defect on the distal surface of the second molar is important for successful treatment during third-molar surgery. The preoperative anatomic relationship with the second molar also is a critical factor.

Age is a main contributing factor. Subjects 25 years or younger exhibit fewer postoperative intrabony pockets. The extent of the intrabony defect on the distal of the second molar also is a critical parameter. Dental plaque affects the wound healing of older patients.

A   Kugelberg's Risk Index M3 is an index predicting the risk for periodontal defects. A value of 1 indicates no risk, 2 is low risk, 3 is moderate risk, and 4 and above is high risk. An index of 0 is correlated with an estimated defect of 2 mm, an index of 2 to an intrabony defect of 3 mm, and an index of 4 to an osseous defect of 4 mm.

B   For patients who on the Kugelberg Risk Index M3 score < 2—patients with no periodontal involvement on the adjacent second molar, patients whose asymptomatic third molars are being removed for orthodontic reasons, or patients with 3 mm or smaller infrabony defects on the adjacent second molar—no membrane therapy is neccessary.

C   For patients who on the Kugelberg's Risk Index M3 score > 2—with deep pockets and narrow, deep infrabony defects on the adjacent second molar—the possibility of closing the flaps completely over the third-molar extraction socket determines whether a resorbable or nonresorbable membrane should be used. If full coverage of the membrane is possible, a resorbable membrane should be employed for GTR. In all other instances a nonresorbable membrane is necessary.

D   For patients with a Kugelberg's Risk Index M3 score > 2—those with deep pockets and deep, wide infrabony defects—a nonresorbable membrane with titanium reinforcement is employed to avoid membrane collapse.

The use of reinforced membranes is well established for wide intrabony defects and guided bony regeneration around implants. The blood clot is well protected from membrane collapse if a titanium-reinforced membrane is used, but the outcome and advantage for comparison with conventional ePTFE membranes have yet to be validated for third-molar surgery and wide spaces.

Treatment modalities will evolve with resorbable membranes (Resolut). These membranes, made of polymers, are well integrated within the soft tissue, but they collapse in wide defects. If an optimal bone level is desired, ePTFE membranes are better.

GTR is an appropriate way of treating periodontal diseases associated with horizontally impacted third molars.

Additional Readings

Kugelberg C. Third molar surgery: oral and maxillofacial surgery and infections. Curr Opin Dent 1992;2:9.

Pecora G et al. The effects of guided tissue regeneration on healing after impacted mandibular third-molar surgery: 1 year results. Int J Periodontics Restorative Dent 1993;13:397.

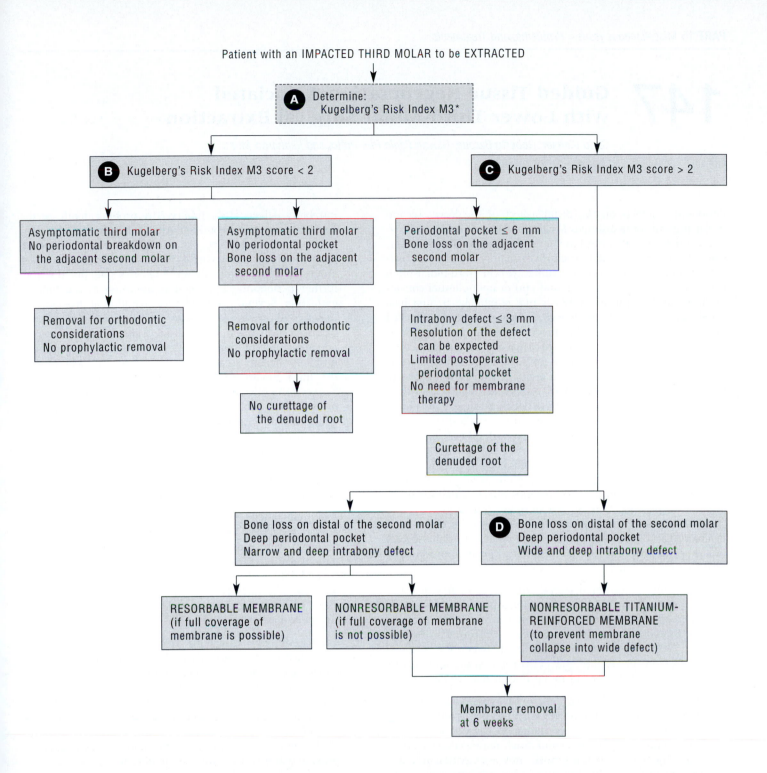

Patient with an IMPACTED THIRD MOLAR to be EXTRACTED

A Determine: Kugelberg's Risk Index M3*

B Kugelberg's Risk Index M3 score < 2

C Kugelberg's Risk Index M3 score > 2

Asymptomatic third molar
No periodontal breakdown on the adjacent second molar

Asymptomatic third molar
No periodontal pocket
Bone loss on the adjacent second molar

Periodontal pocket ≤ 6 mm
Bone loss on the adjacent second molar

Removal for orthodontic considerations
No prophylactic removal

Removal for orthodontic considerations
No prophylactic removal

Intrabony defect ≤ 3 mm
Resolution of the defect can be expected
Limited postoperative periodontal pocket
No need for membrane therapy

No curettage of the denuded root

Curettage of the denuded root

Bone loss on distal of the second molar
Deep periodontal pocket
Narrow and deep intrabony defect

D Bone loss on distal of the second molar
Deep periodontal pocket
Wide and deep intrabony defect

RESORBABLE MEMBRANE
(if full coverage of membrane is possible)

NONRESORBABLE MEMBRANE
(if full coverage of membrane is not possible)

NONRESORBABLE TITANIUM-REINFORCED MEMBRANE
(to prevent membrane collapse into wide defect)

Membrane removal at 6 weeks

*Kugelberg's Risk Index M3. Each of the following criteria has a value of 1: on distal second molar: (1) plaque, (2) pocket depth > 6 mm, (3) intrabony defect > 3 mm, (4) root resorption; third molar: (5) sagittal inclination < 50°, (6) widened follicles < 2.5 mm; (7) large contact area between third and second molar, (8) smoker.

147　Guided Tissue Regeneration Associated with Lower Third-Molar Surgical Extraction

Carlo Clauser, Roberto Barone, Giovan Paolo Pini-Prato, and Leonardo Muzzi

Periodontal defects on the distal aspect of the lower second molar present some distinctive features that include the following: (1) the associated third molar hinders the periodontal diagnosis, (2) the periodontal prognosis is mainly based on statistical data derived from previous studies, (3) the third molar often must be extracted (for periodontal and nonperiodontal considerations) and may leave a defect that should be treated in a timely manner, (4) the periodontal diagnosis may be checked and refined during surgery immediately after the third-molar extraction, (5) the site is exposed surgically at the extraction, providing a unique opportunity for surgical periodontal treatment without additional surgical sessions, (6) surgical access to the lingual side of the second molar presents a significant risk of interfering with the lingual nerve during surgery including reentry procedures after guided tissue regeneration (GTR) procedures with nonresorbable barrier material, and (7) periodontal maintenance distal to the second molar is always difficult, especially if a third-molar extraction is indicated, and the second molar has little space. The correction of morphology to facilitate hygiene is of paramount importance for effective maintenance; this is a strong indication for periodontal regeneration.

Third-molar extraction should be followed by periodontal evaluation and treatment of the associated defect on the second molar if indicated. The treatment may best be accomplished by GTR in selected cases.

A　The communication between the pericoronal space and oral cavity is assessed visually using a periodontal probe or indirectly from the presence of pericoronitis. The probe is used to contact the third-molar crown through a discontinuity in the mucosa. Distinguishing between the penetration of the probe into the pericoronal space and correct insertion into the second-molar pocket may be difficult.

B　If no communication with the oral cavity exists, the third molar does not communicate with the periodontal crevice on the distal of the second molar. In these cases a distal bone dehiscence on the second molar may be detected during extraction of the third molar; however, reattachment is expected because the root surface has not been exposed to the oral environment. These cases therefore are not candidates for immediate GTR; they should be followed in the postoperative period to detect late periodontal defects amenable to standard periodontal therapy, including GTR.

C　Patients who need emergency extractions during acute infection are not candidates for immediate GTR because the barrier membrane cannot be covered adequately. For the same reason, patients with partially erupted third molars are not candidates for immediate GTR because masticatory mucosa and gingiva in the area usually are minimal.

D　Many cases of third-molar extractions heal without significant periodontal defects on the second molar without any additional treatment. Few cases treated before age 25 have

intrabony defects after surgery. The probing depth on the distal aspect of the second molar often is related to the presence of a pseudopocket. Patients older than 25, however, have intrabony defects in 44% of all cases. In the older group the dentist must identify high-risk patients in whom further periodontal treatment is indicated at the time of extraction. Several risk factors for periodontal problems on the second molar have been documented: preoperative plaque accumulation on the distal of the second molar, preoperative probing depth greater than 6 mm, preoperative intrabony defects greater than 3 mm, sagittal inclination of the third molar greater than 50°, a large contact area between the second and third molars, resorption of second-molar distal roots, pathologically widened (more than 3 mm) follicle mesial to the third molar, and smoking habits. Deep intrabony defects (larger than 4 mm) are expected if five or more risk factors are present. These findings are crucial because GTR is an expensive treatment modality and becomes cost effective only if it is predicted to be successful and the alternative entails a predictably poor prognosis.

E　The predictability of GTR procedures is affected by patient and local factors. Local factors cannot be fully evaluated preoperatively; this fact should be communicated to the patient. Patient factors should be evaluated before surgery. A candidate for GTR must have good oral hygiene compliance, no systemic diseases, no smoking habits, no risk for endocarditis or endarteritis, and absence of rapidly progressive periodontitis.

F　The flap design is crucial for GTR procedures. All the available masticatory mucosa should be preserved to ensure adequate coverage of the membrane. Care must be taken to reflect all the tissue behind the second molar without lacerations. The flap also should involve the interdental space between the first and second molars to allow for the passage of a suture. The dentist also should preserve as much of the *linea obliqua externa* of the mandible as possible to provide better support for the membrane.

G　Immediately after the extraction the distal aspect of the second molar is inspected to discover whether calculus is present (which confirms a poor periodontal prognosis if the needed steps are not undertaken) and determine the tridimensional shape of the defect.

H　The principles of GTR are applied as in the treatment of any angular bone defect. The dentist should make the choice between resorbable and nonresorbable materials keeping in mind that sharp dissection may be required to remove a large nonresorbable membrane. In this case, some risk of damaging the lingual nerve is present. A resorbable material is preferred. After the extraction a large bone cavity remains resulting from the periodontal defect, empty third-molar socket, and any bone resection needed for extraction.

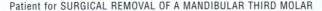

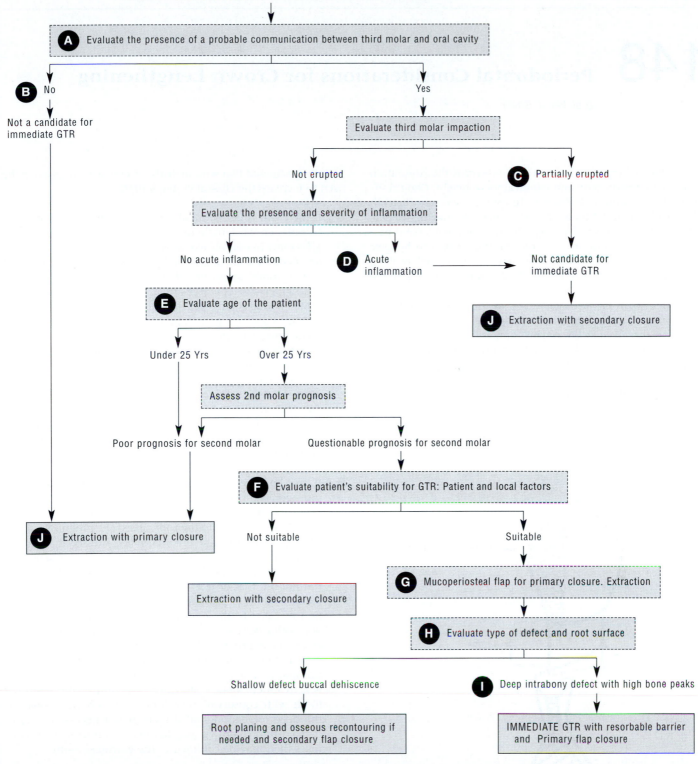

Patient for SURGICAL REMOVAL OF A MANDIBULAR THIRD MOLAR

A Evaluate the presence of a probable communication between third molar and oral cavity

B No → Not a candidate for immediate GTR

Yes → Evaluate third molar impaction

Not erupted → Evaluate the presence and severity of inflammation

C Partially erupted

No acute inflammation

D Acute inflammation → Not candidate for immediate GTR

J Extraction with secondary closure

E Evaluate age of the patient

Under 25 Yrs

Over 25 Yrs → Assess 2nd molar prognosis

Poor prognosis for second molar

Questionable prognosis for second molar

F Evaluate patient's suitability for GTR: Patient and local factors

Not suitable

Suitable

J Extraction with primary closure

Extraction with secondary closure

G Mucoperiosteal flap for primary closure. Extraction

H Evaluate type of defect and root surface

Shallow defect buccal dehiscence

I Deep intrabony defect with high bone peaks

Root planing and osseous recontouring if needed and secondary flap closure

IMMEDIATE GTR with resorbable barrier and Primary flap closure

The membrane should be large enough to cover all the bone cavity and several millimeters of intact bone around it. Both the membrane and fixing device (suture or built-in ligature and knots) must remain covered with tissue. If a membrane with built-in ligature is used, the knot should be a simple square one positioned behind the second molar, making the ligature go all around the tooth.

I Primary closure of the surgical wound is needed for nonattachment and for regenerative procedures. It is contraindicated in cases of infection, in which secondary closure provides better comfort and plaque control.

Additional Readings

Ash MM, Costich ER, Hayward JR. A study of periodontal hazards of third molars. J Periodontol 1962;33:209.

Kugelberg CF. Periodontal healing 2 and 4 years after impacted lower third molar surgery. A comparative retrospective study. Int J Oral Maxillofac Surg 1990;19:341.

Kugelberg CF. Third molar surgery: current science. Oral Maxillofac Surg Infect 1992;2(3):9.

Kugelberg CF et al. Periodontal healing after impacted lower third molar surgery in adolescents and adults: a prospective study. Int J Oral Maxillofac Surg 1991;20:18.

148 Periodontal Considerations for Crown Lengthening

Gretchen J. Bruce

One of the challenges of restorative dentistry is the restoration of teeth with insufficient supragingival tooth height. Clinical situations that require a decision to restore or extract such teeth are (1) short clinical crown, (2) root caries, (3) subgingival perforation, (4) fractures, (5) retrograde wear, and (6) altered passive eruption. If teeth are restored without regard to biologic principles, the periodontium may develop increased probing depths, problems with respect to plaque control, and a swollen cyanotic appearance.

Biologic width has been described as the space occupied by the junctional epithelium and connective tissue attachment coronal to the alveolar crest. This dimension is approximately 2.04 mm. An additional millimeter representing the gingival crevice is combined with this figure to permit the establishment of an intracrevicular restorative margin (Figure 148-1). A minimum of 3 mm of sound tooth above the alveolar process is necessary if a restoration or fracture approaches the crest. Violation of the biologic width may result in inflammation and bone resorption. Surgical procedures such as gingivectomy and

apically positioned flap with or without osseous surgery may be used to increase the clinical crown length.

A If the tooth is periodontally healthy or affected by gingivitis only, crown lengthening may be accomplished by gingivectomy in cases of excess gingiva. This approach requires an adequate zone of attached gingiva with at least 3 mm of sound tooth structure above the crest of bone. If a mucogingival problem is anticipated, use an apically positioned flap to retain the available gingiva and lengthen the crown. A gingival graft is performed in instances of inadequate attached gingiva.

Electrosurgery or laser surgery, as alternatives to gingivectomy, are quick methods for reducing excess tissue and providing good control of hemorrhage. Care must be taken to avoid contact with the bone. Even minimal contact with the alveolar process may result in overcoagulation, necrosis, resorption of bone, and gingival recession. In most circumstances, use of a blade is preferable to use of an electrosurgical unit or dental laser.

B If the bone level is normal with no root fracture, use mucogingival-osseous surgery to expose at least 3 mm of root beyond where the restorative margin is to be placed. If a fracture extends into the root, assess the prognosis, accessibility, and esthetics before proceeding further. If a fracture compromises a furcation, root resection is a consideration. Extraction is indicated if the fracture extends to the middle third of the root or jeopardizes the support of the adjacent teeth. If the root fracture occurs in a more favorable location (coronal to the mid-third of the root), use a gingival flap with osseous surgery to expose the fractured area and create the appropriate biologic width.

Maintenance of esthetics is a major concern in the anterior and premolar region. Orthodontics or forced eruption is a treatment option allowing extrusion of the fractured tooth with conservation of bone and esthetics; however, the need for periodontal surgery is not necessarily eliminated. Minimal crown lengthening to correct osseous contours then may be confined to the extruded tooth.

C If the tooth requiring crown lengthening has periodontal pockets, assess the degree of periodontal support, strategic value, and prognosis using the same criteria as outlined in **B**. Initial therapy is performed before crown lengthening to decrease inflammation and promote better hemostasis. Use mucogingival-osseous surgery to eliminate the periodontal pockets and lengthen the crown.

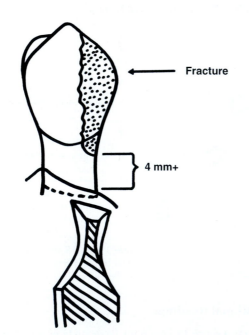

Figure 148-1 When crown lengthening is performed where a fracture extends apically into the root, bone must be removed to expose a minimum of 2 mm of root structure apical to the ultimate margin of the restoration.

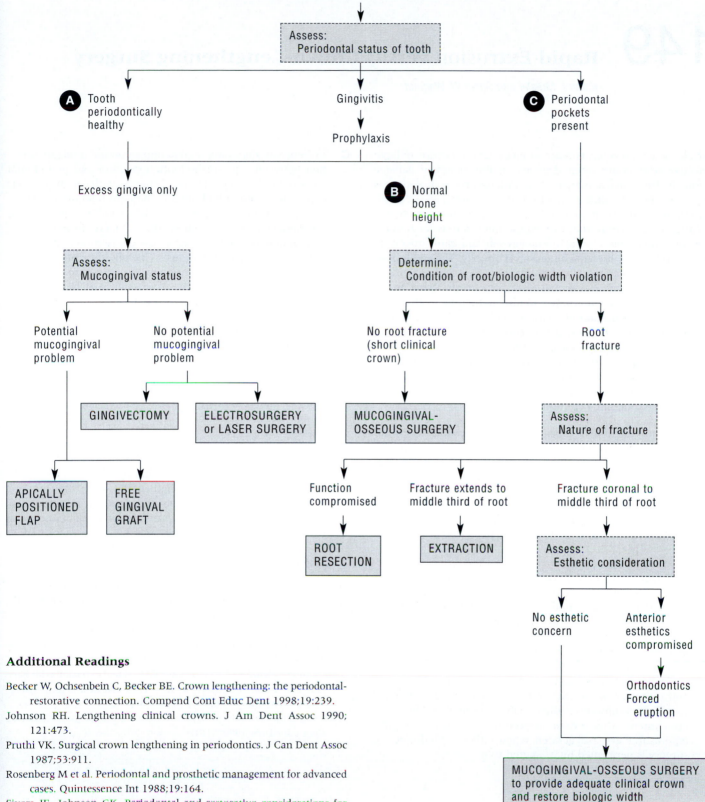

Patient with TOOTH REQUIRING CROWN LENGTHENING

Assess:
Periodontal status of tooth

A Tooth periodontically healthy

Gingivitis

↓

Prophylaxis

C Periodontal pockets present

Excess gingiva only

Assess:
Mucogingival status

B Normal bone height

Determine:
Condition of root/biologic width violation

Potential mucogingival problem

No potential mucogingival problem

No root fracture (short clinical crown)

Root fracture

GINGIVECTOMY

ELECTROSURGERY or LASER SURGERY

MUCOGINGIVAL-OSSEOUS SURGERY

Assess:
Nature of fracture

APICALLY POSITIONED FLAP

FREE GINGIVAL GRAFT

Function compromised

Fracture extends to middle third of root

Fracture coronal to middle third of root

ROOT RESECTION

EXTRACTION

Assess:
Esthetic consideration

No esthetic concern

Anterior esthetics compromised

↓

Orthodontics
Forced eruption

MUCOGINGIVAL-OSSEOUS SURGERY
to provide adequate clinical crown
and restore biologic width

Additional Readings

Becker W, Ochsenbein C, Becker BE. Crown lengthening: the periodontal-restorative connection. Compend Cont Educ Dent 1998;19:239.

Johnson RH. Lengthening clinical crowns. J Am Dent Assoc 1990;121:473.

Pruthi VK. Surgical crown lengthening in periodontics. J Can Dent Assoc 1987;53:911.

Rosenberg M et al. Periodontal and prosthetic management for advanced cases. Quintessence Int 1988;19:164.

Sivers JE, Johnson GK. Periodontal and restorative considerations for crown lengthening. Quintessence Int 1985;16:833.

Wagenberg B, Eskow R, Langer B. Exposing adequate tooth structure for restorative dentistry. Int J Periodontics Restorative Dent 1989;9:323.

149 Rapid Extrusion versus Crown-Lengthening Surgery

Kathy I. Mueller and Galen W. Wagnild

Salvage of teeth severely compromised by caries, fracture, or large defective restorations often depends on the extent of damage below the free gingival margin. A tooth-lengthening procedure is required when significant structural degradation has occurred. Periodontal crown-lengthening surgery is a one-step tooth-lengthening procedure that can expose most defects for restorative correction. This approach removes soft and hard supporting tissues and moves the attachment level apically. The tooth position remains unchanged. However, this surgery may affect esthetics or the maintenance potential of adjacent teeth. Rapid orthodontic extrusion is an alternative tooth-lengthening method that also facilitates restoration of compromised teeth. This procedure moves the residual tooth structure coronally while the soft and hard supporting tissues remain in their pretreatment locations. Orthodontic rapid extrusion is indicated when esthetic considerations are critical or when the anatomy of an adjacent tooth and adjacent coronal restorations would be jeopardized by the surgical apical repositioning of periodontal tissues.

A To be successful over time, restorative procedures must not invade the attachment apparatus. There must be adequate sound tooth structure between the lesion and the coronal extent of the junctional epithelium to place a restorative margin. The margin generally requires 2 mm of sound tooth structure coronal to the attachment. Operative invasion of the attachment often results in gingival recession, periodontal pocket formation, or chronic gingival inflammation.

B Retention of the severely damaged tooth requires critical pretreatment evaluation. Accurate prediction of post-treatment crown-to-root ratio is mandatory. Sufficient periodontal attachment for the tooth to withstand functional forces must remain after the procedure. With all other variables equal, rapid orthodontic extrusion provides a more favorable post-treatment crown-to-root ratio than does periodontal crown-lengthening surgery.

Cylindrical root form greatly enhances the functional and esthetic components of tooth lengthening. A tapered root form compromises the remaining periodontal ligament attachment after either procedure. Likewise, gingival embrasures are exaggerated when either orthodontics or surgery is performed on a tapered root.

C Esthetic variables have a great impact on the modality selection between rapid orthodontic extrusion and periodontal crown-lengthening surgery. Patients with great esthetic expectations and a high lip line may not tolerate the deformity produced by surgery. This defect will be apparent on the damaged tooth as well as adjacent teeth, in most cases.

Maintenance of free gingival margin symmetry could dictate that surgery be expanded to include the entire anterior sextant. This surgical expansion exposes root structure on all included teeth. These significant sequelae may be avoided by using orthodontics to correct the defect.

D The selected modality should not solve one problem while creating others. Short root trunks or significant developmental grooves on adjacent teeth may be exposed by surgery and therefore require the damaged tooth to be extruded. These anatomic findings render a tooth more difficult to maintain if the attachment level is moved apically using a surgical technique.

E Existing coronal restorations on adjacent teeth also influence the selection of extrusion or surgery. Intracrevicular margins on adjacent teeth are exposed using conventional periodontal surgical techniques to lengthen the tooth. Restorations that do not need replacement and demand intracrevicular margins for esthetics are indications for orthodontic rapid extrusion of the damaged tooth.

Additional Readings

Biggerstaff R, Sinks J, Carazola J. Orthodontic extrusion and biologic width realignment procedures: methods for reclaiming nonrestorable teeth. J Am Dent Assoc 1986;112:345.

Kozlovsky A, al H, Lieberman M. Forced eruption combined with gingival fiberectomy: a technique for crown lengthening. J Clin Periodontol 1988;15:534.

Pontoriero R, Celenza F, Ricci G, Carnevale G. Rapid extrusion with fiber resection: a combined orthodontic-periodontal treatment modality. Int J Periodontics Restorative Dent 1987;5:30.

Rosenberg E, Garber D, Evian C. Tooth lengthening procedures. Compend Cont Educ Dent 1980;1:161.

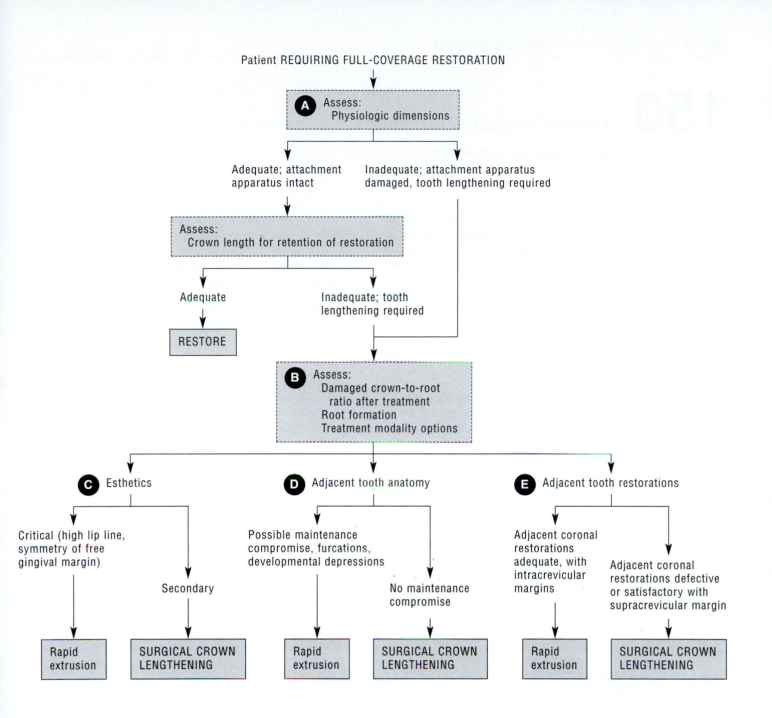

Patient REQUIRING FULL-COVERAGE RESTORATION

A Assess:
Physiologic dimensions

Adequate; attachment
apparatus intact

Inadequate; attachment apparatus
damaged, tooth lengthening required

Assess:
Crown length for retention of restoration

Adequate

Inadequate; tooth
lengthening required

RESTORE

B Assess:
Damaged crown-to-root
ratio after treatment
Root formation
Treatment modality options

C Esthetics

D Adjacent tooth anatomy

E Adjacent tooth restorations

Critical (high lip line,
symmetry of free
gingival margin)

Secondary

Possible maintenance
compromise, furcations,
developmental depressions

No maintenance
compromise

Adjacent coronal
restorations
adequate, with
intracrevicular
margins

Adjacent coronal
restorations defective
or satisfactory with
supracrevicular margin

Rapid
extrusion

SURGICAL CROWN
LENGTHENING

Rapid
extrusion

SURGICAL CROWN
LENGTHENING

Rapid
extrusion

SURGICAL CROWN
LENGTHENING

150 Crown Margin Placement

Kathy I. Mueller and Galen W. Wagnild

The marginal periodontium includes the area in which the fields of restorative dentistry and periodontics become intimately related. This area, although small, is operated in daily by restorative dental practitioners and requires definitive, logical decisions regarding margin location to facilitate long-term, predictable results. Although controversy exists, recent literature supports movement away from margins deep within the gingival crevice and toward shallow intracrevicular or supragingival placement.

A Evaluate the tooth in need of restoration on both structural and esthetic levels before determining margin location.

B Clinical findings such as caries, an existing restoration, fractures, cervical erosion, and uncontrollable root sensitivity may dictate restoration placement below the level of the free gingival margin. Extension of the preparation into the gingival crevice may engage enough additional tooth structure to provide the restoration with adequate retention and resistance form, secure sufficient sound tooth structure for margin placement, and minimize root sensitivity of nonendodontic origin. The physiologic zones or biologic width present in the area of intracrevicular subgingival margin placement must meet minimal guidelines (Figure 150-1). Attempts to modify the tooth preparation by apical positioning of the restorative margin are limited by this fragile tissue complex. Violation of this width may result in gingival inflammation, loss of crestal bone, and pocket formation or apical migration of the marginal tissue. If structural problems cannot be solved without destroying the integrity of

the biologic width, surgical lengthening of the clinical crown or orthodontic extrusion is indicated to reestablish this zone.

C Esthetic requirements may dictate intracrevicular (subgingival) margin location despite other clinical findings that may allow supragingival placement. Determine margin location with respect to esthetics using a combination of factors including tooth position, visibility of margin area during function, and the patient's understanding of the objectives of the restorative effort. If esthetics are important, the crevice should be entered minimally, with the restoration usually from 0.5 to 1 mm apically to the free gingival margin. A restorative attempt to hide a metal collar within the anatomic confines of a shallow, healthy crevice often is not possible without compromising esthetics or sacrificing biologic width. Such conflicts between esthetics and tissue health may best be resolved by minimal entrance into the crevice and use of a porcelain shoulder margin or a margin supported by metal but without a visible metal collar. If esthetics are secondary and structural evaluation permits, locate restorative margins outside the gingival crevice. Such margins are more accurately prepared, predictably registered, and accessible for evaluation, finishing, and patient maintenance. Patients who require restoration after periodontal therapy that apically repositions gingival tissue pose additional complexities. If esthetics are important, the restorative practitioner must first carefully establish that a gingival crevice has indeed reformed postsurgically; placing a restorative margin under the tissue level if no crevice exists may lead to breakdown of the tissue complex, pocket formation, and apical migration of the gingiva. Second, an attempt to locate margins within the gingival crevice of an elongated tooth requires additional axial wall reduction with possible pulpal encroachment. If possible, postsurgical margins should be left above the treated tissue level and exposed furcations.

Additional Readings

Nevins M, Skurow HM. The intracrevicular restorative margin, the biologic width, and maintenance of the gingival margin. Int J Periodontics Restorative Dent 1984;3:31.

Schluger S et al. Periodontal disease. 2nd ed. Philadelphia: Lea & Febiger; 1990. p. 586.

Shillingburg HT, Hobo S, Whitsett DL. Fundamentals of fixed prosthodontics. 2nd ed. Berlin: Quintessence Publishing; 1981. p. 79.

Wilson RD, Maynard G. Intracrevicular restorative dentistry. Int J Periodontics Restorative Dent 1981;4:35.

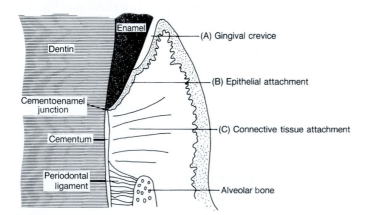

Figure 150-1 Restorative margins located apically to the free gingival margin must terminate, as in **A**, enter into **B**, or they may cause breakdown of the attachment apparatus (**C**).

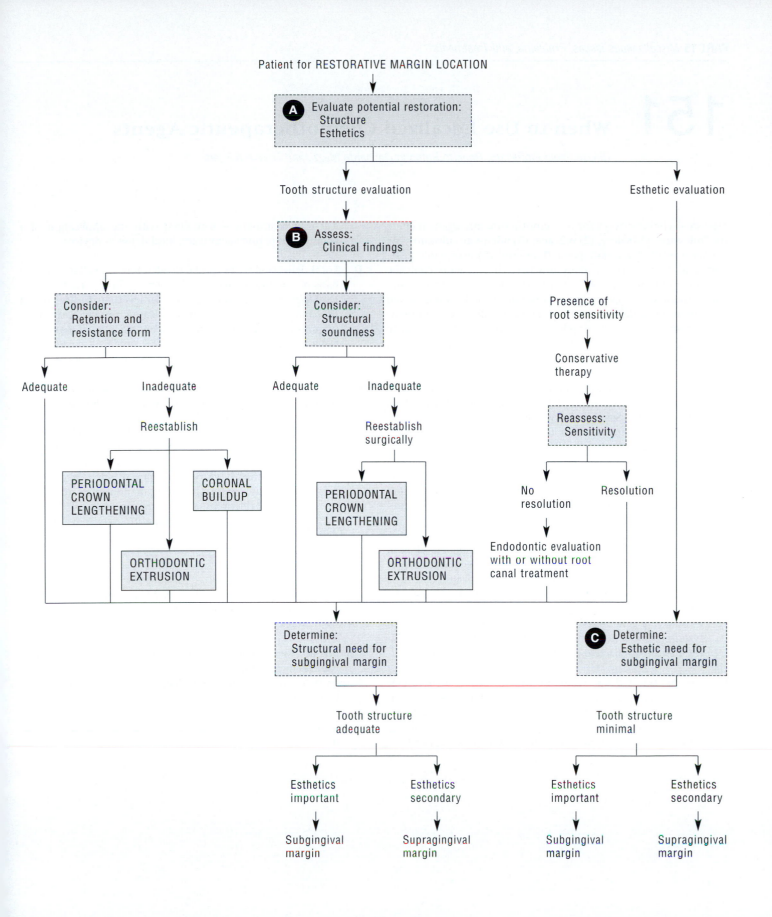

Patient for RESTORATIVE MARGIN LOCATION

A Evaluate potential restoration:
Structure
Esthetics

Tooth structure evaluation

Esthetic evaluation

B Assess:
Clinical findings

Consider:
Retention and
resistance form

Consider:
Structural
soundness

Presence of
root sensitivity

Adequate   Inadequate

Adequate   Inadequate

Conservative
therapy

Reestablish

Reestablish
surgically

Reassess:
Sensitivity

PERIODONTAL
CROWN
LENGTHENING

CORONAL
BUILDUP

PERIODONTAL
CROWN
LENGTHENING

No
resolution

Resolution

ORTHODONTIC
EXTRUSION

ORTHODONTIC
EXTRUSION

Endodontic evaluation
with or without root
canal treatment

Determine:
Structural need for
subgingival margin

C Determine:
Esthetic need for
subgingival margin

Tooth structure
adequate

Tooth structure
minimal

Esthetics
important

Esthetics
secondary

Esthetics
important

Esthetics
secondary

Subgingival
margin

Supragingival
margin

Subgingival
margin

Supragingival
margin

151 When to Use Localized Chemotherapeutic Agents

Giovan Paolo Pini-Prato, Roberto Rotundo, Leonardo Muzzi, and Tiziano Baccetti

The ideal characteristics for a chemotherapeutic agent include the following: (1) safety; (2) efficacy; (3) adequate substantivity; (4) specific effect on pathogenic flora; and (5) acceptable taste, cost, and ease of use. In daily practice, these agents could be administered locally or systemically. In periodontics, the chemotherapeutic agents that are used are usually administered employing local delivery devices. These localized chemotherapeutic agents release the drug into the tooth pocket and achieve and maintain effective concentration of the active agent for the period required to control the subgingival infection.

A Localized chemotherapeutic agents should be used only in conjunction with adequate measures to disperse the bacterial plaque biofilm. Scaling, root planing, and, if necessary, surgical therapy are needed for this. An appropriate supportive periodontal care program must be in place to control the plaque accumulation after the surgical or nonsurgical therapy. During this phase, the patient is regularly recalled so that the level of plaque control can be evaluated, with scaling and root planing appointments when signs of inflammation are present. Patient motivation and performance are critical.

B Systemic antibiotic therapy seems to be most beneficial as an adjunct to mechanical therapy to control infections at generalized residual deep pockets in patients with persistent disease or in patients who continue to lose attachment, despite the periodontal therapy performed. Cases of juvenile periodontitis or severe generalized adult periodontitis may benefit from systemic antibiotic therapy—which represents a more efficient and cost-effective choice of therapy in these cases.

C Patients selected for treatment with localized chemotherapeutic agents are adults who have been treated for periodontitis and are now enrolled in the maintenance phase presenting with isolated nonresponding sites that show a pocket depth over 5 mm and that bleed on probing. Mechan-ical root treatment is combined with the application of a chemotherapeutic agent using local delivery devices.

D Local delivery devices can be divided into two classes on the basis of the time it takes for the agent to be released: (1) *sustained delivery devices* (drug release for less than 24 hours) and (2) *controlled delivery devices* (drug release for more than 1 day). At present, only five chemotherapeutic agents are commercially available: tetracycline fibers, metronidazole gel, minocycline ointment, chlorhexidine chip, and doxycycline polymer.

E A periodontal abscess is defined as a lesion with severe periodontal breakdown, occurring during a limited period, with easily detectable clinical symptoms and localized accumulation of pus within the periodontal pocket. There is not enough scientific evidence to provide a unique treatment regimen for periodontal abscesses. Different therapeutic approaches have been proposed, such as drainage and débridement, systemic antibiotic administration with or without débridement, surgical approaches, or débridement with localized chemotherapeutic agents using local delivery devices.

Additional Readings

American Academy of Periodontology. Position paper: the role of controlled drug delivery for periodontitis. J Periodontol 2000;71:125.

Drisko CH. Nonsurgical periodontal therapy. Periodontology 2000 2001;25:77.

Hancock EB, Newell DH. Preventive strategies and supportive treatment. Periodontology 2000 2001;25:59.

Herrera D, Rolàn S, Sanz M. The periodontal abscess: a review. J Clin Periodontol 2001;27:377.

Tonetti MS. The topical use of antibiotics in periodontal pockets. Proceedings of the 2nd European Workshop on Periodontology; 1996. p. 78–109.

A Patient for WHOM A CHEMOTHERAPEUTIC APPROACH IS BEING CONSIDERED

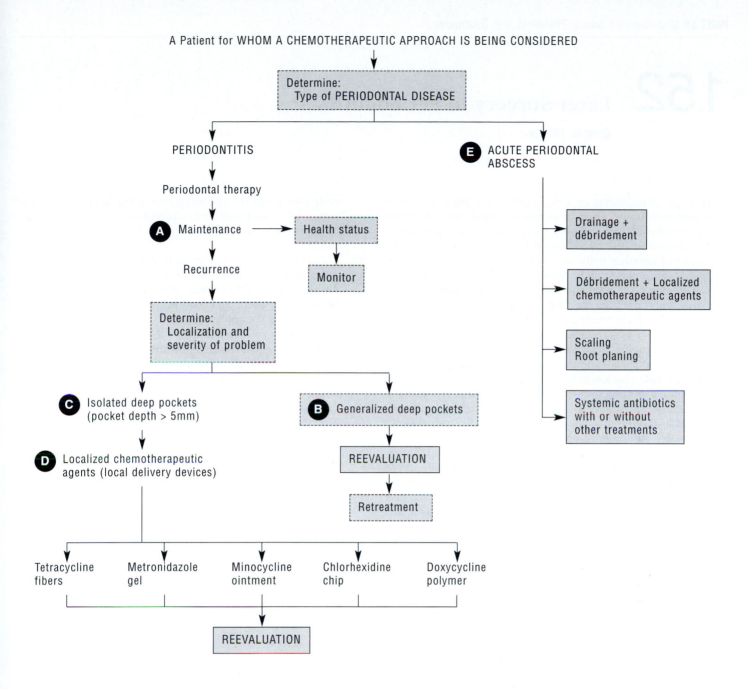

Determine:
Type of PERIODONTAL DISEASE

PERIODONTITIS

E ACUTE PERIODONTAL ABSCESS

Periodontal therapy

A Maintenance → Health status

Recurrence

Monitor

Determine:
Localization and
severity of problem

Drainage +
débridement

Débridement + Localized
chemotherapeutic agents

Scaling
Root planing

C Isolated deep pockets
(pocket depth > 5mm)

B Generalized deep pockets

Systemic antibiotics
with or without
other treatments

D Localized chemotherapeutic
agents (local delivery devices)

REEVALUATION

Retreatment

Tetracycline
fibers

Metronidazole
gel

Minocycline
ointment

Chlorhexidine
chip

Doxycycline
polymer

REEVALUATION

152 Laser Surgery in Periodontics

Scott W. Milliken

Since their introduction in 1962, lasers have been attractive alternatives to scalpel surgical techniques involving soft-tissue procedures (which are the only procedures universally recognized as legitimate periodontal uses of lasers at this time). The use of a surgical laser has many advantages over traditional scalpel surgery for a number of periodontal procedures. Treatment with carbon dioxide (CO_2) and neodymium:yttrium-aluminum-garnet (Nd-YAG) lasers has been shown to be advantageous in soft-tissue removal and in recontouring procedures.

During laser surgery, bleeding is almost completely eliminated, creating a dry field with optimal visibility. This may, in many cases, reduce operating time greatly. Lymphatic vessels in the surgical field also are sealed during laser procedures, resulting in limited postoperative swelling. Lasers are significantly easier than is the scalpel in negotiating the curves, contours, and folds of the mouth, which also may reduce surgical time. Postoperative pain is reduced or eliminated 90% of the time, apparently because of sealing the peripheral nerve fibers. Lasers cause minimal or no scarring, and suturing is almost never needed. Bacterial counts in a laser field are reduced, which may minimize the chance of infection. A laser can cut, coagulate, and vaporize or ablate tissue, depending on the power-setting focus.

A   Treatment of generalized or localized gingival enlargement may be facilitated with a surgical laser. Laser gingivectomy offers several advantages over scalpel surgery such as less bleeding, no packing needed, better postoperative contours, and a blood-free field. A smoother postoperative course may be a big advantage for treatment of mentally challenged or handicapped patients.

B   Lasers may be well suited to crown-lengthening procedures needed because of excess soft tissue and uneven gingival margins. Excessive tissue may be removed quickly and easily with a laser to expose additional tooth surface for restorative needs or esthetic demands. The practitioner must take care not to violate the biologic width. This may be prevented by sounding for the position of the alveolar crest relative to the proposed new tissue level. If the biologic width space will be compromised, traditional crown-lengthening techniques must be used.

C   The repositioning or elimination of an aberrant frenum is a procedure extremely well suited to the laser. Surgical time for maxillary midline frenectomies is dramatically reduced because the laser vaporizes the tissue and eliminates the need for sutures and hemostasis. Postoperative pain medications are eliminated in nearly 100% of the cases, and no postoperative scarring is encountered. Laser frenectomies often are completed in 30 seconds as the skill and comfort level of the surgeon increases.

D   Laser biopsies may be performed as alternatives to scalpel biopsies in all instances. The principles, treatment goals, and protocols regarding tissue sampling and pathologic analysis are the same as they are for scalpel procedures. Potential seeding of malignant lesions may possibly be reduced with the laser. The hemostatic nature of lasers is particularly advantageous for biopsies involving highly vascular areas such as the tongue and buccal mucosa. Biopsies often may be done faster, but deep lingual resectioning requires suturing. An interesting note is that lasers offer relief from painful aphthous ulcers. This does not speed healing, but patients report pain relief after low-power laser application. The need for local anesthetic remains.

Additional Readings

Carranza FA Jr, Newman MJ. Clinical periodontology. 8th ed. Philadelphia: WB Saunders; 1996. p. 591.

Pick RM, Pecaro BC, Silberman CJ. The laser gingivectomy: the use of CO_2 laser for the removal of phenytoin hyperplasia. J Periodontol 56:492.

Pogrel MA, Yen CK, Hansen LS. A comparison of carbon dioxide laser, liquid nitrogen cryotherapy and scalpel wounds in healing. Oral Surg Oral Med Oral Pathol 1990;69:269.

Patient for LASER SURGICAL TREATMENT

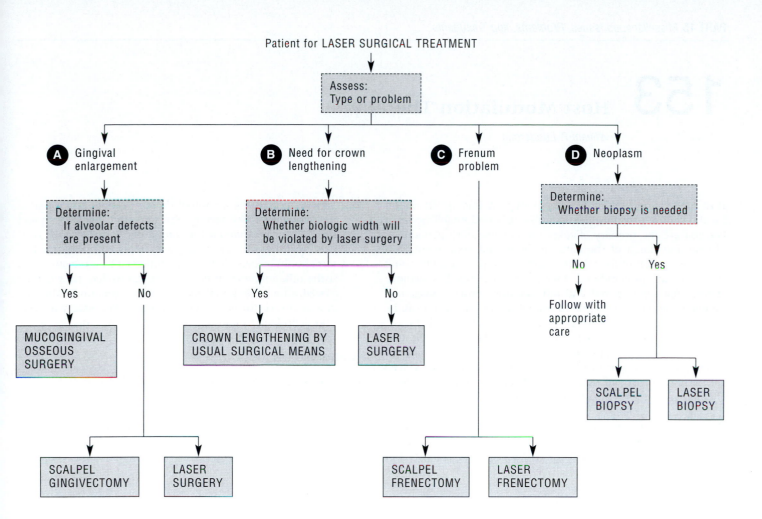

153 Host Modulation Therapy

William P. Lundergan

Host modulation therapy is a relatively new therapeutic option for the clinician treating periodontitis. It is well established that bacteria are the primary etiology for inflammatory periodontal disease, but much of the damage (bone and attachment loss) occurs as a result of the release of cytokines, prostaglandins, and matrix metalloproteinases by the host. Research has demonstrated that nonsteroidal anti-inflammatory drugs, collagenase inhibitors, and bisphosphonates (inhibit bone resorption) can be useful adjuncts in controlling inflammatory periodontal disease; however, at this time, only one host modulating medication (Periostat) has been approved as an adjunct to scaling and root planing for the treatment of periodontitis. Periostat has received the American Dental Association Seal of Acceptance as a chemotherapeutic product to slow or arrest periodontitis.

A Periodontal maintenance patients that are not well controlled should be considered for host modulation therapy. Periostat (20 mg doxycycline) is a collagenase inhibitor and is generally taken twice daily for a period of 3 to 9 months.

B Patients presenting for initial therapy should be evaluated for periodontal risk factors. Smokers and diabetics should certainly be considered for combining Periostat with conventional débridement therapy. Patients with low-risk factors should be débrided initially followed by a reevaluation. If the inflammatory disease is well controlled, they can be placed on a periodontal maintenance program. If the disease is not controlled, then combining Periostat with further débridement and/or surgery should be considered.

Additional Readings

Caton JG et al. Treatment with subantimicrobial dose doxycycline improves the efficacy of scaling and root planing in patients with adult periodontitis. J Periodontol 2000;April:521.

Waller C et al. Long-term treatment with subantimicrobial dose doxycycline exerts no antimicrobial effect on the subgingival microflora associated with adult periodontitis. J Periodontal 2000;September:1465.

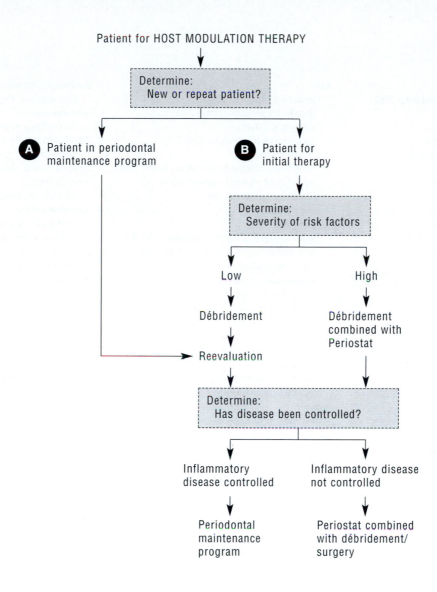

Patient for HOST MODULATION THERAPY

Determine:
New or repeat patient?

A Patient in periodontal maintenance program

B Patient for initial therapy

Determine:
Severity of risk factors

Low

High

Débridement

Débridement combined with Periostat

Reevaluation

Determine:
Has disease been controlled?

Inflammatory disease controlled

Inflammatory disease not controlled

Periodontal maintenance program

Periostat combined with débridement/ surgery

Index